From Manual Evaluation to General Diagnosis

Assessing Patient Information before Hands-On Treatment

Alain Croibier, DO, MRO(F)

Foreword by Jean-Pierre Barral, DO, RPT, MRO(F)

North Atlantic Books
Berkeley, California

Upledger Institute Enterprises
Palm Beach Gardens, Florida

Published by
North Atlantic Books
Huichin, unceded Ohlone land
Berkeley, California
and
Upledger Institute Enterprises
11211 Prosperity Farms Road
Palm Beach Gardens, Florida 33410

Cover art © iStockphoto.com / O'Luk
Cover and book design by Brad Greene
Printed in the United States of America

From Manual Evaluation to General Diagnosis: Assessing Patient Information before Hands-On Treatment is sponsored and published by North Atlantic Books, an educational nonprofit based in the unceded Ohlone land Huichin (Berkeley, CA) that collaborates with partners to develop cross-cultural perspectives; nurture holistic views of art, science, the humanities, and healing; and seed personal and global transformation by publishing work on the relationship of body, spirit, and nature.

North Atlantic Books's publications are distributed to the US trade and internationally by Penguin Random House Publisher Services. For further information, visit our website at www.northatlanticbooks.com.

Library of Congress Cataloging-in-Publication Data

Croibier, Alain.
    From manual evaluation to general diagnosis : assessing patient information before hands-on treatment / Alain Croibier ; foreword by Jean-Pierre Barral.
        p. ; cm.
    Includes bibliographical references and index.
    ISBN 978-1-58394-319-9
    1. Osteopathic medicine. 2. Diagnosis—Methodology. I. Title.
    [DNLM: 1. Diagnostic Techniques and Procedures. 2. Osteopathic Medicine—methods. WB 112]
    RZ341.C76 2012
    615.5'33—dc23   2011016254

3 5LP 24

North Atlantic Books is committed to the protection of our environment. We print on recycled paper whenever possible and partner with printers who strive to use environmentally responsible practices.

Acknowledgments

Even when it is the reflection of work, practice, and personal research, a book is never written alone. The information I have received, the encounters I have had, and the exchanges I have made along the way have inevitably left their impressions. This book is written encompassing that input.

Whenever possible, and when reasonably possible, I have acknowledged the sources of specific ideas. Occasionally it was simply impossible to cite the originator of a concept, and I accept the blame for not remembering.

I would especially like to thank my esteemed colleague, Jean-Pierre Barral. For many years we have worked together on several kinds of research; we have written several books and articles together, and we have taught courses together.

Although he has not directly contributed to the drafting of this book, his immense clinical experience, observation skills, and higher perspective, along with some of his comments as well as numerous reflections, have contributed greatly toward progress in our field. I thank him from the bottom of my heart for all this shared experience and for his friendship and generosity.

Likewise, my gratitude goes to my companion, Dr. Francoise Coullet, MD, DO, for her whole-hearted support and also for her attentive and patient proofreading. Her considerable advice and shrewd contributions have helped clarify certain passages.

Thanks to my friend Olivier Bazin, DO, MRO(F), for his thorough proofreading and pertinent observations that helped to create the original French text.

Thanks to those who assisted with this English-language version: Cassie Williams, PhD, RPOB, CST, for her translation work; George Lord Jr., DC, and Ann Hoeffel, MT, who also assisted with the translation; and Annabel Mackenzie, RST, BI-D; Dawn Langnes and Mark Bookhout, PT, MS, FAAOMPT, for editing.

Finally, I would like to thank everyone that I have approached over the last few years who have contributed more or less directly to the realization of this work through their instruction, reflections, encouragement, presence, exchanges, or testimony:

Jean-Pierre Amigues, DO, MRO(F)
Jean Arlot, DO, MRO(F)
Martine Auran, DO, MRO(F)
Vincent Benedetto, DO, MRO(F)
Elie Beringuier, DO, MRO(F)
Georges-Charles Bex, DO, MRO(F)
Philippe Bourdinaud, DO, MRO(F)
Marc Bozzetto, DO
Paul Chauffour, DO, MRO(F)
Philippe Cievet, DO, MRO(F)
Daniel Courthaliac, DO, MRO(F)
Christian De France, DO, MRO(F)
Jean-Pierre Dessaint, DO, MRO(F)
Bruno Ducous, DO, MRO(F)
Viola Frymann, DO, FAAO
Alain Gassier, DO, MRO(F)
Ali Guermazzi, DO, MRO(F)
Jean-Pierre Guiliani, DO, MRO(F)
Bernard Hamm, DO, MRO(F)
Gerard Kokotek, MD
Jean-Paul Krimm, DO
Roselyne Lalauze-Pol, DO, MRO(F)
Jean Lambrou, DO
Francois Laurent, DO, MRO(F)
Serge Leveque, DO
Alain Lignon, DO, MRO(F)
Serge Majal, DO, MRO(F)

Robert Mesle, DO, MRO(F)

Bernard Minaudier, DO

Bernard Mohr, MD

Gerard Montet, DO, MRO(F)

Serge Paoletti, DO, MRO(F)

Gerard Pacault, MD

Jean-Jacques Papassin, DO

Jean-Luc Payrouse, DO

Robert Perronneaud-Ferre, DO, MRO(F)

Jean Peyriere, DO

Christian Pons, DO, MRO(F)

Claude Porion, DO

Didier Pratt, DO

Bernard Quef, DO, MRO(F)

Nadine Racano, DO

Andre Ratio, DO, MD

Louis Rommevaux, DO, MRO(F)

Michel Roques, DO, MRO(F)

Jean-Paul Saby, DO, MRO(F)

Raymond Solano, DO

Gerard Sueur, DO, MRO(F)

Pierre Tricot, DO

John E. Upledger, DO, OMM

Frank Willard, PhD

Serge Xilberman, DO

Thanks to the patients who had confidence in me and to the students who worked with me. All have provided many stimuli for me to advance and find the answers to their many questions.

This book was "in the works" for over ten years and will no doubt be relevant for a long time. The impetus to finish the project came from Peter Schwind, a colleague from Munich, and Rolf Lenzen of the German branch of the Elsevier publishing house. The difficulty was not as much the idea of writing it as in the achievement of the work undertaken. Osteopaths' computers overflow with intricate course materials; the pain of the outcome of the work, however, is such that very few have the opportunity to be published without external and earnest encouragement.

To the osteopaths of the whole world:
    Fond memories for those of yesterday!
    Godspeed to those of today!

Table of Contents

Foreword

For many years, Alain Croibier and I have joined our efforts in osteopathic research. Working in the field, we also know the confusion of patients who suffer for not investing themselves in us enthusiastically to try to ameliorate and improve their treatment. Before caring for them, one needs to decipher, evaluate, and carry out a diagnosis. The efficacy of osteopathic therapy depends as much on manual techniques as on diagnostic precision based on indications. Our diagnoses have some points of convergence with traditional medicine, both claiming a unique characteristic: the appreciative work of the hand.

It is necessary to be able to guarantee to patients that your actions are harmless. Assure them that *primum non nocere* ("first, do no harm") is of primary importance; only then can we let our hands perform.

It is also essential that the osteopathic culture is supported by some solid foundations; it is from this body of knowledge that we can develop.

Alain Croibier has had the conviction and courage to assemble into one work some elements of diagnostic reasoning and proper tests of our art. We salute this synthesis, which will allow future generations of osteopaths to have a manual exclusively devoted to osteopathic diagnosis.

—Jean-Pierre Barral, DO, RPT, MRO(F)

Introduction

Many European countries are making progress in formally recognizing osteopathy. In each case, lawmakers are posing serious questions regarding the competence of osteopaths and are concerned with the issue of patient safety. Therapeutic techniques are only one component of osteopathy. The framework and scope of diagnosis is of the utmost importance. The skill of the practitioner is closely linked to his or her ability to analyze and reflect before forming a diagnostic conclusion. No health profession can have a position of responsibility without a reliable system of diagnosis.

Nevertheless, among osteopathic publications, books on therapeutic techniques are numerous, but texts concerning diagnosis remain rare. Osteopathic assessment is based principally on clinical manual investigation. Thus, for many experienced osteopaths, diagnosis goes without saying: they consider that, above all, it is a question of common sense. For them, there is no need to detail and explain, much less to write on the subject. As long as the need to communicate is not considered indispensable, diagnosis may remain a private process. However, it is necessary to exchange views with others to effectively formulate how we organize our diagnosis.

My experience in teaching osteopathy has given me perspective on the evaluation process used in our clinical practice. This work is the result of many years of reflection, research, and note-keeping in the course of daily professional consultations. I have tried my best to answer the numerous questions posed by the most inquisitive students: those who are anxious at the prospect of establishing a clinical diagnosis.

In osteopathy, as in all medical disciplines, diagnosis is more an art than a science. Concealed behind its apparent simplicity are complexity and a great many principles. There is no typical procedure. Practitioners must be methodical in the application of an intricate, precise, and specific body of knowledge. The problems of diagnostics often come down to one key element: all examination must be done at the same time—look, listen, palpate, understand, and observe.

Also, as practitioners we sometimes must divide the indivisible. For example, we must be able to separate the psychoemotional from the physical, which can nevertheless be intimately linked. The true difficulty is to define and organize all these elements within the allotted consultation time.

While the opportunity to acquire new therapeutic techniques holds tremendous appeal to students and professionals alike, diagnosis often does not become a preoccupying concern until the end of their course of study. It is the demands of clinical reality that make them acutely aware of their inevitable shortcomings in this area.

Conventional medicine identifies disease, and the diagnosis determines the course of treatment. Generally medication or surgery is prescribed. In osteopathy, the therapeutic response is different, and so too is the diagnosis. However, while the outcome is not the same, the evaluation process is of a comparable importance. The objective of this book is to provide an extensive educational framework for the examination of patients.

A practitioner must be an excellent clinician to be able to analyze subtle signs in a patient. A thorough command of symptomatology and pathology is vital if one is to avoid pitfalls in the course of everyday practice. Some aspects of a patient's condition may have to be evaluated using a more global approach to the individual's constitution and personality. A section of useful practical clinical knowledge pertaining to this is provided.

An osteopath must endeavor to be a general practitioner, not a specialist. Rather than impose our own favorite techniques, it is wisest to choose the approach best suited to the needs of each specific patient. An accurate diagnosis is the surest way to devise a truly individualized treatment and thereby achieve the best possible results.

Theory and Fundamentals of Diagnosis

Chapter 1

The Concept of Diagnosis

One must learn to recognize exactly the constitution of every season and of every disease; and to recognize what positive and negative elements are found in common in a given constitution or a given disease.

— HIPPOCRATES

Definitions and Etymology

While the origins of the term *diagnosis* are Greek, it is difficult to understand them fully. The prefix *dia* implies going through or across, or dividing; the rest of the word derives from the verb *gignoskein*, which means "to learn" or "to know." *Gnōsis*, which comes from *gignoskein*, has the meaning "knowledge" or "knowing," and can have a spiritual or religious connotation. The word *diagnostic* is thought to be derived from *diagnōstikos*, meaning "having the ability to recognize." For Hippocrates, the term meant "possessed of discernment." Currently, the term comprises two aspects:

- The part of medical practice that aims to determine the nature of the disease being observed. It is the art of recognizing and identifying diseases by their symptoms and of distinguishing them from one another. Although the diagnosis can be reconsidered at any moment, the time taken to make such a determination is indispensable for establishing a prognosis and a choice of therapy.

- By extension, the word *diagnosis* is also used to refer to a process of reflection in order to identify the nature of a dysfunction or of a difficulty prior to taking action.

Accordingly, the reader will understand that a single Greek word, *diagnōsis,* has simultaneously held the meanings of medical discernment, decision-making, and diagnosis. For Jean-Charles Sournia (1995), the term *diagnosis* designates both the intellectual steps taken to identify a disease and the decisions reached as a result of taking these steps.

SUMMARY

Diagnosis is on one hand an effort of reflection and of gathering facts and data, and on the other, as a result of this effort, expressed as concisely as possible in terms that are part of an existing coordinated system of knowledge.

The Need for Diagnosis

The true imperatives of diagnosis are identifying a dysfunction and making decisions accordingly. The impact of these decisions underlines the importance of the quality of discernment needed by the practitioner who will perform therapy.

It is not actually necessary to have an already-formulated diagnosis in order to provide a certain degree of care to a patient. There are numerous care-giving disciplines, many of them supplementing medical practice, that provide care within a therapeutic framework that is predefined by another practitioner.

A practitioner who undertakes a considered action rather than simply providing service by rote, however, *can and must diagnose.* Performing an evaluation differentiates the professional practitioner from a simple care provider. Let me state clearly that this distinction in no way implies a value judgment. It refers to technical aptitudes and requirements rather than to the quality of humanity of the caregiver or the practitioner. This quality of humanity should, in principle, be the same for the skilled practitioner and the supplementary caregiver. If we had to choose just one attribute in common for practitioners, caregivers, and by extension educators, *kindness* would seem to be basic and essential. Francis Peabody, MD, wrote in *Caring for the Patient*, as quoted by Harrison (1995):

> The significance of the intimate personal relationship between physician and patient cannot be too strongly emphasized, for in an extraordinarily large number of cases, both the diagnosis and the treatment are directly dependent on it. One of the essential qualities of the clinician is interest in humanity, for the secret of the care of the patient is in caring for the patient.

COMMENTS

An osteopath is a *single practitioner* who both evaluates and performs manual treatment. This dual role of knowledge-based practitioner and therapist highlights the idea that osteopathy is not merely palliative but is a bona fide autonomous healing art whose concept is both diagnostic and specifically therapeutic.

An osteopathic diagnosis requires a solid scientific and technical grounding.

Some therapists choose to *be* osteopaths who practice this challenging art exclusively, respecting the principles of evaluation and therapy. Others claim to "do" osteopathy through the application of certain techniques taken to a greater or lesser degree out of their original contexts. Some such practitioners even have a degree of success with this approach.

Undertaking a Diagnosis and Evaluation

In European osteopathy's struggle for formal recognition, the associations that defend and promote our profession have often focused on enumerating the differences between medical and osteopathic forms of diagnosis. Some of these organizations have even chosen to abandon the term *diagnosis* so as not to ruffle feathers.

This is not the forum to judge the soundness either of the arguments they put forward or the political merits of such choices, but it seems clear that no profession can claim a high level of competence if it does not have a system of diagnosis worthy of the name. It is clear that we can emphasize the differences in diagnosis as practiced by a variety of medical specialties. The greater challenge is to establish their similarities. My reflections and research on the subject brings up the situation of one patient receiving many different diagnoses based on the specialty of each practitioner (fig. 1.1).

I believe that in most of the major medical systems, the work of diagnosis follows an identical path. Approaches differ according to context, of course; they depend on the medical doctrine and set of potential therapeutic responses particular to each system. We should not forget, however, that despite notable differences, the patient remains the central element in a diagnosis. Depending on the chosen viewpoint, a single patient may be thought about and examined in many different ways. The various approaches to diagnosis may observe a single clinical reality but do not consider it in exactly the same manner. Whatever the specialty, each practitioner can only see the advisability of accepting a patient into care through the lens of his or her own knowledge and understanding of health and disease.

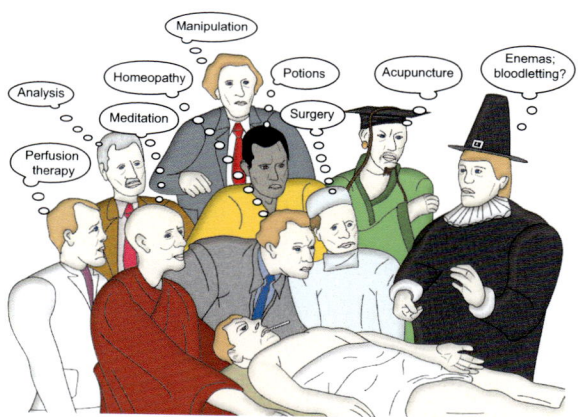

Figure 1.1. Different diagnostic points of view.

When all is said and done, *a diagnosis is a point of view expressed by a health care practitioner relative to a patient's situation.* The practitioner must take into account the patient's general state of health and fitness, the seriousness of his or her condition, and the appropriateness or of a given therapeutic response.

The diagnosis is just one facet of the reality of the patient and of his or her pathology. Regardless of the therapeutic framework, every step of a diagnosis rests on three key points:

- a *positive diagnosis,* which seeks to identify some abnormality or dysfunction present in the patient. The idea of "normal" can vary greatly according to the context. The very nature of the abnormality or dysfunction that the practitioner seeks to identify is thus closely linked with the concept of therapy.
- a *differential diagnosis,* which is an attempt to distinguish between similar conditions and possibilities yielded by the positive diagnosis. By performing a differential diagnosis, the diagnostician eliminates the less likely hypotheses and comes to focus on the most plausible one(s), thus achieving greater clarity about possible contraindications or precautions to be observed.
- an *etiological diagnosis,* which aims to discover factors that may be causing the dysfunction diagnosed. This determines what might be considered an objective cause, a predisposing factor, or a tendency that might incline the patient toward developing the condition. When possible, effective treatment of such causative factors can prevent recurrence.

Certain authors, such as Thomas (1999), compare this tripartite division to reasoning according to Aristotelian logic, consisting of thesis, antithesis, and synthesis (fig. 1.2).

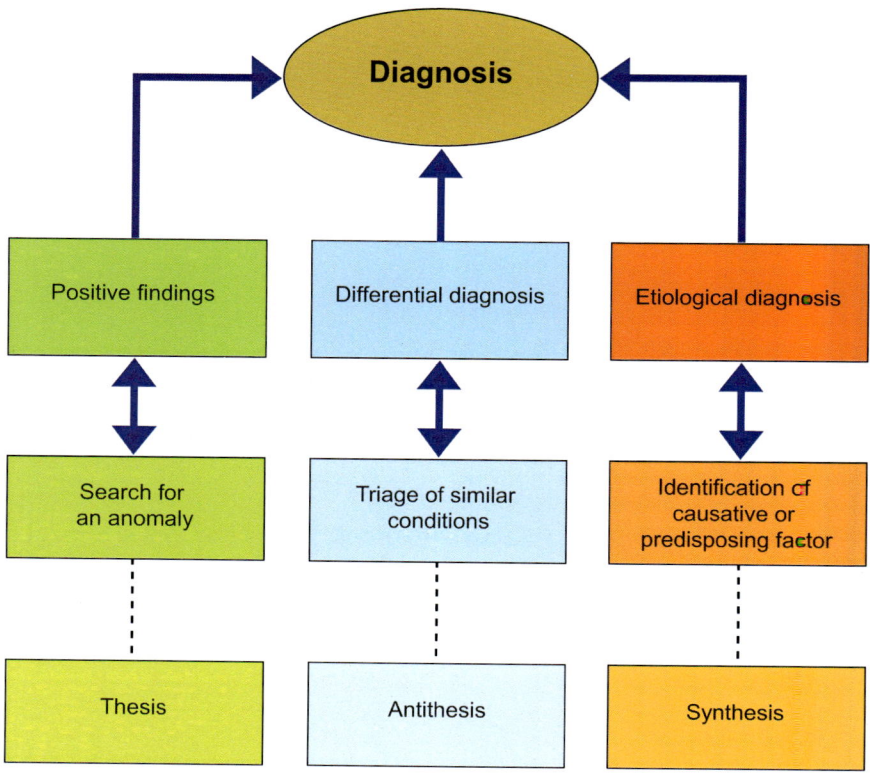

Figure 1.2. General approach to diagnosis.

The Foundation of Diagnosis

The ideas of diagnosis and therapy are closely linked. As a general rule, if we can find only what we look for, we will only look for things for which we have an available response or therapeutic approach. Whatever the subject, things that are beyond our comprehension do not interest us. This fact of life holds true for diagnosis, which is accordingly subordinated to the application and potential of the therapeutic intervention. At the same time, diagnosis is the precursor for this therapeutic application and action.

Based on this fact, pretherapeutic evaluation or diagnosis is a very specific element of a given therapy. The degree to which a given diagnosis made by a practitioner of a healing art will be understood by a person who does not share the same technical and semantic foundation will vary. The difficulties arising between members of a profession and laypeople come about, to a large extent, as a result of this specificity. The issue can also arise between newcomers to a discipline and experienced practitioners, or among practitioners of different therapies. Technical jargon often suffers as it passes from one area of specialization to another.

According to the practitioner's skill level and the therapeutic approach, the notion of diagnosis varies as much in its methodology and goals as in its means and principles. Allopathic medicine may be what first comes to the Western mind, but other medical traditions also exist, each of which goes through its own particular series of diagnostic steps. Through comparison, we will see that diagnosis according to these different traditions involves entirely different elements, and that the term *medical* has many different meanings.

NOTE

A diagnosis is a highly specific aspect of a given specialty; it is only fully understood by a practitioner of the same school or of a closely related discipline. As such, a given diagnosis is often incomprehensible to anyone lacking the same foundation as the practitioner who made it.

Forms of Diagnosis

Allopathic medicine is so deeply rooted in our culture that current usage tends to designate it simply "medicine." That is to say, allopathic diagnostic and therapeutic methods are considered in Western societies to be a kind of standard. To a greater or lesser degree, our minds are conditioned by the allopathic "brand" that has been imposed since the Middle Ages. It is even difficult at times to convince people of the existence of other approaches to health and disease, and other methods of observing or evaluating patients.

Preliminary Diagnosis

In Allopathy

According to Garnier and Delamare (1995), the definition of diagnosis is "the act by means of which the physician, gathering into a group the symptoms of disease displayed by the patient, associates them with an illness that exists in the catalog of diseases." Diagnosis rests on a collection of objective elements considered as a whole, which makes it possible to identify a disease entity. A diagnosis emerges from information about the patient gathered by means of:

- history
- clinical examination
- supplementary examinations and tests

This makes it possible to assemble symptoms into an established framework and usually leads the diagnostician to identify this collection as a *disease* or a *syndrome*. This identification is arrived at within what is called the nosological framework. Nosology is the system of the classification of disease, and nosography is the systematic description of disease. The kind of diagnosis based on the patient's symptomatology as it relates to this framework is termed a "nosographic" or "pathological" diagnosis.

Contemporary medicine addresses the consequences of the disease process or the process itself. It focuses its diagnostic search on the physiological mechanisms of the body's decompensation. Therapeutic action usually relies on an external force opposed to the symptoms. This force is usually chemically based: medications. Occasionally, medicine uses a mechanical force or agent: surgery. At others times it resorts to a physical force, as in radiation therapy.

In Osteopathy

With its basis in anatomy, visualization of structures in motion, and observation of nature, osteopathy is an original therapeutic system that attempts to restore the body's proper relationship with the universal laws of health. Osteopaths seek to remove the causes of the patient's symptoms by treating the imbalance that is at their origin. We focus our diagnostic efforts on anatomical disorders and on the compensations that the body creates in response to them. We identify the *mechanical dysfunctions* that the patient presents and then determine which ones have a direct connection to the problem.

As in classical medicine, the osteopathic version of diagnosis rests on two fundamental elements: patient history and clinical examination. Clinical examination is more thorough, with precise palpation playing a bigger role in osteopathy. In addition to the search for classical clinical findings, osteopaths add an examination and an evaluation of the mechanical abilities of the body's various structures. Osteopaths are more concerned with the mechanical conditions of good health than with their intrinsic expression in a disease process. Our goal as osteopaths is primarily to restore the conditions of good health within the patient's body, drawing to the greatest extent possible the patient's powers of self-healing and self-regulation.

Osteopathic diagnosis is not based on a process of reflection within a nosological framework. In no way is it connected with the identification of a defined disease or condition. While it rests on knowledge of anatomy, biomechanics, physiology, and the signs of normal or abnormal structure and function, osteopathic diagnosis is based on *perceptions*. Osteopaths seek to learn through their hands, from a biomechanical point of view, the origin of an impairment of the mobility of the bodily structures. This kind of diagnosis, which identifies the mechanism responsible for a given patient's symptomatology or pathological decompensation, is called "pathogenic" or "nosogenic" diagnosis.

Differential Diagnosis

In Allopathy

According to Garnier and Delamare (1995), differential diagnosis consists of "the elimination of similar conditions by means of ratiocination from that condition that the physician seeks to identify." From the point of view of methodology, one of the first steps of differential diagnosis is to consider all possible hypotheses. Some of these are more likely, others less so. Every possible disease entity is passed through a filter without deductively giving preference to or having any prejudice against any one of these candidates in the process. It's not a matter of adding weight to the most likely presumed diagnosis but rather of not excluding other possibilities. This first step is not one of reflection but of objectively classifying the various possible pathologies.

The second step involves a process of discussion that leads the practitioner to consider each hypothesis as more or less likely. Examinations and supplementary tests are performed as needed, allowing a leading hypothesis to be chosen. This second step of differential diagnosis is driven by reflection.

In Osteopathy

The first step of differential diagnosis explores the notions of indication and contraindication. Depending on the severity of the case, it may or may not be advisable to accept a patient for osteopathic care.

In the taxonomy of the healing arts, osteopathy is located in the branch that might be called the "iatromechanical" medicines. Osteopaths add nothing to the body that wasn't already there; we "rearrange" its mechanics. We have no great effect on problems caused by genetics, heredity, or deficiencies. We must be perfectly able to identify anything outside of our area of competence.

It is imperative that osteopaths be thoroughly familiar with the signs of the principal clinical syndromes. This knowledge allows us as practitioners to consider the contraindications, both absolute and relative, to our therapeutic approach. It is not always easy to define the exact nature of an osteopathic differential diagnosis. Even if a familiarity with nosography is required, in no way does that imply arriving at a nosological diagnosis. The precision required by allopathic diagnosis has no relevance in the appropriate practice of our art.

The other tier of differential diagnosis has to do with an attempt to detect the pattern of the patient's mechanical dysfunctions. This is, in fact, the point at which the patient's particular pathogenesis is determined. From an anatomical and physiological point of view, numerous interactions exist. A visceral dysfunction can cause back pain, and a somatic dysfunction can give rise to visceral problems. A cranial disturbance can bring about headaches with pain radiating into the neck, while a dysfunction in the cervical spine can cause lancinating pain in the cranial vault. There is no shortage of examples demonstrating this interdependence of biomechanics and symptomatology. Sorting out this tangle is the second tier of differential diagnosis.

Etiological Diagnosis

In Allopathy

According to Garnier and Delamare (1995), etiological diagnosis is the "search for the causes of pathological conditions." In classical medicine, this is a task of preventive medicine or public health medicine that aims to discover an objective material cause for the patient's condition. Its concern is both for the individual and for society. For the individual, its aim is primarily the prevention of recurrence. For society, it seeks to prevent the spread of the condition to others, to improve its treatment, and to prevent its occurrence.

This third reflection takes place at a point in time that can be considerably later from the time when the positive and differential diagnoses are established. Medical treatment is often begun prior to this stage of diagnosis, which generally requires extra clinical examinations, the results of which can sometimes be long (days or weeks) in coming. In fact, the true etiology of conditions is rarely discovered, since irrefutable anatomical, physiological, and statistical proofs are required to fully confirm the etiology.

If etiology is not formally determined, a disease is generally classified as "idiopathic." About seventy percent of diseases are currently considered idiopathic.

13

	Positive diagnosis	Differential diagnosis	Etiological diagnosis
Allopathic diagnosis	Identification of a pathogen	Examination and discussion of hypotheses	Search for etiology of pathology
Osteopathic diagnosis	Determination of a pathology	Discussion of indication(s) and hypotheses	Search for etiology of pathology

Figure 1.3. Comparison of diagnostic approaches.

In Osteopathy

The etiological diagnosis of osteopathy seeks to determine how the original mechanical disturbance came about. (At times, however, we must settle for identifying those factors that perpetuate the dysfunction.) The origin of the imbalance is discovered either by means of follow-up studies, specific tests, or with the aid of the practitioner's knowledge of functional semiology and the laws of nature.

Our principal aim is to prevent a recurrence of the condition. If its root cause is eliminated or if we can take effective action against its direct consequences, the chain of dysfunction should no longer negatively affect the patient's health. The goal of treatment is to obtain a lasting result, not make patients dependent on our manipulations; this is the most important reason for this essential stage of diagnosis.

Trauma, malpositions in utero, and difficult births constitute the triad of preeminent biomechanical pathogenesis. Postural habits and repetitive actions done with poor body mechanics, stress, anxiety, emotional upsets, unhealthy lifestyle, and intoxication can be equally prolific sources of mechanical dysfunctions and of the loss of the equilibrium that health depends on.

Summary of the Steps in the Diagnostic Process

The parallels between modes of diagnosis are summarized in figure 1.3. The osteopathic and medical approaches to diagnosis follow generally similar courses, with each organizing itself according to its own outlook and methodology.

NOTE

- Osteopathy is not a mere adjuvant or supplementary technique susceptible to a greater or lesser extent to integration into another approach to healing. It is, rather, a true medical art, complete in itself, with its own systems of logic, diagnosis, and therapy, and its own particular set of indications and contraindications.
- Without claiming omnipotence for the osteopathic approach, it is important to stress that it is risky to mix it with classical medical practice. The two disciplines have neither the same scope nor the same principles. Finally, they take very distinct views of physiopathology.

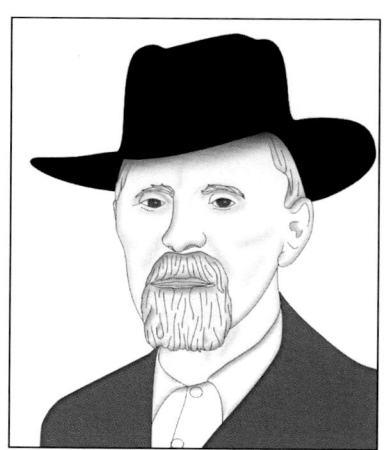

Figure 2.1. Andrew Taylor Still.

Chapter 2

The Osteopathic Paradigm

I do not claim to be the author of this science of Osteopathy. No human hand framed its laws; I ask no greater honor than to have discovered it.

— ANDREW TAYLOR STILL

History

Osteopathy was founded in the United States in the second half of the nineteenth century by Dr. Andrew Taylor Still. Disappointed by the results and the theories of the way medicine was practiced at the time, he decided to focus not on the illness but on the conditions necessary for health.

Firm in his religious convictions, Still started from a belief in the principle that God had created man as perfect. From the mechanical point of view, he felt that if the structures of the body were in correct alignment and functioning properly, and if the flows of blood, lymph, and nerve impulses were free of interference, good health would inevitably follow.

In Still's view, an osteopath practicing appropriately should be content with allowing the *vital principle* to come to the tissues of the periphery. To do this, the practitioner must remove every mechanical obstacle to the free circulation of the vital forces.

From this theoretical basis, using the anatomical and physiological knowledge of the time, Still worked systematically to understand the functioning of the body's frame and its contents. Working with his hands, he freed joints and released muscular tensions.

Nevertheless, in Still's mind, osteopathy was not limited to musculoskeletal problems. He accepted patients suffering from severe mechanical problems, but he also occupied himself with patients presenting a wide variety of ailments.

His therapeutic success owed much to his philosophy of avoiding medications and instead simply working with his hands and applying basic, simple, and hygienic measures.

Old Europe and the New World

The way that the osteopathic profession has evolved in Europe is quite different from its evolution in the United States. It was brought to Europe by one of Still's own students, John Martin Littlejohn, who created the first school of osteopathy in Great Britain in 1917. From there, the concepts of osteopathy spread and gradually took root in continental Europe.

It can be said that in Europe, osteopaths practice outside of the realm of conventional medicine; in the United States, osteopaths are also trained as medical doctors. Consequently, American osteopaths have ready recourse to allopathic medicine and surgery in their practices, while in Europe osteopaths remain faithful to the tradition of manual therapy.

Osteopathic Philosophy and Principles

Still's Concept

Initially, Still's primary focus was on osteoarticular mechanics. Several attempts have been made to systematize his thinking. The osteopathic concept is quite simple in its basics; expressing it as a formula, however, can be a complex challenge. One example of the difficulties involved is the task of making all of Still's original writings available to the general public.

According to the osteopathic concept, health does not depend on an external remedy of any sort but rather on perfect biomechanical harmony. Osteopathy is sometimes compared with the art of bonesetting—therapy for the joints. While there are parallels between the two therapeutic approaches, the clearest distinction between osteopathy and bonesetting is the former's scientific foundation and its holistic view of health. It should be emphasized that the central concept in osteopathy is that good health depends on the ability of all bodily structures to move freely, rather than on an idealized posture or alignment of the joints.

Principles of Osteopathy

The principles of osteopathy are the elementary general and theoretical rules that guide its practitioners' conduct. These general principles govern a group of phenomena, and their validity is proven by the predictability of their therapeutic results.

- The body is an indivisible whole.
- Structure and function are interdependent.
- The body is endowed with a high degree of perfection, which gives it the abilities of self-regulation, self-defense, and self-healing.
- Life is movement.
- The movement of fluids is essential to health.
- The nervous system plays a central role in controlling the body's fluids and the exchange of information.
- An osteopath must try to distinguish effects from causes.

The Goals of Osteopathy

These goals concern a set of ideas that osteopaths have in mind in connection with providing treatment, i.e., our objectives, intentions, and desired results:

- to correct mechanical disorders
- to restore the mobility of mechanical structures
- to stimulate the body's autoregulatory mechanisms
- to optimize the body's capacities for self-defense and self-repair
- to repair the body's damaged ability to adapt when environmental changes have overwhelmed the capacity of autoregulation, leaving it susceptible to disease
- to fight certain disease processes that are not just symptoms of the illness but are also factors contributing to its continuation or to further damage
- to bring the body's *vital principle* to the periphery in order to awaken the *inner physician*

Osteopathic Tools and Techniques

These techniques focus more on therapy than on diagnosis, and consist of technical interventions that allow the practitioner to act and to do something specific for the patient. It is implicit in osteopathic thinking that osteopathic intervention can optimize the chances of improving the patient's health.

- Manipulations are carried out precisely on the structures that are limited in their mobility.
- The manipulation must focus on or be aimed at the structures responsible for the body's principal imbalance.
- It is useless, or even dangerous, to manipulate a structure that is unrelated to the mechanical disorder, even if symptoms present themselves at that location.

Elaboration of the Original Concept

Still's original concepts were further developed and augmented by other practitioners in such a way that these additions have now been fully accepted and incorporated into the osteopathic art.

The Craniosacral System

William G. Sutherland extended Still's concept to the sutures (articulations) of the cranium. The cranial sutures persist throughout life and make the cranium behave rather like a dynamic, moldable puzzle. Sutherland's discoveries and clinical observations made it possible to add cranial treatment to the corpus of osteopathic practice. For Sutherland, normal cranial mobility corresponded to good health, while cranial restrictions were either the result of trauma or systemic disease.

Sutherland set out or described the following precepts and functional units:

- the existence of a functional unity between the cranium and the sacrum;
- the anatomical and physiological components of the *primary respiratory mechanism*—the subtle, slow pulse involved in regular cranial and sacral motions;
- the significance of this mechanism in directing and controlling major functions of the body, at once attesting to and playing an active role in the maintenance of good health;
- the physiological action of the cerebrospinal fluid, which acts like a tide, transported throughout the body by the vast network of fascial microtubules.

Manipulation of the cranium and its meninges often yields very interesting results in the treatment of newborns, children, and adolescents. It is also indicated in treating adults following trauma or when certain chronic pathologies are involved.

- The craniosacral system is a point of connection among the developing brain, spinal cord, and sensory organs. Psychomotor development depends on it functioning properly.
- It plays a significant role relative to the otorhinolaryngological sphere, to the eyes, and even to visceral functioning.
- Through its influence on the brain, it plays a key role in the qualities of sleep, rest, and recuperation.

- Because of the pituitary's location at the very heart of the cranial system, the cranial system's mechanical functioning plays a key role in the quality of sleep and the individual's ability to rest and recuperate.
- In view of the central location of the pituitary gland, in the very heart of the cranial system and at the "hinge" of the sphenoid and occipital bones, the cranial mechanism provides support to the endocrine system.
- The craniosacral system also helps to mediate spinal posture and mechanics.

The Visceral System

Still's writings indicate that manipulation of the viscera formed part of the way osteopathy was practiced even by its founder, who incorporated these structures into the biomechanical whole. Subsequently, various practitioners of the art have developed a systematic understanding of the mechanics of the organs and an approach to visceral manipulation. One notable American osteopath who helped to develop these approaches was Percy Hogan Woodall, who in the early twentieth century set out a set of principles of urogenital mechanics. In Europe, more recently the works of Jacques Weischenck, Jean-Pierre Barral, and Pierre Mercier have contributed greatly to the development of a systematic approach to the viscera and the role they play in the body's mechanical management.

Visceral manipulation is used to improve the position, circulation, and motion of organs in a wide range of dysfunctions and visceral problems. The techniques are particularly effective in issues involving the digestive tract and the pelvic organs.

- Visceral mechanics support many physiological functions relating to homeostasis:
  - The organs of elimination contribute to the maintenance of the health of the body and its ecology.

- The autonomic nervous system has plexuses located within or close to the viscera.
- The immune system has numerous relaying or connecting points in various organs.
- The endocrine system plays a contributing role in the visceral system.

■ Visceral mechanics influence parietal mechanics and posture—*visceral* refers to the organs themselves; *parietal* refers to the body "walls" that surround the viscera or the body cavities that contain them.

■ The viscera are major targets for emotions; they therefore play a role in relaying mental influences.

Chapter 3

Basic Principles of Osteopathic Diagnosis

At a time when many fields of health care claim the label of osteopathy, it would be highly presumptuous of me to present myself as the keeper of osteopathic orthodoxy. On the other hand, it is of primary importance to state that no diagnosis can be authentically osteopathic in nature unless it conforms to Still's conceptual and philosophic principles.

This chapter will serve as a brief reminder—a summary of the origin and evolution of osteopathy. This will provide a clearer understanding of the specifics of osteopathic diagnosis as it relates to our profession's concepts and philosophy. We will see that the rules of the art of osteopathy must not be confused with the rules of diagnosis.

The Framework of Diagnosis

In his writings, Still speaks almost exclusively about philosophy. He tells us the proper frame of mind to cultivate and how to evaluate the body, beginning with normal in order to understand what is abnormal or pathological. However, he gives little practical or technical guidance. At one point in his writings, Still (1892, 33) uses the image of a mechanic repairing a machine. For him, "repair" means:

> an adjustment from the abnormal condition in which the machin-
> ist finds it to the condition of the normal engine.... As osteopathic

machinists we go no further than to adjust the abnormal conditions back to the normal. Nature will do the rest.

Today, with osteopathic knowledge becoming more and more complete, it is becoming clear that a synthesis is required. Seeing the individual as a whole allows us to take a specific approach to health care. How can we teach the diagnosis and treatment of each part without losing sight of the whole?

Progress in the state of our art has allowed for increasingly precise cataloguing of manipulations, which leads to complexity. It is no longer enough for us to know the various therapeutic tools. We must also be able to use them in a way that meets the requirements of the situation. We must be able to explain them clearly and intelligently according to the case at hand. The range of available osteopathic therapies is much greater than it was initially. We acquire the many and varied techniques slowly because they need to mature. This slow pace in acquiring techniques often impairs the development of a holistic view of things. The osteopathic concept is consistent with a great deal of scientific knowledge that now exists. Practitioners may be strongly tempted to place knowledge above hands-on learning and the development of manual skill. The increasing complexity of the osteopathic healing art undoubtedly explains the common phenomenon of losing one's conceptual bearings. Many practitioners turn to other therapeutic concepts or philosophies in order to create their own systems of diagnosis.

We need to find coherence in our art. The work of diagnosis allows us to reconnect with the conceptual basis of osteopathy in its various aspects. A therapeutic intervention is a powerful tool, but alone it is not enough—it must also be used in the best interests of the patient. There is no miracle technique that can be applied systematically to everyone. When not indicated, a technique has no intrinsic value. The best technical ability in the world won't make up for a lack of insight in diagnosis.

Principles of Diagnosis

Osteopathic diagnosis explores the quantitative and qualitative aspects of human biomechanics. Osteopathy is a mechanically based healing art. It is a full-fledged system of thought that has its own set of standards. For the osteopath, health can only be maintained within the context of the whole and perfectly balanced biomechanism.

The term *mechanism* should be understood in the broad sense. It does not involve the neuromusculoskeletal system alone but also all the tissues and elements that exert a mechanical influence in the body. Pressure, tension, support, and constraint of every sort exist throughout the body, and the scale of their action ranges from the body as a whole to intracellular relationships. Osteopathic diagnosis evaluates the integrity of these biomechanical systems, from the densest to the most subtle. *The mechanism of the body is whole and indivisible.*

Osteopathic diagnosis is not concerned exclusively with the spinal column and the joints. It seeks to determine, as specifically as possible, the mechanical causes of dysfunction or disease, wherever they may be. Osteopathy is not spinal therapy; it is not limited to spinal manipulation, and osteopathic thought does not come down to a simple reflexive explanation of pathology. This is in no way meant to minimize the significance of the spinal keyboard that commands and regulates numerous bodily functions through the intermediary of the autonomic nervous system. It would, however, be reductionist in the extreme to assign the spine full responsibility for mechanical dysfunctions and to place it alone at the center of osteopathic diagnosis and treatment.

Osteopathy is the science of mechanical interactions throughout the human body. For the osteopath, the proper functioning of this mechanism depends not only on the skeletal elements and their articulations but also on everything that can act on these parts. The soft tissues are of the greatest significance. Originally considered as a whole component, they have become the object of increasingly minute and precise examination.

For the osteopath, every anatomical element is a potential mechanical vector that can act, for good or for ill, on the body as a whole. *Osteopathic diagnosis explores the relationships between structure and function.* All of the structures of the body exist in mechanical interdependence. It follows that the functions they support are also interdependent. Structure governs function, and function produces reverberations on structure. Every structural disturbance can give rise to functional disturbances. Diagnosis seeks to identify the faulty structure that is responsible for the functional disorder. It also takes into account the resulting adaptations and maladaptations throughout the body.

Osteopathic diagnosis takes place in the present: it is here and now. The patient is structured like an onion, and our diagnosis corresponds to the layer being examined. This implies, among other things, that we treat the patient and not our idea of the patient. We should not attempt to treat deep, hypothetical, or invisible layers without first freeing up more superficial, concrete, and visible ones. Diagnosis takes account of this idea of the present moment: it is the result of what the therapist can discover and what the patient allows to be revealed in the moment.

Osteopathic diagnosis is global: it respects the concept of the wholeness of the person. One of the great principles of osteopathy is the unity and oneness of the human being. The body does not function as an ensemble of separate units but rather as one harmonious entity. The interests of the whole are most important, and every constituent part works to support the whole. Conversely, every part that does not function properly creates repercussions in the whole.

Chapter 4

Positive Diagnosis in Osteopathy

Life is short, art is long, opportunity fleeting, experiment treacherous, judgment difficult. The physician must not only do what is appropriate, but also make the patient, the assistants, and external things cooperate.

— HIPPOCRATES

The Nature of Osteopathic Diagnosis

Diagnostic research is always governed by exposing things that aren't right, that don't fit—in a word, things that are abnormal. The ability to distinguish between what is normal and what is pathological constitutes the central pillar of positive diagnosis. Depending on the context, the idea of normality can take many different forms. Traditional medicine usually requires a biological or radiographic abnormality to confirm a diagnosis. For the osteopath, abnormality is found primarily in a bodily structure's loss of movement. Osteopathic diagnosis is mechanical in nature.

From Physiology to Pathology

Norm and Normality

What is the basis of the notions of "normality" and "norm"? According to Henri Laborit (1979), in medicine, as it is taught in medical schools, an individual is considered to be *organically normal* if he or she falls within a certain range on a Gaussian bell curve (box 4.1) in which all phenomena and all biological values are represented. We can then say whether a given individual is diabetic, uremic, or hyperthermic, and whether or not he or she possesses an organic lesion. An individual is considered *psychologically normal* if he or she conforms to a Gaussian curve in which human behaviors in a given society are plotted, according to the historical epoch and the range of values established. In both cases, the why or how of abnormality is rarely considered. On this level, the individual can only be considered without taking the environmental and sociocultural context into account. Therapy for such individuals is generally limited to attempts to bring them into conformity, and to do so as quickly as possible. Efforts are rarely made to adapt the environment so that the subject can find what is normal and balanced for him or her as a person.

From a therapeutic point of view, different approaches exist. The first tries to treat patients to bring them into conformity with the Gaussian curve. The second seeks to harmonize patients or their environment to help them recover, or discover, their own individual normality and balance. Generally speaking, the former method is a short-term approach. It may constitute a symptoms-based response or be used to address the most urgent matters first in an emergency. The second strategy is more long-term. It attempts to modify the environmental factors and requires time for the body to react and adjust to the changes. These two approaches are not mutually exclusive but rather can complement each other in a useful way.

Box 4.1. Gaussian Curves and the Classification of Normal

In a given population, if individuals are ranked according to a specific characteristic (height, weight, IQ, blood-sugar level), most individuals are found at points closest to the mean. Conversely, with increasing distance from the mean, fewer individuals are found. At the two extremes of the curve, there are almost no individuals. The graphical representation of this is called a Gaussian function, and it has the shape of a bell curve (fig. 4.1). This curve expresses the density of probabilities of a group of random variables. Use of the bell curve may be the

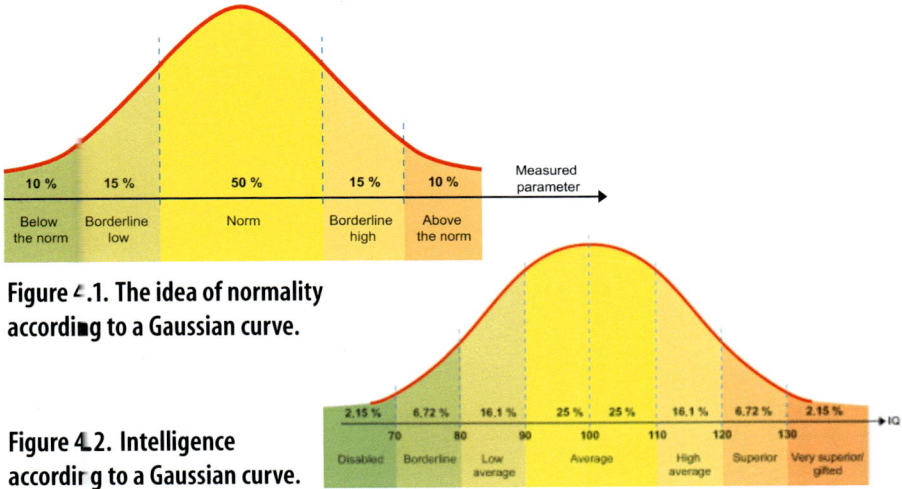

Figure 4.1. The idea of normality according to a Gaussian curve.

Figure 4.2. Intelligence according to a Gaussian curve.

reason for a number of biases, and its application to human beings creates a kind of tyranny of the majority. For example, considering foot size, female patients wearing sizes 4½ and 10½ are at opposite ends of the bell curve. Even if we agree that for marketing purposes these women are somewhat rare, anatomically speaking, does it follow that they are less normal than those who wear size 7½? Should we then decide that the well-being of these women is unimportant because they are less numerous? Along the same lines, assessment of intelligence using the idea of an intelligence quotient (IQ) has been the source of many evaluation errors.

The Normal and the Normative

It is important to remind ourselves of the omnipresent normative ness—the conformist tendency—of our Western societies. More generally speaking, nearly all societies tend to impose developmental and social norms. To give just one example, for children there is a general rule that by a certain age they must be well-groomed, and at other specific ages they must be able to speak, walk, read, and so on. None of this takes into account the individual child's particular speed of development or temporary or constitutional difficulties or challenges.

In a society, the norm represents the rule of the dominant. At our level as therapists, in addition to doing our job as technical practitioners, we can try to bring some balance to this tendency. We often need to reassure those who fall outside a traditional norm, and to disrupt prejudices that they may have toward themselves while reminding them that "normality" is just a particular point of view. Sometimes we just need to avoid accepting and reinforcing a ready-made formula or diagnosis based on a given ideal, rather than feeding the psychological power of an ideal that patients often feel they should conform to.

Different Types of Disorders

A distinction is often made between *functional pathology* and *organic pathology,* which can lead us to think that pathology is clearly divided into two different types. The reality is a bit more subtle. Léon Vannier (1965) defines three types of disorders that, when taken together, give each patient's pathology its own distinctive appearance:

- lesional disorders
- functional disorders
- sensory disorders

Lesional Disorders

Lesional disorders result from damage to an organ's anatomy These are the best-understood problems of organs, since they provide a clear record of the development of the disease process and make for a relatively easy diagnosis. Such pathologies are often termed *organic*. This kind of disorder is usually confirmed by clinical and supportive investigations. The patient with an organ thus affected is no longer considered to be *organically normal.*

Functional Disorders

Functional disorders are expressions of an alteration in the functioning of an organ. When the organ's functioning is disordered, reactions appear that differ according to the affected organ and to the particularities of the patient. It is often impossible to establish a diagnosis of a disease or to put a label on this collection of clinical facts. Even if the group of symptoms cannot objectively be assigned a diagnosis by the classical methods of imaging and biological analyses, they are of great significance diagnostically.

Allopathic medicine can find itself powerless in the face of functional disorders when they do not correspond to a recognizable clinical picture. Osteopathic manual diagnosis generally allows the practitioner to find a localized site of dysfunction and to identify the mechanical disturbance that is its likely cause. The practitioner can thereby trace the origins of functional disorders linked to malfunction of glands, organs, plexuses, or nerve ganglia.

Sensory Dysfunctions

Sensory dysfunctions arise at the beginning of every disease or, to be more precise, at the beginning of every condition leading to disease. They constitute the "state of malaise" that precedes the appearance of functional and lesional dysfunctions. The way in which these individual manifestations appear is in accord with the character of the affected person, whose psyche and sensitivity are modified by them. Each such pattern is strictly individual.

At this point, there is an absence of organ damage and of lesional dysfunctions. The functioning of the organ has not changed, and functional changes have not yet manifested. Sensory changes are the only signs of dysfunction. These signs, however, often discourage the patient and confuse the therapist.

Differences between individual psyches and sensitivities are numerous. At times, these are the only signs that reveal the existence of a disease process in a patient, manifesting an inner state of imbalance or disorder, or a lack of synchronization with the external world. They sometimes accompany an established group of symptoms of a recognized disease or a clinical syndrome. This gives an individualized expression that is characteristic of that person's response to the disease.

Chronologically, when any disease process begins, symptomatology often progresses from the surface to the depths following these stages:

- psychosensory
- functional
- somatic or lesional

Healing progresses in the opposite direction. Osteopathic diagnosis must identify what stage the patient's dysfunction is currently in. By identifying the nature and stage of the presenting dysfunctions, we can judge the seriousness of the disease. The prognosis and the therapeutic choices depend greatly on a proper understanding of the stage of the disease, and this understanding also dictates the other actions the therapist needs to take.

Osteopathic Dysfunctions

Physiopathology

From an osteopathic point of view, any mechanical disturbance, whatever its location in the body, can be detrimental to the patient's general energy management and consequently to his or her health. Through manual diagnosis, the osteopath detects the anatomical elements whose movement is defective. This alteration of motion can cause changes in the local biomechanics and create local symptoms. Via various pathways it may also cause repercussions at a distance and give rise to symptoms far removed from the original imbalance.

As we have seen, the osteopathic art represents an indivisible approach to three major biomechanical systems: the musculoskeletal, visceral, and craniosacral systems. Each of these systems is in constant interaction with the others. The physiopathological intricacies of these interactions can be difficult to untangle. From the mechanical point of view, none of these systems has more importance than the others. Only a rigorously performed diagnosis can determine which system plays the greatest role in the pathological process of any given patient.

Terminology

Dysfunction

The osteopathic profession has chosen the term *somatic dysfunction* to refer to the musculoskeletal domain. This term replaces the formerly used *osteopathic lesion*, as the word *lesion* can cause confusion. For the other major systems, we have chosen to continue the use of the term *dysfunction* in the mechanical sense, but we indicate the specific context as *visceral dysfunction* or *craniosacral dysfunction*.

Designation of Dysfunctions

As a general rule, the designation assigned to a dysfunction is based on the degree of mobility that the affected structure retains. For example, a vertebra with a flexion dysfunction has lost its ability to extend relative to the vertebra beneath it, but it can flex correctly. A right torsion dysfunction of the sphenobasilar synchondrosis (SB joint) means the joint is unable to make a left twisting motion, but torsion to the right is still possible. An inspiration dysfunction of the liver refers to the situation in which the liver cannot move properly on expiration, although it moves correctly during inspiration.

Primary and Secondary Dysfunctions

Every patient presents unique biomechanical dysfunctions that they have an easier or harder time tolerating, as each dysfunction causes different degrees of harm or inconvenience. As a general rule, dysfunctions show a certain level of organization and interdependence. Of particular significance is the *primary dysfunction,* which can potentially cause the greatest imbalance for the body and for health in general. This may be the oldest dysfunction or the one that gives rise to the greatest number of secondary dysfunctions. *Secondary dysfunctions* represent a phenomenon of adaptation and compensation in the body in response to a primary dysfunction.

- An *adaptation* is a spontaneously reversible pattern of rebalancing. *Whether it is painful or not, it is essential for the practitioner to recognize it for what it is, because there is nothing to be gained by treating it.*
- A *compensation* is a chronic fixation existing as part of a pattern of adaptation. Compensations are spontaneously irreversible and constitute an actual secondary dysfunction. Treatment them is only indicated if they remain after the primary dysfunction has been successfully addressed.

Adaptations and compensations are two processes by which the body attempts to restore balance in a group of biomechanical disturbances that are secondary to a primary dysfunction.

Physiological and Nonphysiological Dysfunctions

Dysfunctions are called "physiological" when they respect the normal axes and planes of movement of the articulation involved. They are generally articular fixations situated within the limits of normal motion for the surfaces involved. For instance, the limitation of motion of a vertebra that rotates to a normal extent in one direction but not in the other in the transverse plane, or that has extension within normal limits but does not flex properly, is a physiological dysfunction.

On the other hand, nonphysiological dysfunctions do not respect the normal axes or planes of motion of the structure. These generally result from hits or other traumatic injuries. They can also occur as complications of physiological dysfunctions that have evolved under the influence of additional mechanical factors. Translational vertebral malposition, for example spondylolisthesis and lateral sacral flexion, are examples of nonphysiological dysfunctions.

Chains of Dysfunction (Formerly Lesional Chains)

For reasons outlined above, the term *chain of dysfunction* has replaced the phrase *lesional chain*, which was used in the past. It refers to the concatenation and organization of the dysfunctions that have brought the patient into the general biomechanical predicament found at the time of examination.

Somatic (i.e., Musculoskeletal) Dysfunctions

According to osteopathic terminology, somatic dysfunctions consist of alterations or modifications in the components of the musculoskeletal system and their attachments. These dysfunctions affect not only the frame of the body—skeletal, articular, and myofascial structures—but also the vascular, lymphatic, and nervous elements that connect to it.

Numerous hypotheses have been put forward on somatic dysfunction and have been debated in as scientific a way as possible. In any case, the notion of somatic dysfunction in the body is very familiar to osteopaths, who discern it precisely. The osteopathic understanding of somatic dysfunction specifically differs from the understanding of other manipulative therapists. This concept rests on a multitude of clinical signs and is actually an original clinical entity.

A somatic dysfunction consists of a change in the normal functioning of an articulation or joint, and it is diagnosed according to specific criteria. Eileen Di Giovanna (1997) uses the mnemonic RATS for these criteria:

- R for *restriction of motion* within physiological limits. The affected articulation does not have perfect freedom of movement, and its range of motion is less than normal. The restriction affects one or more planes of movement. In most cases, it involves minor movements of a given articulation. It is detected by tests of mobility designed to evaluate the degrees of freedom in joints.

- A for *asymmetry*. The position of the vertebrae, other bones, or other structures is generally asymmetrical.
- T for changes in *tissue texture*. The soft tissues around an articulation presenting with somatic dysfunction undergo palpable changes. These changes are produced in the skin, the fascia, and/or the muscles.
- S for *sensitivity*. Although it can be difficult to interpret, palpation of the tissues elicits tenderness in places where normally there would be none in the absence of somatic dysfunction.

Not every somatic affliction is a somatic dysfunction according to this classification. Fractures, sprains, and degenerative and inflammatory processes do not constitute somatic dysfunctions. According to Fred Mitchell Jr. (1979), the term *somatic dysfunction* implies the notion that manipulation is an appropriate, effective, and sufficient treatment for this condition.

Visceral Dysfunction

Most of the internal organs are surrounded by envelopes whose movement is aided by serous lubricant. This liquid is contained within a cavity that is sealed on all sides. The organs can therefore slide against one another and against the walls of the cavities that contain them. In many respects, this arrangement is comparable to what is found in musculoskeletal articulations. Barral and Mercier (2004) give the following definition for the concept of visceral articulations. They use an implicit analogy with syssarcoses, which is an arthrological term having to do with the glide planes necessary for the movement of certain structures. Visceral movements originate in a number of different ways:

- Locomotion and musculoskeletal activity. Our movements and bodily positions affect the position and movements of our organs.

For example, moving the trunk causes changes in the geometry of the walls of the visceral cavities as well as the fluid pressure within them. These changes within the cavities in turn lead to adaptations in the forms of the viscera and cause them to move and situate themselves accordingly.

- Involuntary and automatic muscular contractions:
  - Pulmonary respiration, with 20,000 to 25,000 movements per day, represents a very large source of movement.
  - The other automatic movements, such as cardiac contractions and the various kinds of visceral peristalsis, also generate movement.
- Intrinsic visceral activity. In addition to the movements listed above, Barral and Mercier describe low-amplitude visceral movements and deformations, to which they assign the term *motility*. In medical or physiological language, motility usually refers to movements such as intestinal peristalsis. Barral and Mercier note that the movements they describe possess their own rhythm, axes of motion, and amplitude. Motility in this sense is not a passive extrinsic motion that the organ experiences but rather an intrinsic movement arising within the organ itself. Motility seems to result from processes taking place within the constituent cells of the organ's tissues. Embryology clearly offers a key for the understanding and study of this phenomenon, given the similarity between the planes and axes of these movements and those of the migration of the organs in the course of their development during gestation.

We can define visceral dysfunction as alteration or modification in the components of the mechanics of the viscera. Visceral dysfunction affects the mobility and/or the motility of organs. It may or may not give rise to visceral symptoms. It can also cause referred pains in the neuromusculoskeletal system. These dysfunctions can have a disruptive effect on the organs' ability to slide, on the ligamentous system of the organ, and/or on the organ's motility:

- The *visceral sliding mechanisms* are disturbed whenever a fixation is created by excessive sticking between two contiguous serous membranes. This is termed a *visceral fixation*. This sticking can come about as a sequela of dessication, as is the case in many inflammatory processes (infections, allergies, etc.), or from adhesions secondary to surgeries, wounds, or hemorrhage into the serous cavity.
- The *visceral ligamentous system* can be affected in its basic tone:
  - Ligaments that are too lax or improperly adapted to the organ's mechanical context frequently allow *ptoses* to occur.
  - Ligaments that are too tight or insufficiently elastic hamper and limit the play of the viscera; this is called *ligamentous fixation*.
- Motility can also suffer. This generally involves states of irritability that affect either visceral muscle cells or the metabolism of organs. Organs are the "full" parenchymatous structures such as the liver, kidney, or spleen. Viscera are the "hollow" structures shaped like tubes or pockets, such as the intestines, stomach, or bladder.
  - In the case of viscera, it is often noted that disturbances in motility are accompanied by spasms.
  - In the case of the organs, diminished motility is often associated with disturbed cellular or metabolic activity, acute or chronic intoxication, a decrease in vitality, and reactions to psychological or emotional shocks.

Any somatic dysfunction can produce negative effects in visceral function, which is dependent on the circulation of blood and lymph and the functioning of autonomic nerves. This is one of the basic principles of osteopathy. The links of cause and effect between the viscera and the greater organism do not, however, run in only one direction. The organs and viscera are tethered to osseous, muscular, and/or fascial structures that form the walls of the trunk. As a result, every visceral dysfunction can directly disturb parietal mechanics. *Parietal,* from the Latin *paries,* refers to wall-like structures such as the parietal bones of the skull or the walls of the trunk. For example, the lung is surrounded by two thicknesses of pleura: the visceral pleura, which covers the lung directly and moves with it, and the parietal pleura, which lines the part of the thoracic wall that forms the cavity occupied by the lung. Increased tension or pressure from a visceral dysfunction can throw off the axes of motion or inhibit the mobility of certain parts of the trunk. Vertebral mechanics are therefore subject to visceral constraints. In these cases, viscera do not cause actual misalignments of individual vertebrae, but the biomechanical context of certain sections of the spine undergoes a general distortion. In certain cases this translates into chronic or chronically recurring spinal pain. At times this state of affairs produces violent muscular reactions with acute symptomatology such as lumbago or torticollis.

Visceral ligaments also contain numerous proprioceptors providing a constant stream of feedback to the cerebellum relating to their states of tension. They thereby participate in the regulation of posture and can affect it negatively in cases of dysfunction.

According to Barral (2004), "the purpose of visceral manipulation is to recreate, harmonize, and increase proprioceptive communication in the body to enhance its internal mechanism for better health."

Craniosacral Dysfunctions

Following Sutherland's discoveries, osteopaths now believe that the sacral and cranial structures work together as a biomechanical unit that they call the *craniosacral system.* This unit consists of a variety of subtly arranged anatomical and functional elements whose organization gives rise to what is called the *primary respiratory mechanism* (PRM). This mechanism is based on five components:

- fluctuation of the cerebrospinal fluid (CSF)
- the meninges, or reciprocal-tension membranes
- the central nervous system and its inherent motility
- the articular mobility of the cranial mechanism
- the articular mobility of the sacrum between the ilia

"Craniosacral dysfunction" refers to anything that impairs the PRM. Harold I. Magoun (1951) says that this is a result of the corruption of structure, functioning, or interrelations among any parts of the PRM. He distinguishes three major kinds of dysfunctions:

- dysfunctions involving liquids: any alteration of rhythm, volume, speed of fluctuation, composition, or availability of the CSF
- sutural dysfunctions: any alteration in the structure, position, or motion of one or more cranial bones
- soft tissue dysfunctions: any alteration of structure or function of the meninges or nervous tissues

Close observation of the PRM is a rich source of information. It is both an indicator of and a player in the general vitality of the body.

The craniosacral unit is the jewel box of the neuromeningeal system. The PRM allows for a certain amount of CSF to be diffused throughout the body, meaning that the PRM allows for "respiration" in the very heart of the tissues and is a means of maintaining homeostasis.

The network of peripheral nerves, sometimes called the peripheral nervous system, is mechanically continuous with the tissues of the central nervous system. Any mechanical dysfunction affecting one of these divisions of the nervous system can have repercussions for the other division and create symptoms in it.

My own experience and my work with Jean-Pierre Barral have allowed me to catch a glimpse of the dynamics of the nervous system, with the nerves and meninges acting as elements that play an integral and integrating role in the craniosacral unit. The origins of a great many symptoms, even ones appearing a great distance away, can often be traced to it.

Chapter 5

Differential Diagnosis in Osteopathy

Osteopathic physicians must be able to give a reason for the treatment they give, not so much to the patient, but to themselves.

— ANDREW TAYLOR STILL

There are two primary aspects to differential diagnosis:

1. A search for possible contraindications or precautions to be taken when accepting a patient, and
2. The classification and triage of dysfunctions brought to light by the positive diagnosis. This classification is made according to the seriousness of the conditions, the likely benefits of osteopathic treatment, and any foreseeable downside or risks.

Contraindications to Osteopathic Treatment

"Diagnosis to rule out" is a key step in the process of osteopathic diagnosis. In performing an examination, osteopaths may become aware of one or more conditions that exceed our competence or go beyond our scope of practice. But how is a contraindication defined? There is a set standard of behavior or code of conduct for many clearly defined situations. These are based on the nature of the emergency at hand or the extent to which the situation is serious or critical. Apart from such clear-cut situations, there is a wide variety of conditions for which different practitioners, depending on their experience, will realize very different results.

Alternative and Supplementary

It can be challenging both to understand the concept of contraindications and to decide that one exists for the situation at hand. That is, nearly identical situations can either constitute a major contraindication to care or an indication for care with cautions. An example: a patient comes to your office with dorsolumbar vertebral pain. You learn from your history and examination that his general condition has deteriorated and that he has been experiencing weight loss, asthenia, and loss of appetite. Everything seems to indicate a serious pathology. Your responsibility is clear: you must refer this patient to a specialist who can do a full workup, make a precise diagnosis, and establish a treatment plan for the patient's most significant problem.

Now imagine that the same patient comes to you with the same complaint of vertebral pain. This time, he tells you that he is suffering from and being treated for liver cancer. In coming to you, he is seeking relief for his back pain. In this case, you can certainly accept the patient in the hope of helping him, but you make certain accommodations to adapt to his situation.

Although the complaint is the same, the circumstances surrounding the two visits are not: in fact, the difference is huge. In the first case, no diagnosis of his serious condition has been made. The patient coming to an osteopath as the first health care professional he has seen, cannot rely on our competence and abilities alone. Since our therapeutic approach is not the one considered optimal for the treatment of his problem, accepting him as a patient might be a waste of his precious time. Treating him is therefore absolutely contraindicated in this scenario.

In the second case, a medical diagnosis has already been made. We have to take into account any risks that the patient's pathology might entail, but we can make a reasonable attempt to help him. This is not a matter of trying to treat his cancer but focuses more modestly on reducing his back pain. With treatment that has been adapted to take the underlying pathology into account (leading us to choose certain approaches and avoid others), the condition is now only a relative contraindication.

There is therefore neither an absolute limit to contraindications nor a comprehensive scale that can be used in every case to determine which patients are appropriate to accept for care and which are not. The issue is nuanced and requires insight; it depends on whether the osteopath is being considered the provider of *alternative* therapy, as in the first situation, or of *supplementary* therapy, as in the second. Between these two examples there is a large difference in risk, and management of the same patient can differ radically.

Absolute Contraindications

There are a certain number of clinical manifestations for which pure osteopathic treatment is not appropriate. These are:

- Any condition requiring emergency surgery or other emergency medical treatment: situations in which a patient's status is critical, whether a matter of life or death or just a question of functional ability, requiring resuscitation, emergency medical intervention, or surgery.

  I don't mean to imply that osteopathy can never play an appropriate role in the management of such cases, but it would be improper to take on the management of such a patient without his receiving prior or simultaneous care from others, who can provide medical, surgical, or even lifesaving care.

  These cases include fractures, decompensating metabolic pathologies, cancer, etc.

- Conditions that will probably not respond adequately to purely osteopathic treatment are: conditions for which allopathic therapy, or some other therapy, is known to be much more effective, and conditions for which there is no clear osteopathic course of action (intense or refractory pain, anaphylaxis, allergies in the acute phase, etc.).

Principles for Determining Suitability of Treatment

Finally, determining the suitability of treatment is a matter of common sense. Here are some principles to remember:

- *Immediate or long-term dangers of the treatment itself.* Our treatments must be totally free of danger to the patient. Any time that our manipulations or treatment might cause harm to the patient, we must abandon the course of action. The primary factors for increased risk are:
  - risk of hemorrhage or vascular accident (e.g., arterial dissection, aneurysm, or compression)
  - congestive heart failure (risk of cardiac decompensation)
  - risk of ischemia caused by a hazardous manipulation
  - risk of neurological injury
- *Wasting the patient's time:* in cases of a progressing pathology or of a medical or surgical emergency, it can be of utmost importance to take immediate appropriate action. In addition to the problems associated with a bone fracture, some fractures can also pose severe danger to blood vessels and nerves. A fracture or a severe sprain are good examples of pathologies requiring referral to a surgeon.
- *Ineffectiveness* of treatment or *lack of benefit* from it: why make a patient wait for nonosteopathic treatment if it is better suited to his condition? For example, many cases of acute pain respond very well to strong analgesics. The difference here is often between a disease in the acute or active phases and a disease in a less active phase. Kidney stones or gallstones can be good indications for

treatment in the "cold" state: the therapist may make an attempt to affect the conditions that might be promoting calculus formation. By contrast, either of these problems in an acute stage is a definite contraindication to treatment.

Principal Contraindications

It is not possible for a list of principal contraindications to be exhaustively complete, but it is an attempt to give an overview of a number of common situations or conditions. Contraindications to accepting a patient for osteopathic care should not be confused with contraindications to the use of a given technique or kind of technique. The osteopathic toolkit is sufficiently well stocked with therapies and comprehensive enough to allow the practitioner to accept many patients who present contraindications to certain kinds of osteopathic treatment, and not others.

Osteoarticular Manipulation

Clinical contraindications to osteoarticular manipulation are numerous. There is a general consensus, at least regarding manipulations of the spinal column. Technical contraindications vary somewhat according to a practitioner's experience and manual skill. Certain maneuvers may be questionable for new therapists, while their use by expert practitioners can be very helpful and effective.

A few examples of cases where prudence is essential: patients on anticoagulant therapy, those with osteoporosis, and those whose spines are not yet fully developed. These can be called "relative contraindications." The key word for accepting these patients is *gentleness*. You must not manipulate bony articulations if your technical ability does not allow you to do so gently; "manipulating" does not mean "traumatizing." A therapist who knows how to stay tuned in to the tissues throughout the manipulation can be both very effective and gentle at the same time.

For the majority of the contraindications listed, manipulation has to be considered a mistake, even if it will not necessarily lead to disastrous consequences. Certain cases are risky. The benefit that the patient may realize from manipulation is very clearly not as great as the risk it can pose.

For many conditions, the primary diagnostic challenge is in the beginning stage. Symptoms can be atypical, and X-rays can still appear normal, given the gap that frequently exists between the actual state of the spinal column and a lesion's appearance in scans. Only a quality clinical examination, complemented as needed by lab tests and imaging studies, can allow us to form a sufficiently clear clinical picture of a person's condition and of the appropriateness of accepting him or her as a patient.

Contraindications to High-velocity, Low-amplitude Manipulative Techniques (Thrusts) on the Vertebral or Peripheral Level

- trauma:
  - recent traumas that have not been investigated through conventional imaging
  - fractures, vertebral compressions with or without associated dislocation, ligamentous tears with vertebral instability
  - osseous or ligamentous avulsion
- neoplasms:
  - primary or secondary tumors (metastases in bones)
  - Paget's disease
  - osteoid osteoma (a very painful benign tumor; risk of manipulation is low but the patient's chances of getting relief as a result are also very low)
- infections:
  - spondylodiscitis and rheumatoid arthritis
  - spondylitis
  - tuberculosis
  - osteomyelitis

- inflammatory processes:
  - rheumatoid polyarthritis
  - rheumatoid spondylitis
  - Scheuermann's disease
- vascular and hematologic dysfunctions:
  - arteriopathy
  - vertebrobasilar insufficiency
  - vertebral angioma
  - aortic aneurysm with slow dissection, or other arterial aneurysm
  - arteriosclerosis with aortic calcifications
  - severe arterial hypertension
  - venous thrombosis
  - myocardial infarction (possibly accompanied by angor animi)
  - hemophilia
- anatomical anomalies (congenital or acquired):
  - malformation of the craniospinal hinge
  - anomalous lumbosacral transitional segment(s)
  - spondylolisthesis (relative contraindication)
  - isthmolysis (of a vertebra)
  - congenital or acquired fused vertebra (relative contraindication)[1]
  - agenesis of all or part of a spinal segment (e.g., hemivertebra)
  - spina bifida
  - advanced spondyloarthrosis (relative contraindication)
  - vertebral osteosynthesis and arthrodesis
  - extreme scoliosis or kyphosis (relative contraindication)

---

1. Attempts to realign one part of a fused vertebra relative to another by use of high-velocity, low-amplitude thrust manipulations are, of course, fruitless, and while the entire block can be gently manipulated relative to the rest of the spine using other techniques, osteopaths consider thrust techniques directly on fused vertebrae to be contraindicated. However, unfused vertebrae in the same spine may be manipulated in the absence of other specific contraindications.

- conditions of metabolic origin:
  - osteoporosis (relative contraindication)[2]
  - osteomalacia
  - metabolic osteoarthropathies (gout, chondrocalcinosis)
- neurological conditions:
  - herniated disc (relative contraindication; avoid manipulation at the affected level)
  - meningitis and meningeal syndrome (reactive cervicalgia)
  - cauda equina syndrome
  - peripheral entrapment neuropathy (relative contraindication)
  - hyperalgesia: temporary contraindication to direct structural techniques in all cases of hyperalgesia involving gross muscular reactions and a tendency to massive contractures, which cause a serious loss of precision in such techniques if no muscular barriers have been created

---

2. Osteoporosis is a cause of spinal pain, and patients who are affected by it frequently consult us about it. This condition requires great caution for osteopaths. Generally, it should be considered a contraindication to direct structural techniques. Exceptions can be made based on the practitioner's technical abilities and the severity of demineralization. However, it should not be subject to a blanket exclusion rule. There are possibilities for action with gentler techniques to diminish stresses on the vertebral column. Certain manipulations of the dura mater, of vertebral ligaments, or of the attachments of the central tendon (described below) are especially useful and appropriate in these cases. Manipulating certain organs involved in the metabolism of calcium and phosphorus can also yield the possibility of physiological improvement. Other therapies that can contribute to improvement of the bodily environment and remineralization of the skeletal system, such as diet, should also be considered. This is the case with homeopathy and naturopathy.

The central tendon or "core link": This term refers to the heterogeneous fascial ensemble that mechanically suspends the center of the thoracoabdominal diaphragm from the cervicothoracic hinge and the base of the cranium—i.e., the pericardial ligaments, the posterior mediastinal splanchnic plexuses, the attachments of the pleura to the mediastinum, diaphragm, and cervical spine, and the visceral sheath of the neck. Some specialists even view it as a deep chain for maintaining equilibrium in the body.

- emotional and psychological conditions:
  - psychosis
  - hysteria and other obsessive neuroses; some authors raise concerns about "manipulation dependency" in these patients.
- general concerns:
  - cancer affecting the skeleton, e.g., by metastasis
  - bones in growth phase (relative contraindication)
- medication-related:
  - anticoagulant or antivitamin K therapy; can pose a major risk of hemorrhage, even with minor impact or short stretching.
  - chronic corticosteroid therapy. The concerns here are osteoporosis, an increased danger from ligamentous fragility, and that there are certain antibiotics that have been implicated in tendon rupture.
- long lever techniques (general osteopathic treatments, not necessarily high velocity or low amplitude):
  - fracture of the appendicular or axial skeleton
  - total hip, knee, or shoulder prosthesis
  - surgical fixation of a fractured member, preconsolidation
  - vertebral osteosynthesis
  - Barré-Lieou syndrome
  - arterial aneurysm with slow dissection

Direct Manipulation of the Viscera

Absolute Contraindications

Absolute contraindications are any organic lesions in which manipulation can promote the dissemination of neoplastic metastases, increase the risk of perforation, or cause vascular rupture.

- recent thoracoabdominal trauma—avoid any risk of secondary visceral rupture or of hemorrhage, including slow hemorrhage
- aortic aneurysm
- right-sided cardiac insufficiency (beware of visceral manipulations that have a strong impact on the circulation and those that decongest

certain organs, as they can overwhelm the heart through an increase in circulating blood volume)

- pulmonary subedema; left ventricular insufficiency
- active-phase inflammatory or infectious processes (appendicitis, acute ulcers, hepatitis, etc.)
- tumors of the digestive tract—any mass or indurated area that raises suspicion when palpated requires careful and thorough evaluation.
- acute pancreatitis
- cholestasis
- visceral cysts (hydatid cysts or renal cysts)
- intrahepatic hemangioma (increased risk in patients taking oral contraceptives)
- contraindications to recumbency: gastroesophageal reflux disease (GERD), right-sided cardiac insufficiency, acute pulmonary subedema

Precautions and Relative Contraindications

- severe diabetes mellitus (because of increased fragility of the vascular system)
- anticoagulant therapy
- superficial venous dilatation of the abdomen
- recent history of radiation therapy
- pregnancy
- long-term corticosteroid therapy
- Regarding pleural or pulmonary manipulation, certain severe pathologies can constitute relative or absolute contraindications based on the fact that manipulation may require significant support from, or pressure on, the ribs:
  - Emphysema causes fragility of the pulmonary parenchyma.
  - Recurrent pneumothorax indicates greatly increased vulnerability of the visceral pleura.
  - By increasing the risk of rib fracture, severe osteoporosis raises questions pertaining to the use and "dosage" of pleural or pulmonary manipulations or of vertebrocostal techniques.

Craniosacral Manipulation

It is illogical to maintain that cranial osteopathy is utterly harmless and can be practiced on any patient at any time with no restrictions and without specific indications. Contraindications to craniosacral manipulation exist, and we should keep them in mind. These contraindications relate to any serious condition in which variations in the pressure of cerebrospinal fluid (CSF) can be problematic, such as:

- recent cranial fracture
- intracranial hemorrhage
- intracranial neoplastic processes
- a recent blow or trauma to the cranium
- recent cerebrovascular accident (CVA; i.e., stroke)
- intracranial hypertension
- intracranial aneurysm
- acute meningitis
- recent shaken-baby syndrome

SUMMARY

The practice of osteopathy must be totally harmless, or as harmless as reasonably possible. The actions that we take must be effective and must never cause iatrogenic conditions. Our therapeutic actions must be adapted to the case at hand and must produce only beneficial results.

Professional Competence

Competence is defined as the ability to make good judgments and decisions. For any therapist, regardless of the field, the most important aspect of competence, and perhaps the only one, is knowing one's limitations. Once we accept the importance of this condition of self-awareness, we can also admit that the limitations imposed by relative contraindications can and do vary from one osteopath to the next. My colleague and friend Vincent Benedetto once said, "Osteopathy has no limitations; only osteopaths do." His point is that we need an appropriate degree of humility regarding our own abilities as therapists and technicians, distinct from the potential of osteopathy as a profession overall.

The decision to accept a patient must always be subject to one key question: what is the likelihood that he will benefit from your treatment? If your experience and your toolkit of therapeutic techniques bring you to a sincere belief that you have the ability to help this patient resolve his problems, then you may accept him. Conversely, every time you first approach a pathology with which you have no experience, great caution is required. I am not implying that no effort should be made to bring the patient relief; the point is that you must be sufficiently clear and sincere with him. It is usually possible to undertake a therapeutic trial, but results are key. After two or three treatments, improvement is the main indication of effective treatment, and stagnation is a sign that treatment is ineffective. If the patient does not respond to your efforts, you owe it to him and to yourself to refer him to practitioners or doctors who are more competent than you for the situation at hand, or to help him investigate other therapeutic approaches that may better suit his needs and his path to recovery.

Here again, the concepts of "global" and "holistic" can mislead us in our evaluation of patients' needs. We must be extremely broad-minded as to the possible causes for the deterioration in our patients' health. In no case can we believe, or claim to others, that we have the therapeutic solution to every problem. We must be able to distinguish what is properly within the scope of our competence and what is not.

To say that our approach is "global" does not mean incorporating a large number of eclectic therapies into our practice; nor does it mean that we can claim omniscience. It implies, simply, awareness: we must be aware of our own limits, of promising and not-so-promising indications for therapy, of contraindications to specific therapies, and of our responsibility to refer to others who are better suited to manage the case of any particular patient when necessary.

NOTE

On another level, competence is proportional to the degree of satisfaction we feel in our own abilities. It is never a waste of time to ask ourselves regularly about our attitudes about our function as therapists. We must never forget that we are simply fulfilling a social function or role. We must carry out this role conscientiously, and we must never consider ourselves to be vested with a special mission, nor think that we possess some kind of extraordinary power. We are, in fact, powerless over the suffering of other people, and even more so over other people themselves. Losing sight of these limitations and lacking this mental grounding is often the first step away from the path of professional responsibility, the first step toward drifting in a haze as we start to entertain illusions of being a guru, self-appointed or otherwise.

Triage and Classification of Conditions

The other aspect of differential diagnosis involves understanding the pattern of the patient's dysfunction. In the beginning stages of the therapeutic relationship, the practitioner, as part of the diagnostic process, has created a complete inventory of the dysfunctions that afflict the patient. Not all of these are pathogenic, and some are of limited interest. We must make a quick classification or triage of these dysfunctions so that we can then do the best possible job of focusing on the ones that have the greatest impact on the patient's health and proper functioning.

The mechanics of the human body are complex, and so are the ways in which dysfunctions interact. Our differential diagnosis must determine which dysfunction is primary or, in any case, which is least ancillary. Numerous methods exist to allow us to decode the pattern of the patient's dysfunction and to pinpoint the primary or key problems. None of these is sufficient by itself, but rather this operation results from a convergence of various elements. For this reason, the phrase *diagnostic convergence* is often used.

A general understanding of classic signs and symptoms is important, as is a grasp of those that are more specific to the functional pathology in question. Symptomatology, however, is not always enough to differentiate between two related conditions. In some cases, additional diagnostic work is needed to lead us to a proper diagnosis. Here again, our manual skills play a paramount role. The art of osteopathy specifically makes extensive use of tests of inhibition and mechanical aggravation. Using our hands, we can compare two dysfunctions in order to determine which of them is more significant.

The hierarchical classification of the seriousness and nature of the patient's needs and conditions results from our consideration of the information gleaned from: the interview and examination; the therapeutic focus that we then adopt based on this initial diagnostic work; and, possibly, supplementary tests that may be needed to help us fine-tune our understanding of the mechanical interactions involved.

The elements of the interview, which is an essential part of this process of classification, are primarily the patient's complaints, symptoms, and any history of prior complaints as well as their chronology. The therapist's intellectual tools are knowledge of anatomy and signs and symptoms; experience; knowledge of global patterns of health and disease in the body; and logic and reasoning. This list would be incomplete if it did not include intuition and the ability to reason by analogy. Touch is clearly one of the therapist's most important sensory tools, but information transmitted by all the other sense organs is also important. When considered as part of overall sensory data, qualitative information from palpation shows its importance.

Chapter 6

Etiological Diagnosis in Osteopathy

> To find health should be the object of the doctor. Anyone can find disease.
>
> — ANDREW TAYLOR STILL

Osteopathy is a system of therapy that focuses on the long term, which is to say that it modifies the patient's landscape and his ability to adapt to the environment. Given this context, we can only discuss causation if we consider some fundamental concepts. A few of these key ideas are *care, health,* and *healing.*

Health

Contrary to many systems of belief, health is not uniquely associated with or dependent on ingesting medications. Established allopathic medicine studies health in all its forms but in the final analysis pays little attention to the circumstances that contribute to good health. Medical-school thinking is deeply rooted in Louis Pasteur's germ theory of disease. Accordingly, studies done in medical schools tend to be much more interested in sick human beings than in ones who are well, or in the conditions that good health requires.

Professor Jean-Charles Sournia (1995) relates that in response to the question "What is a healthy person?" a young American interr once answered, "A healthy person is one who has not yet been fully examined." It is insidious in our medicalized societies that health seems to have become a precarious state that portends no good. Health ministries and departments pay hardly any attention to anything but disease, and public "health" budgets are, for the most part, sickness budgets.

Definitions of Health

Health means the state of someone who is healthy and whose faculties are intact. According to the World Health Organization, "health is a state of complete physical, mental, and social well-being and not merely the absence of disease or infirmity."

According to René Dubos and Maya Pines (1971, 10), health is

the ability to function effectively within a given environment. And since the environment keeps changing, good health is a process of continuous adaptation to the myriad microbes, irritants, pressures, and problems that daily challenge man.

This correlates with the osteopathic idea of health: the ability to adapt to diverse conditions and numerous brutal stresses and strains.

Principles of Health

Every human being has needs that must be satisfied to live. But what differences are there among living, surviving, and being healthy? Listed below are a number of principles that human beings must follow in order to enjoy good health, based on the ideas of Adam J. Jackson (1996) and Nadine Delchambre (2000). For Jackson and Delchambre, health is not a matter of destiny or luck but of universal laws that control every phenomenon of nature and every manifestation of life. According to these principles, health results from living in sync with these laws, while illness is the result of living out of sync with them. Many other authors confirm variations on the same points. The following seem to be the main routes, as it were, of health. Some concern the body and others the mind.

Bodily Powers and Functions
Breath and Respiration

Deep breathing is essential for good health. It is an instinctive, entirely natural, and vital process. A sedentary lifestyle, confinement within buildings, and air-conditioning have caused many people to lose this instinct. Once it is lost, it is a great challenge for people to regain it and to breathe correctly.

The human body can live for weeks without food and for days without water, but deprived of oxygen, it dies after a few minutes. Breathing is an essential component of health and of the process of natural healing. It assists the delivery of nutrients throughout the body and facilitates the creation of energy. It helps the circulation of blood and lymph. (The lymphatic system is primarily activated by two things: exercise and deep breathing. Some studies have shown that a little exercise combined with the practice of deep breathing can multiply the flow of lymph fifteen times.)

Breathing eases mental and emotional stress, relaxes the thoracic musculature, and calms the nerves. It nourishes, cleanses, and relaxes the whole body as it calms the mind.

Nutrition and Hydration

According to the principles of healthy eating, we are what we eat, the times we eat, and the way we eat. We need to chose foods that are whole, fresh, unrefined, and preferably organic.

Good nutrition requires good digestion, which means it is important to chew well, to eat in a relaxing environment, and to avoid eating late at night and nibbling between meals. We should also never eat too much.

It is also important to drink enough water, which is a major constituent of our cells. Water consumption needs to be emphasized specifically, and we shouldn't consume excessive amounts of other drinks. Seventy percent of the foods we eat should also be rich in water.

As much as possible, we should make an effort to avoid substances that are destructive to our cells, such as refined sugar, table salt, tea, coffee, and alcohol, and to avoid excessive consumption of meat, dairy products, and to a lesser extent, fish.

Exercise

Regular exercise improves blood circulation and cardiac and respiratory function. Physical exercise improves the circulation of fluids in the joints, preventing the development of arthritis and related phenomena. It strengthens the muscles and maintains the bones in good condition while preventing calcium loss.

Exercise is also important for mental well-being; it helps to ease disorders such as anxiety and depression. In the brain, exercise brings about a release of beta-endorphins, which promote a feeling of emotional well-being. According to the neuroscientist David Servan-Schreiber, MD (2003), studies done at Duke University have shown that physical exercise is more effective than antidepressants. People who walked briskly for thirty minutes three times a week have results comparable to those taking antidepressants for a period of a few weeks. After one year, the rate of recurrence of depression symptoms was over thirty percent in the antidepressant group and just eight percent in the exercise group.

Elimination

It is as important to eliminate wastes as it is to get proper nutrition. The role of the organs of elimination is to remove every sort of undesirable or dangerous compound of both endogenous and exogenous origin. Good intestinal transit, good elimination of urine, and moderate elimination through the skin are signs that the body's self-cleansing system is functioning well. Conversely, poor elimination leads to a state in which the body becomes autointoxicated and as a result becomes an excellent host for opportunistic diseases. We can think of this group of functions as a variable influenced by a variety of factors, such as nutritional habits, the use of toxic substances, stress, and worry, among others.

Rest

Social and professional pressure is often considerable, work days often seem endless, and some people find it very difficult to relax. Some take refuge in alcohol as a way of calming their stress or in stimulants so that they can accomplish even more. Still others use chemicals to help them adapt to a speed or rhythm of life that threatens to leave them behind. It is odd to think that in an era when we have so many time-saving machines (the Internet, telephones, fax machines, washing machines, dryers, vacuum cleaners, computers, cars, airplanes, etc.), people never have enough time. Without doubt, their lives are more hectic now than ever before.

It is a well-known fact that many people neglect their need for sleep. Doing so, however, makes people carry over one day's stresses to the next day. The resulting agitation lays the foundation for chronic diseases and stress-related pathologies. Every living being needs rest. If the body and mind do not get enough rest to keep them refreshed and rejuvenated, good health will remain out of reach.

Rest is essential for our physical and emotional health. Mental relaxation reduces the heart's burden by thirty percent, lowers arterial tension, and reduces the body's oxygen needs by fifty percent. Rest also reduces the amount of lactic acid in the blood. Lactic acid and related substances are associated with physical exertion but also with anxiety, neurosis, and arterial hypertension. Rest improves mental functioning: it yields more regular EEG readings and improves alertness, reaction time, and short- and long-term memory.

Body Mechanics

Proper body mechanics, both at rest and in motion, are key to managing our energy. As a result of walking upright, human beings wage a constant battle against the effects of gravity on the structures of their bodies. This battle takes place on several organizational and anatomical levels. Good posture and proper body mechanics are essential for good health. Less-than-perfect mechanical interconnections can hinder the circulation of bodily fluids or cause irritation to the nervous system. This in turn can form the root of various dysfunctions. Similarly, our posture affects our mood and our emotions. The brain is stimulated by our posture and mechanical functioning.

At the same time, and conversely, the dynamics of our thoughts act on our posture. Depressive people tend to lean forward, hunch their shoulders, and lower their gaze. Optimistic and happy people tend to hold their heads up and walk in a more upright way.

Good posture must never be restrictive. It can come from self-awareness and the decision to stand up straight, but it is more often the reflection of harmonious mechanics of the various parts of the body. Poor body posture at work, carrying small children, and asymmetrical exercise are examples of influences toward abnormal posture that are best avoided. Traditionally, it is thought that holding the body in inappropriate ways sooner or later leads to imbalance.

Accidents, serious falls, and the resulting traumatic injuries can cause considerable sequelae and produce long-lasting negative effects on body mechanics. A large part of human mechanical capacity is often compromised well before adulthood, however. The way that we arrive in the world can make a big difference in our ability to be balanced later in life. Good body mechanics depend on good gestational life and a good birth experience. Excessive constraints on the fetus in utero or during birth leave a significant amount of evidence in the tissues. ' False folds" of tissue show up quite early in life as, for example, neonatal plagiocephaly, strabismus, repeated occurrences of otitis media with seromucous secretions, scoliosis originating in childhood or adolescence, and migraines in adults. These difficulties, which are amplified by the forces of growth, are powerful causes of profound asymmetries and imbalances that create areas of weakness throughout life. Preventative osteopathic therapy for newborns, toddlers, and children that is focused on increasing their chances for future good health is therefore a high priority for many parents.

Environment

It is difficult if not impossible to enjoy good health in an unhealthy environment. Fresh, unpolluted air and natural light are building blocks of a healthy environment. Spending several hours a day in artificial light can be the cause of severe imbalances, especially in the neuro-endocrine system. Living or working in an atmosphere of confined or recycled air day after day is not conducive to good health.

Electromagnetic radiation given off by machines at the office (computers, photocopiers, fax machines, monitors) or at home (televisions, mobile phones, microwave ovens) can alter the normal magnetic fields that have always been part of the human environment and can thus have a negative effect on our health.

Sometimes we must consider things inside the body. The wide variety of metals (amalgam fillings, crowns, pivots, bridges) that can be present in the mouth, where they are bathed in saliva, can actually generate minuscule electrical currents, causing a constant disturbance for the body's internal environment. In some sensitive individuals, these phenomena can create a constant imbalance in the autonomic nervous system and can give rise to numerous symptoms of dystonia.

It is important for us to arrange things in such a way that the places where we work and live are beneficial to our health. Plants are the best purifiers of the home and work environment.

Nonphysical Qualities and Powers

Mind and Spirit

It is a common misconception that the mind and spirit have to do only with our mental health and emotions. In fact, they constitute the emotional and physical foundations of health. Our bodies are actually controlled by our thoughts, and our thoughts depend on the mind and spirit. The power of thought can be used to stimulate the immune system, relieve pain, and clear up skin problems. Professor André Trifaud (2001) asserts that the power of thought is such that it can account for "unusual," "unforeseeable," and "inexplicable" remissions and cures of certain diseases that are classified as incurable by medical science in its present state.

Mind and spirit are at the very root of both health and disease. They are powerful forces that influence our actions and behavior and control every organ and cell in our bodies.

Faith

Faith is spiritual conviction that, far more than intellectual ability alone, allows us to accomplish the impossible. It connects the human spirit with a higher power. Faith is recognition of the vital forces that hold the living world together. For our health to flourish, earthly food is not enough; as human beings we need spiritual food as well.

Faith gives confidence and peace to the spirit. It releases power that can sometimes accomplish miracles. Many physicians believe that faith plays a major role in the phenomena of healing, especially in patients with serious illnesses who recover despite their prognosis. Claude E. Forkner, MD, former president of the New York Cancer Society, once said: "Very often we do not know what it is that brings about the recovery of the patient. I am sure that often it is faith that is the most important factor" (Jackson 1996, 108). Dr. Elmer Hess, president of the American Medical Association, writes: "A physician who walks into a sickroom is not alone. He can only minister to the ailing person with the material tools of scientific medicine—his faith in God does the rest" (Jackson 1996, 108).

Faith is a veritable reservoir of energy from which a person can draw the strength needed to achieve a desired goal. Worry, doubt, fear, anxiety, and anguish are the opposite of faith, and all are destructive to health.

Although they are often equated, a distinction must be made between faith and belief. Belief is the result of the development of a thought process. Faith is more a biological process than a creation of the mind. Faith usually precedes knowledge or belief, and its roots develop from positive personal experiences. Faith is entirely distinct from religion; it is something that an individual possesses personally. There is no need to associate with any religious organization whatsoever to feel connected to a superior spiritual power or a higher order of things.

Love

Love overcomes many difficulties. It is important for health because it is the essence of life. Without it, life loses its meaning, and a person deprived of it can easily sink into depression. Hatred, egotism, anger, and resentment are some of the forces opposite to love. These negative feelings cause the body to produce poisons that can kill just as effectively as the most toxic chemicals. From the beginning of time, love has always been a force for healing. As a feeling, it is very close to faith, and showing love is an act of faith.

Love nourishes the body and the spirit. It has been shown that people who feel loved heal more quickly than others. Feeling it increases the activity of the immune system, stimulates the release of hormones that help fight stress and pain, and modifies and improves the body's condition in general. Love is not only a factor in healing but is also essential in maintaining health.

Paule Salomon (1997) lists four "pillars" of love: the need to be loved; the need to love others; the need to love oneself; and the need to love life. Fulfilling these requirements enables us to avoid internal and external conflicts. Daniel G. Amen, MD, of Los Angeles, whom I know well, is a specialist in SPECT imaging of the brain. Dr. Amen (2002) has identified a number of objective changes brought about by feelings, including love, in five areas of the brain: the prefrontal cortex, the anterior cingulate gyrus, the basal ganglia, the temporal lobes, and the deep limbic system. He brings together information from numerous studies of psychosomatic medicine that have long shown that certain factors, including isolation, rejection, family or work conflicts, and the loss of self-esteem, were major factors in the development of somatization. Each of these conditions has an injurious effect on one or more of Salomon's four pillars of love.

Laughter

Laughter has an extraordinary power to affect the body. It helps reduce pain: at the level of the brain, it stimulates the production of endorphins, which are natural painkillers and also strengthen the functioning of the immune system. Laughter also promotes increased respiration and stimulates the heart and lungs. It stimulates gastrointestinal functioning through its massaging effect on the abdominal organs and tissues. Laughter also has a beneficial effect on our frame of mind. Various studies have shown that people concentrate better after a good laugh. Laughter reduces the effects of stress by decreasing blood levels of adrenaline and cortisol, which are marker hormones for stress.

In short, the conditions that pertain to health are on many different planes or levels that range from the densest to the most subtle, from the physical plane to the spiritual by way of the emotional, energetic, and environmental.

SUMMARY

Health is feeling content within yourself, feeling happy about your life and about where you live, feeling good in your body, in your relationship with your significant other, in your family, in your heart, in your mind, and on the planet.

Balanced Health

The Scales of Health

Health is a matter of dynamic balance. In my book *Trauma: An Osteopathic Approach* cowritten with Jean-Pierre Barral, we represent health as a balance (fig. 6.1). One scale bears the weight of the factors that are favorable to good health, and the other has those favorable to disease. This approach allows us to visualize how an imbalance can come about as a result of even minute traumas. Considering the various possibilities that can cause a loss of balance, on one scale are all the negative and deleterious influences, and on the other are those factors that the body has at its disposal and which are best able to counterbalance them: the abilities to adapt, to compensate, to eliminate wastes, and to repair itself. In the bag on the left scale of the balance are listed the principal negative factors that arise in people's lives. Each factor represents a greater or lesser weight or burden, according to its intensity or severity.[1]

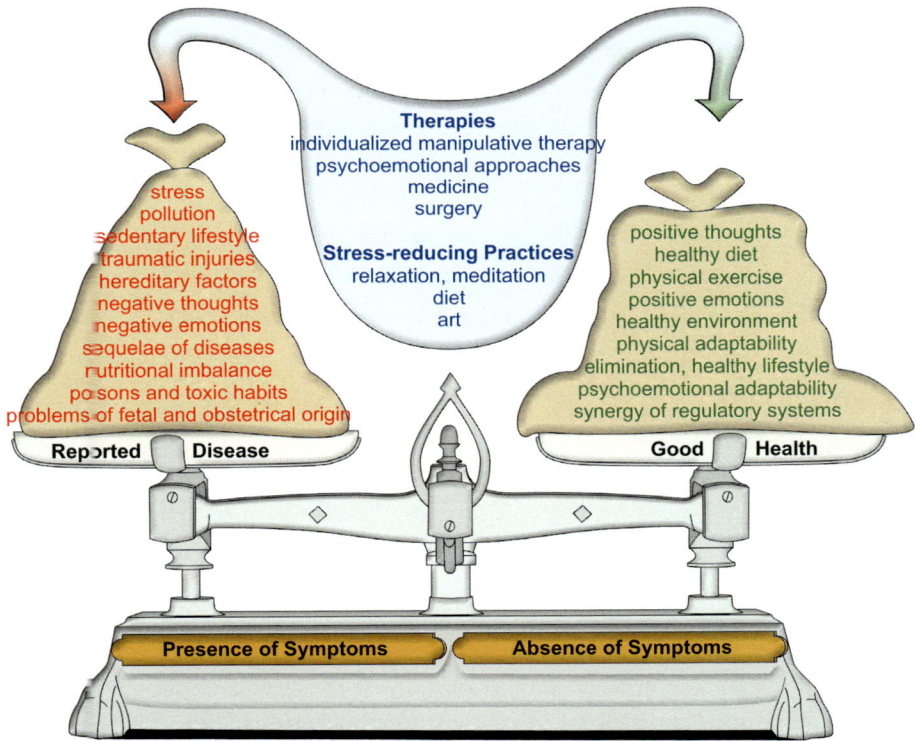

Figure 6.1. The Balance of Health.

---

1. I place vaccinations among the negative factors because certain vaccinations can be problematic in predisposed individuals. For example, I have seen numerous patients who have been utterly destabilized after being vaccinated for yellow fever. The liver becomes totally fixated, the metabolism is strongly affected, and they present severe pain in the spine and the right scapula. The necessity for precautions applies more and more to certain kinds of vaccinations, which also proves that there is no guarantee that the relationship between risks and benefits is entirely clear.

On the right side are all the factors that have a positive effect on health. A patient's forces of good health depend variously on his or her constitution, mental state, healthiness of lifestyle, etc. Good health does not mean having empty scales; it means having a good balance between the two sides in real time. The negative factors must be well balanced by the positive ones.

Body mechanics and the ways they can be disrupted are some of the causative factors of particular interest for the osteopathic physician, but they are not the only ones that can be addressed in osteopathic practice. As for the negative factors, a great many of them can be treated or improved through osteopathy. To cite the most obvious ones: fetal constraint and its consequences, the sequelae for the mother of a difficult childbirth, the aftereffects of traumatic injury, and certain psychological and emotional stresses that can be released by working on the body. Osteopathy also works to improve the patient's energy levels by strengthening the body's mechanical adaptability and/or by helping to improve elimination.

Scales Out of Balance

Life presents us with all kinds of challenges to health, and no one is immune to them. On the other hand, as long as our ability to compensate and adapt are intact and functioning, we can remain in good health despite these challenges. We are said to be *in apparent good health,* or free of symptoms. If the challenges exceed the limits of the forces of compensation and adaptation, even a very small negative factor can cause a disease process to be unleashed. The expression "the straw that broke the camel's back" expresses this idea. The load on the left side of the scales may be at the point where adding a small weight can upset the balance of the scales and send the patient into a clear state of disease. This explains why a small chill can degenerate into pneumonia or pleurisy, the simple act of picking up a pin from the ground can provoke acute lumbago, or a mild disappointment can send a predisposed person into severe depression.

In an individual who still has significant reserves of adaptation and compensation, social stresses do not necessarily lead to health issues. On the other hand, if she is at the limit of her ability to cope, being laid off from work may cause her to develop an ulcer, a case of depression, acute lower back pain, or an infectious disease.

Care, Healing, and Self-healing

People often confuse the concepts of "healing" and "providing care." The meanings of these expressions are actually very different. It is important not to confuse the two if we hope to have reasonable therapeutic objectives.

Providing care or *caring for* consists of providing the treatments that a patient may need in order to recover. These treatments are the means by which the caregiver attempts to optimize conditions for the restoration of the patient's health. The idea of "care" also implies attention given to the patient.

Healing means the disappearance of a disease or the return of health. It consists of the complete cessation of a physical or mental disease. It is the positive outcome to a pathological process with a return to the prior state of health. Healing is the process by which balance and integrity are restored to our being.

Dr. Walter Bradford Cannon was the father of the concept of homeostasis. According to this concept, when there is pathology, regardless of what it is, the body knows, based on its own norms and standards, what steps it needs to take to stop the progression of the disease and to reestablish balance. When the body is not able to restore balance on its own, intervention by a therapist is needed.

The pattern or scheme of an individual's health is written in the ensemble of the elements that form our physiology. This pattern is an integral part not only of our biological and neurophysiological activities but also of the particular behaviors, constructive or not, of our tissues.

Finally, *caring* comes from the caregiver, while *healing* comes from the patient. Caring is a matter of *doing* and is subject to its own limitations and, sometimes, inability to bring about desired change; healing is in the realm of *being* and draws on the immeasurable possibilities of that realm.

As caregivers, we must always remain humble. While we must do whatever we can to help our patient, we have to remain aware that caring has no power of its own. All our treatments may be needed in order for healing to occur, but all our therapy will not necessarily bring it about. If the patient's inherent healing abilities are insufficient, even the best techniques may fall short. Jacques Andreva Duval (2004) writes:

> Every time a sick person is "healed," it is his own resources that heal him, regardless of the therapeutic method used. What medications or therapists must do is to assist the manifestation of the resources that exist in the body, either by strengthening and guiding them or by removing adverse forces that hinder them from asserting themselves. This concept is, or should be, the keystone of every therapeutic approach.

True healing comes from the patient. This is undoubtedly why Still called it "self-healing." The wonderful capacity for self-healing is an innate capability of the body.

Contemporary medicine is based on an approach to healing that is not holistic. In general, its treatments originate from the outside and use artificial methods, such as surgery, radiation therapy, and medications. There is no denying that certain medications or surgical procedures can be useful at times. We know that they can be indispensable for saving lives in crisis situations. From our perspective, healing is a process that takes place within; nothing external to the body can bring about its healing. The ability to heal is a natural property of the body, which is perpetually in a process of healing.

Take the example of a fracture. However serious it may be, all that the physician or surgeon can do is realign the bone fragments and immobilize them, using a cast or a pin, so that the bone can repair itself as well as possible. Regardless of their level of skill or the complexity of the procedure, the doctors do not cause it to heal. The consolidation of the bone and the healing of the fracture are accomplished by the patient's own inner forces. Depending on the fracture site and the patient's lifestyle, the results will be good or not so good, and the healing process will be rapid or slower. Healing, therefore, does not depend on the quality of care alone.

For the osteopath, the same principle applies: our manipulations help to optimize conditions for the necessary internal healing processes to work. The osteopath's therapeutic approach seeks to awaken what Hippocrates called the "inner physician," meaning the capacity for self-healing. In his preface to *Osteopathy, Research and Practice* (1910), Still declared:

> Man's power to cure is good as far as he has a knowledge of the right or normal position, and so far as he has the skill to adjust the bones, muscles, and ligaments and give freedom to nerves, blood, secretions, and excretions and no farther.

A favorite argument of certain detractors of osteopathy is that the placebo effect explains our results. We cannot prove a negative, but this argument shows a lack of understanding of the principles of healing. There is also the contrary to the placebo effect: a nocebo effect, or "white coat syndrome." Studies on this subject show that people sometimes fall ill, experience other negative effects, or even die after taking a placebo. This is proof, if proof is needed, that disease and health take complex paths. Healing is sometimes assisted by the patient having a realization that helps reset the circuits relating to the self-regulation and self-healing of the body's major systems. The placebo effect has been well demonstrated and quantified in numerous studies. For us, it provides scientific proof of the existence of the wonderful forces of self-healing that are central to osteopathic theory.

Today, ostensibly in the service of objectivity, efforts are being made to deny this effect, and researchers try to eliminate it as a factor in drug studies. Would it not make more sense to try to understand how certain people are better at mobilizing their self-healing powers? Despite moves in the opposite direction, this question represents a very important subject for research. Data that could be priceless for health and healing would certainly be obtained, and the positive repercussions for humanity of the resulting discoveries would be fantastic. But who would finance such a study?

Returning to the subject of healing, it is highly pretentious to attribute to ourselves the ability to heal. Responsible therapists try to find the best treatment they can provide and trust nature to do the rest. Etiological diagnosis—diagnosis of the origins of a problem—must keep this objective in mind. Determining the cause of an imbalance is only helpful if it can lead us to ways of stimulating and improving the patient's ability to self-heal.

Osteopathic Etiology

Among the essential conditions for good health, the place of osteopathy seems clear. As its practitioners, our actions aim to restore good body mechanics and to harmonize posture. This gives us access to one of the great keys to health. But there are others as well.

Visceral manipulation improves the removal of wastes from the body via its organs of elimination, and certain craniosacral or tissue techniques allow us to clear away specific unhelpful emotions. Combining these approaches also allows us to stimulate the defensive capabilities of the immune system. Osteopathy exerts a positive effect on health in a number of ways.

This being the case, it appears clear that, depending on the elements of health that the patient may have compromised, our actions will be effective to a greater or lesser degree. We then need to determine which element we should try to balance first. This is the reason for forming our etiological diagnosis, the diagnosis of causation: we want to determine if there is a mechanical breakdown that can undermine the conditions of good health, or if other systems are at fault.

The discovery of a precise event or an obvious cause that correlates with the dysfunction allows us to be confident in our diagnosis of a mechanical etiology. Returning to the principles of health depicted in figure 6.1, note that each of them can be targeted by one therapeutic approach or another. Each approach—nutritional analysis, laughter therapy, movement therapy, breathing exercises, colon hydrotherapy, therapy addressing aspects of the mind, spirit, or emotions—attempts to restore health where it is failing, to lessen the load on the left scale of the balance, or to counterbalance it on the right. Our role is not to be purveyors of all of these therapeutic responses, but our etiological diagnosis should lead us to consider the possibility that some other therapy might be indicated as a higher priority than osteopathy. Again, a holistic approach does not mean omnipotence. It is not a matter of having the answer to everything but of having the broadest possible understanding of physiological and physiopathological interactions so that we can find the therapy best suited to the patient and the stage of evolution.

We must never lose sight of the fact that health is the result of balance between human beings and the natural environment that surrounds us. The search for causation ultimately comes down to identifying the heaviest burden on the "disease" side of the balance that we are able to remove, and in so doing, restore balance.

Chapter 7

Tools of Manual Diagnosis

When an osteopath explores the human body for the cause of disease he knows he is dealing with complicated perfection. He must master anatomy and physiology and have a fairly good knowledge of chemistry; then he can reason from the effect to the cause that gives rise to the abnormal condition or disease.

— ANDREW TAYLOR STILL

The hand plays a major role in osteopathic diagnosis. All knowledge has importance, but the difference between two therapists who have an equal level of knowledge is in the value of their respective hands. More from a diagnostic point of view than therapeutic, the hand is the supreme tool of the osteopath. It rarely finds indifference.

The Objectivity of Sensations

Inevitably, a reasonable question arises regarding our perceptions. Certain manual sensations in osteopathy cannot be objectified in the scientific sense. Are these sensations not founded in reality? Palpation is a sense that can be trained, as with the other senses. Setting aside the diagnostic approach for a moment, let's reflect on the necessary confidence that we must have for our perceptions. For example, we might forget that the nose is a very delicate sensor, because smelling an odor does not mean much when large quantities of the odor's source are present. An incident that happened several years ago illustrates the sensitivity of our noses. A ship loaded with styrene sank, and the inhabitants of the area reported smelling a strong chemical odor, even though no significant trace could be found even by the most sensitive detectors. First, this implies that at times our senses are more efficient than the sensory devices used to scientifically objectify some of the things we perceive. Second, when we sense something—an odor, perfume, or aroma—we have varying degrees of common perception. Some people have very sensitive or better-trained noses than others. Our impressions alone—"Does that not smell like something?"—allow us to give credit to the sensation without needing to measure the material empirically in micromoles per cubic meter. Why do we not act the same way with all our senses?

We think that education of the senses allows a certain degree of objectivity within a defined framework. My esteemed friend, Jean-Pierre Barral, gives the example of the winemaker, who by appearance, smell, and taste can locate a wine in time and space. This ability most often draws admiration for the skill of the eyes, nose, and educated palate of this specialist.

Doctors talk of *objective signs* arising from information obtained at the time of the clinical examination, in contrast to *subjective symptoms*, those described by the patient. Palpation, inspection, and auscultation call on the senses of the therapist. Apprenticeship and knowledge play a huge role in the reliability of reading sensations and in their exploitation. The ear, extended by a stethoscope, allows a doctor to detect cardiac malfunction, circulatory disturbances, or pulmonary pathology. Give the stethoscope to a sound engineer, even one who is extremely competent in analyzing sound waves, and the conclusion drawn will probably be very different from that of a doctor.

What we say about the education of a sense makes approaching certain phenomena more objective. It does not involve anything transcendent, like a gift or a savant, but simply that training and education may allow extraordinarily keen abilities of perception.

Diagnostic Touch

If palpation is the art of manual examination, certain components of its osteopathic application are special. Osteopathic touch is distinguished by classical palpation from other dimensions. For example, with regard to the diagnostic significance of movement, palpation of structures is rather more dynamic than static. In other respects, much information is gathered by the hands. Deciphering gathered information during the course of a long apprenticeship allows the hands to be used clearly. Finally, osteopathic touch is also a special form of communication, accomplished tissue by tissue.

Touch and the Sense of Touch

"The sense of touch is passive; touch is voluntary," wrote Raoul Tubiana (1980). This illustrates the distinction between the sense of touch and education on touch. While the sense of touch is present in the entire surface of the skin, only the hand touches. The hand is a true tool that we need to learn to control and use. Using the minute portion of the brain that we usually access, the hand is a fabulous treasure of which we only exploit a few possibilities, which are more or less difficult to master.

The most significant are the sensory functions of touch and prehension (grip). It is impossible to dissociate sensitivity and motivity at the level of hand. Their association gives the hand unique powers of information and execution. The hand possesses an exceptional sensory level, and the richness of its cutaneous covering in sensitive corpuscles cannot fully explain its sensitivity. The hand can increase its ability to gather information thanks to kinetic maneuvers of mechanical exploration: manipulation and palpation.

While the other sense organs are controlled by the body, the hand adapts and moves toward an object that it wants to "know," thereby participating in learning about the object's shape. This tactile knowledge gives us access to three-dimensional vision.

The hand is a particularly skilled sensory organ. It doesn't involve adjacent receptors in a hidden sensory apparatus but is a true sensory-motor complex. Specially adapted to psychomotor activity, this complex presents the strongest density of superficial and deep receptors.

Osteopathic Touch

Osteopathic touch can be broken down into several components:

- the parameters of the hand and some tissues
- the parameters of the mind of the observer
- the palpatory parameters to observe

Parameters of the Hand and Tissues

- Position of the patient and body parts. In a general way, it is necessary to respect the patient's optimal position of relaxation. Examination of an element is much easier if the practitioner respects this imperative of muscular resolution of the region approached.
- Position of the hand. The hand is an adaptable tool, malleable and polyvalent. Always adapt it to the cutaneous surface and evaluated element. A hand that offers maximum contact is generous and is well accepted by the tissues.
- Method of approach to the tissues. Injury and identification of superficial elements generally poses little problem. A different approach is needed for the deeper structures. As in surgery, there are true palpatory methods of approach that allow the hand to find the best access to deeper elements. Respecting these paths of deep palpation allows us to avoid superficial structures and to contact deep structures with the least amount of tissular intervention possible.
- The depth of action or perception in the tissues. The pressure the hand exerts on the tissues is determinant. It must always be adapted to the density of the element being palpated. It is necessary that there is perfect agreement between the manual pressure and the density of the investigated structure. It is only possible to perceive if one does not exceed the limits of their sensory receptors.

Parameters of the Mind of the Observer

My friend and colleague, Pierre Tricot, has worked extensively on the parameters of the mind of the person who palpates. I have been greatly inspired by his concepts.

Intention

Intention is what you want to do. Without intention, nothing can be envisaged. Do you want to perceive a form? Heat? Tension? According to your intention, you can sense different things, even without moving your hand. Another aspect of these palpatory parameters concerns your mental state. Your reception will be much better when you have good intentions. If you are there to help, listen, and care for the tissues, the reception of information is greatly facilitated. Intention constitutes the orientation of your mental focus during palpation. Tricot (1992) says: "Life responds to intention, to the force it is subjected to."

Attention

Attention constitutes the setting of the perceptual limits to what you adjust. It is your ability to select, among all of the sensory information attained, what interests you. Attention constitutes the field of conscience in which you place the state of your palpation. It allows you to connect to a vast whole in order to extract your information. You can filter the functional information by its quality or position in space. Attention is the adjustment of the sensitivity and selectivity of your palpatory mental focus. With the same position of the hand, it is possible to place your mental abilities on different anatomical levels to perceive each of them. For example, with your hands embodying the lower part of the thorax, you can sense, at different levels, the ribs and spine, the diaphragm and its ligamentous connections, and the liver and neighboring organs. The difference in perception is due more to your mental state and your attention rather than your hands and their pressure (fig. 7.1).

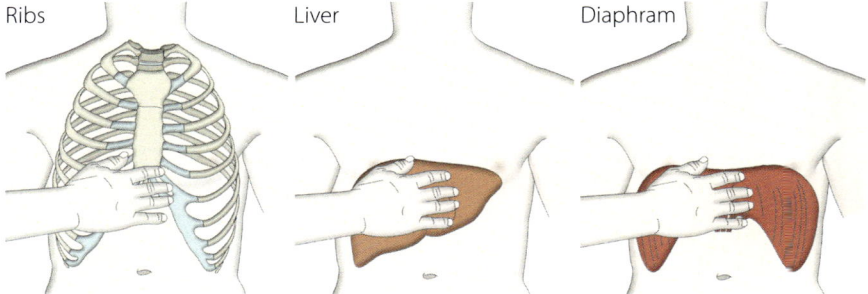

Ribs   Liver   Diaphram

Figure 7.1. The different levels of palpatory attention.

Mental Reproduction

This concerns reproducing mentally the information you attain via your sense organs. The practitioner needs to reinstate the perceived phenomena as faithfully and objectively as possible. It is something like mentally mimicking what your hands perceive without finding it there, using neither reason nor logic. Mental reproduction allows you to decipher the collected sensory information.

Visualization

When you palpate an anatomical element to evaluate or manipulate it, it is necessary to visualize it at all times. The visualization of palpated structures constitutes a palpatory moment that has no substitute.

Visualization is the action by which theoretical anatomy, which is in the domain of the *known,* is united with manual sensations, in the domain of the *perceived.* It results in a particular approach of the palpated element, which may then be learned in three dimensions. This unique state of perception allows an easier evaluation of movements and of the freedom of the anatomical element being considered. Ideally, you must be capable of creating a mental image in three dimensions and also to be aware of your own space. That will sometimes necessitate stretching your spatial anatomical knowledge to redesign that palpated element from a new perspective. That visualization must be made with the tips of your fingers: you should not only see the structure itself but also the induced modifications of your hands that palpate and make it move. If you can add to that a visualization of the mechanical and functional connections of the palpated structure, you will have accessed the essentials of manual diagnosis in record time.

Palpatory Parameters to Observe

Morphostatic Parameters

These are the palpatory parameters that help to identify an anatomical element and to determine if a palpatory object is damaged or if there are structural abnormalities:

- placement
- shape
- volume
- symmetry
- regularity
- consistency
- temperature
- moistness, humidity, or dryness

Concerning temperature, Jean-Pierre Barral has worked a tremendous amount on heat perception. He is the discoverer of *manual thermal diagnosis.* According to his research, the best thermal perceptions are not made by physical contact but at a distance from the skin of the patient. The temperature differences that are useful in diagnosis are best felt about four to six inches from the body. He has established a true map that serves as a reference for all those using this diagnostic tool.

Mechanical Parameters

Mobility is the determining element of osteopathic diagnosis. Evaluate how the element is spontaneously mobilized, or let it be mobilized by the hand.

Histodynamic Parameters

These are felt as modifications from a certain idea of the normality of a tissue undamaged by dysfunction. These are the determinants of tissular functional abnormalities:

- density: analyze all modifications of consistency compared to healthy tissue. Generally a loss of mobility, dysfunction, and lack of energy of a structure are translated as an augmentation of its apparent density.
- tension: analyze the response of the tissues when applying a soft stretch and then releasing it. In the case of dysfunction, the tissues lose their elasticity, which is the generator of mechanical tension.

Painful Parameters

Pain and sensitivity are risky bases for diagnostic interpretation. I must repeat it: do not build your diagnosis on pain, no matter how provoked it is. Keep this in mind so that it does not blind you.

Sensory Abnormalities

- spontaneous
- provoked

SUMMARY

- Diagnostic touch is more than simple palpation. It strives to distinguish clinical elements that are pertinent and significant from qualitative and quantitative points of view.
- The hand should be an extension of the osteopath's mind. It allows us to obtain the palpatory discernment necessary to establish a diagnosis.

Osteopathic Tests

Tests of mobility are indispensable for osteopathic diagnosis. They allow us to observe harmony and disharmonies while linking a structure with its function. Thus we can distinguish two main categories of osteopathic tests:

- tests on the attraction of the mechanical structure
- tests hearing the physiological function or spontaneous movement

Diagnosis is never established on the basis of one test. The convergence of clinical analysis and the coherence of the results of several tests allow us to formulate a viable diagnosis.

Tests Founded on the Study and Observation of the Structure

The Notion of Structure

Structure is a static concept that involves anatomical elements along with their forms and relations that support a function at a given moment. The more normal a structure is, the better its chances of functioning are, and for the body, the better its abilities are to heal or adapt. This is one of the basic postulates of the osteopathic concept: structure governs function.

Structural Tests

In the diagnosis of structure, the practitioner actively palpates a structure, which is then studied in a dynamic manner by mobilizing it. Most often, the practitioner applies a constraint or movement on a part of the patient's body and then manually observes the mechanical response. Thus we get an idea of the connections of position, form, and mobility of the examined elements.

To a great extent, the precision of the test depends on the ability and experience of the practitioner. The most frequent cause of error is an approximate identification or an imprecise palpation of the anatomical references.

Structural tests determine the presence or absence of normality of shape, mobility, and connection among different mechanical chains of the body. If the connections are abnormal, or if the tissues are of abnormal structure, we say that there is a dysfunction. The practitioner estimates:

- the quantity of movement, meaning the fullness of mobility or amplitude of articular play in the degree of the evaluated movement, the course of the organ, or the amplitude of the cranial deformation in one direction. We consider hypomobilities as abnormal. Hypermobilities are generally constitutional or adaptive to the overlying or underlying restrictions of mobility in an articular chain.
- the quality of movement, which is a bit more subtle. It is the more delicate appreciation of certain parameters, such as the ease or annoyance of accomplishing a movement, or more, the quality at the end of the movement. This observation informs us about the elasticity of periarticular structures, motor reactions to mobilization, and the state of the articular interface.

Pain in the course of movement is not a good diagnostic sign because it is too dependent on the ability and softness of the practitioner.

Articular tests at the vertebral or appendicular skeletal levels, visceral tests of mobility, appraisal of tissular gliding with traction, and the evaluation of the elasticity of a structure are also examples of a structural diagnosis.

Tests Founded on the Study and Observation of Function

The Notion of Function

Function is a dynamic concept. It could be said that function is an activity of a structure at a given moment. It is both the actor and witness of a corporal dynamic. Generally, weakness in function displays a lowered overall vitality. Stimulation of function can be a very useful therapeutic vector, via the homeostatic reactions to which it leads. The more the body functions normally, the better its chances are of healing and adaptation.

Not all functions are palpable or observable directly in the course of the examination. Most often, the osteopath is using a technique called listening, with the hand placed on a given part of the body to gather tissular information at a given depth. Viola Frymann (1998), a contemporary American osteopath, declares:

> The term *function* is not only applied to vegetative activities of the organism, such as circulation, respiration, digestion, etc. As well, it includes activities such as thought, sensation, creative expression, meditation, and even spiritual aspiration.

Functional Tests

These tests evaluate the level of activity of one or several parts of the body. The practitioner "listens" to the functioning of the body. Precision isn't really dependent on the practitioner's ability, but it is dependent on how accustomed the practitioner is to diagnostic practice as well as his or her palpatory education. Even though the body is not mistaken in indicating how it functions, that does not necessarily mean that the practitioner is capable of sensing it.

Functional tests place the observed element in optimal conditions so that its functioning and possible imbalances can be sensed. The visceral movements provoked by respiration and motility can be sensed. Somatic dysfunction, spontaneously and noticeably expressed by an articular imbalance, can also be perceived during the test.

This type of test can employ some corporal elements, with function important for the individual's overall activity. The function of an active element is tested according to the primary respiratory mechanism (PRM), thoracic respiration, or its own motility. For example, the practitioner can determine if the rhythmic activity of a body part is normal or abnormal.

Generally, if the tested element presents satisfactory mechanics, with good participation in its function, the movement perceived is free and easy. By contrast, if it is dysfunctional, with mediocre participation in its function, the perceived movement is limited and difficult.

Appraisal using this approach is augmented by a large prognostic value. A patient with satisfactory PRM parameters will be rehabilitated much more quickly that one whose PRM is slow or weak.

From a semantic point of view, body listenings correspond to diagnosis by functions; tests of mobility and routines correspond to diagnosis by structure. These two diagnostic approaches do not oppose each other but usefully complement each other. They do not deliver the same information, but they allow us to improve manual diagnoses and to be precise about the reaction mode of the patient. The art of diagnosis consists of discovering the place where structure and function are in imbalance.

Manual Listening

The notion of manual listening blends some rather varied approaches. Depending on location and pressure, the hand can listen to various tissues at different levels. The awareness, mental state, attention and intention of the practitioner are also important parameters that contribute to the elaboration of different listenings.

William G. Sutherland and Rollin Becker were without doubt the first to utilize this sort of approach. John E. Upledger and Jean-Pierre Barral have developed other types of listening. Each osteopath must strive to construct his or her own frame of reference of listening, adapted to the needs of the practice.

In light of my practice and research, it is possible to distinguish three levels of listening: listening of functions, listening of tissues, and listening of the subtle body. For convenience, I have named them:

- functional listening
- tissular listening
- listening to the subtle body; also called emotional listening

Functional Listening

Functional listening seeks what is called *inherent potential*. Sutherland (1939) summarizes this diagnostic approach by saying that it ought "to permit the internal physiological functioning of manifesting its own unfailing strength rather than utilizing a blind force coming from outside." Most often, this type of listening seeks to sense the movement or rhythmic deformation of an anatomical element or of a coherent mechanical whole. Usually it concerns small amplitudes of movement with variable frequencies that are dependent on the observed function. Among the principal functions suited for this type of evaluation are respiration, the PRM, and visceral motility. Observations of other cellular or tissular activities have been reported with rhythms of very low frequency. The ease of palpation and decoding of these rhythms is proportional to the delicacy and sensitivity of the hand.

A diagnostic tool, the *fulcrum,* is often used to decipher and use this internal potential of the tissues. The therapist creates a fixed point to serve as a point of reference in order to improve perception.

The forces of self-healing envisaged by the osteopathic concept are truly evaluated by this type of listening. The body possesses the aptitude to manifest health across this *inherent potential,* such as the abilities to maintain compensatory mechanisms in response to injuries or diseases, and by the intermediation of different systems. This type of listening observes biodynamic forces within the individual.

Tissular Listening

Tissular listening seeks to discover the seat of major mechanical disequilibrium. The hand is at the crux of all attraction exerted by the contracted tissues. The perception of this attraction seems independent of the physiological rhythms, like that of respiration, and undergoes a bit of modification across its different phases. According to the contracted level and the depth of the evaluated tissues, this sensation can be more or less clear. The direction of the attraction, its strength, and the components that can be perceived allow for a certain amount of deciphering. The brain, by analyzing what the hand feels, allows the practitioner to suspect certain anatomical elements more than others.

The practitioner can use this type of listening to investigate the whole body, a limited topographical area, or a particular mechanical system. This listening relies on the principle of tissular disorganization induced by all osteopathic dysfunctions. Tissular connections, normal operation of increasing and falling pressure, and the phenomena of reciprocal tensions drive and propagate this disorganization. It is possible for a trained hand placed in right areas to perceive these imbalances and to localize their origins.

Emotional Listening

Emotional listening, or listening to the subtle body, is accomplished by a very light touch, at times almost losing contact with the skin. Depending on the therapist's reference system, the hand may search for different sensations. Some practitioners find a vibratory activity, and others find thermal, electromagnetic, energetic, or emotional variations. With this type of listening, it is thought that the mental state of the therapist, her receptivity and availability, allow her to feel via other channels more than just with the hand. For example, with a certain level of empathy, the emotions of a patient are like delicate emanations that can be perceived or interiorized. These ambient perceptions can be made in different ways, and by different means and different representations, according to the developed abilities of each therapist.

REMARKS

For all methods of listening, several remarks are in order.

- It is easy to lose ourselves in this type of approach. From the start, certain practitioners doubt everything, and others doubt nothing. Although this doesn't happen for the same reasons, both of these attitudes are risky.
- Changing hands allows us to verify if a perception is valid. We should feel the same thing when we change sides or change hands.
- A rather simple means to validate or refute a sensation is to use *induction*. Imagine perceiving with your hand a movement or a

counterclockwise attraction. Mentally, try to imagine that your hand encourages and accompanies the tissues in the direction you've felt or believe you've felt. We say that you go *in the direction of the listening,* or that you *follow the listening.* If the tissues accept the encouragement of your hand, your initial perception was correct, and you can consider it valid. If the tissues refuse your encouragement, your initial perception was wrong. It is then necessary to reconsider your initial listening, or to revisit the placement of your hand. Basically, induction is a therapeutic technique; do not abuse it in diagnosis. If the sensations delivered in the listening are real, explanations and theories that arise around them must always be considered working hypotheses and not as truths. It is important not confuse the perception itself with the explanation that we try to give it. As I said earlier, a perception in itself is enough, without the need for "scientific" support to render it more credible.

Routines

Routines are repetitions of a battery of very rapid tests that allow us to detect only lesional localizations. Their goal is to create an assessment of the dysfunctions of the patient, which is uniquely the realization of the *state of mechanical links of the patient.* John Wernham (1995) writes:

> That leads up to the question of the "routine." The routine is of the same nature as our practice. Neither a monotony without end, nor a sense of only offering limitation, but a resolute activity always in search of the highest level of success.

In daily practice, we cannot predict the mechanical dysfunctions that the patient presents, so we use routines, which rapidly investigate the large sectors of the human machine. The musculoskeletal structures, visceral elements, craniosacral system, and neuromeningeal dynamics are all quite mechanically entangled. Pain in one sometimes reflects a dysfunction in another. It seems rather risky to immediately free a specific mechanical sector after only considering limited elements of the interview or listening to the symptomatology of the patient. We prefer to use a system of routines for each patient so that there will be no diagnostic dead end. Surprises can be numerous: a visceral dysfunction is often hidden behind vertebral pain, but the neurovegetative disorder that favors the visceral dysfunction at times may only be an expression of an imbalance of the craniosacral system, or conversely, may be induced by a vertebral dysfunction. As practitioners, each of us has experienced the difficult proof of certain diagnoses at the root of such interactions.

For airplane pilots, there are checklists for everything. Dozens of items are checked before starting, before heading down the runway, before takeoff. None are too complex; at times the checklist has only two or three simple instructions. For example, the pilot has to point a finger or verify electronically when the brake is released, that the flaps are in position, or that the lights are on. It might seem obvious that a professional pilot could remember such basic settings, but the issue is something different: the logic of a routine. *Routine keeps the uncertainties in check,* even for the most elementary things. It allows a feeling of security and calmness. It prevents negative thinking like doubt, which could later place the lives of the passengers in danger. At the moment the plane starts to speed down the runway, the pilot does not have to wonder if the flaps are in place. That was done, and the routine made sure of it. A commercial airline pilot is required to scrupulously follow these numerous checklists. For an osteopath, it is a matter of choice: you can choose to use this approach or not. If you do use routines, at the moment you make your osteopathic decision, you know, like the pilot, that you have verified everything, and the flight will proceed flawlessly.

Chapter 8

Organizing a Diagnosis

One expects a practitioner to proceed with a critical examination and to complete a short report of this examination.

— ANDREW TAYLOR STILL

In office practice, the organization of a consultation is entirely a personal matter. It is necessary that the sequence of events be personalized so that practitioners feel at ease. For many professionals, diagnosis is a matter of course. Each has habits and references, and thinks there is nothing important to say or write about it. However, students and young professionals are often baffled about organizing their findings without becoming overwhelmed and wasting time.

Before going into greater detail, I will begin with an overview of the practical organization of diagnosis as I see it. This framework will be used in the chapters that follow. Even if the practical organization varies from one practitioner to another, the main outlines are comparable, and the main stages are in the same order and share several similar details.

General Examination and Detailed Examination

The organization of an osteopathic consultation has two distinct stages: the general examination and the detailed examination.

General Examination

The general examination requires general questioning, a general clinical examination, and a manual diagnosis (fig. 8.1). It leads to a complete picture of diagnostic possibilities. The *differential diagnosis* usually takes place at the end of the general examination.

Detailed Examination

The detailed examination focuses on the elements that came up in the general examination. The practitioner has already eliminated any possible contraindication and proceeds with the investigation of a mechanical dysfunction. The detailed examination is based on specific questioning, local clinical examination, and specific manual diagnosis (fig. 8.2). A *specific diagnosis* can be arrived at following the detailed examination. An *etiological diagnosis* can be researched once the specific diagnosis has been accomplished.

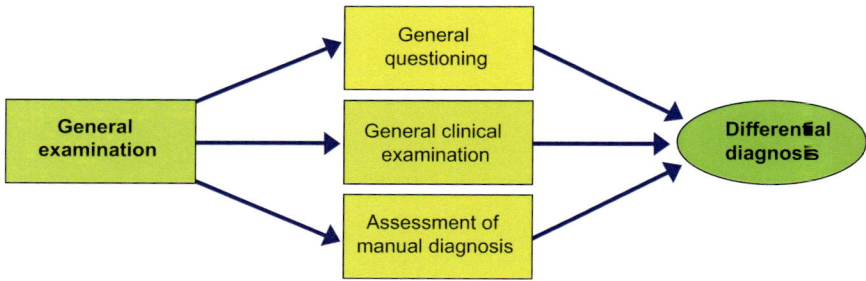

Figure 8.1. General examination.

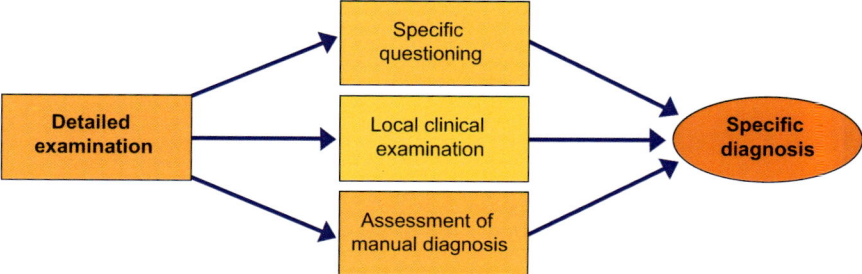

Figure 8.2. Detailed examination.

Direction of the Diagnosis

The different stages of diagnosis proceed in an orderly sequence.

- *General questioning* mainly searches for:
  - the reason for the consultation
  - the circumstances of the appearance of the complaint
  - previous medical surgeries
  - previous medical history
  - lifestyle
  - treatments and medications
- *General clinical examination* is organized around:
  - analytical and global inspection
  - evaluation of symptoms
  - evaluation of the general state of health
  - evaluation of the individual
  - global postural examination
- *Assessment of manual diagnosis* is a rapid evaluation of principal sites of dysfunction. It is based on a methodical and systemic examination consisting of:
  - listening
  - techniques
- The *differential diagnosis:*
  - determines possible contraindications;
  - selects and prioritizes the elements discovered through questioning, general clinical examination, and manual diagnosis;
  - leads to the emergence of a probable diagnosis, which should be confirmed by the specific diagnosis.
- The *specific diagnosis:*
  - evaluates, examines, and tests the elements or structures revealed by the general examination;
  - determines the precise nature of the dysfunction and formulates the course of specific manipulation;
  - more rarely, the specific diagnosis could detect a new problem,

bring to light a missed contraindication, or suggest a precaution to a manipulation.

- The *etiological diagnosis:*
  - synthesizes all the elements brought to light by the general examination and the detailed examination;
  - searches for a possible or probable cause of the identified dysfunction;
  - suggests a path forward that might prevent any recurrence of the problem, and can be useful in advising the patient accordingly.

Summary

It is thus possible to establish a synoptic flowchart (fig. 8.3) summarizing the general organization of the current practical diagnosis.

REVIEW

- Osteopathic diagnosis is based on three elements: *detection, analysis,* and *understanding.* A diagnosis is not only a *point of view* expressed with regard to the patient; osteopathic diagnosis should allow the practitioner to discover where and in what directions the body *structure* and *function* are in *disequilibrium.*
- The true imperative of osteopathic diagnosis is that it be in line with the fundamental principles of osteopathy.
- These principles, originally defined by Andrew Taylor Still, were expanded on by William G. Sutherland and other developers of the diverse disciplines of osteopathic intervention. Osteopathy is a method of completely natural health care without the use of pharmacological substances.
- Conceptually, the osteopathic approach is rather simple: the task is to discover the *roots* and the *causes* of a dis-ease in the *mechanical dysfunctions* of the body.

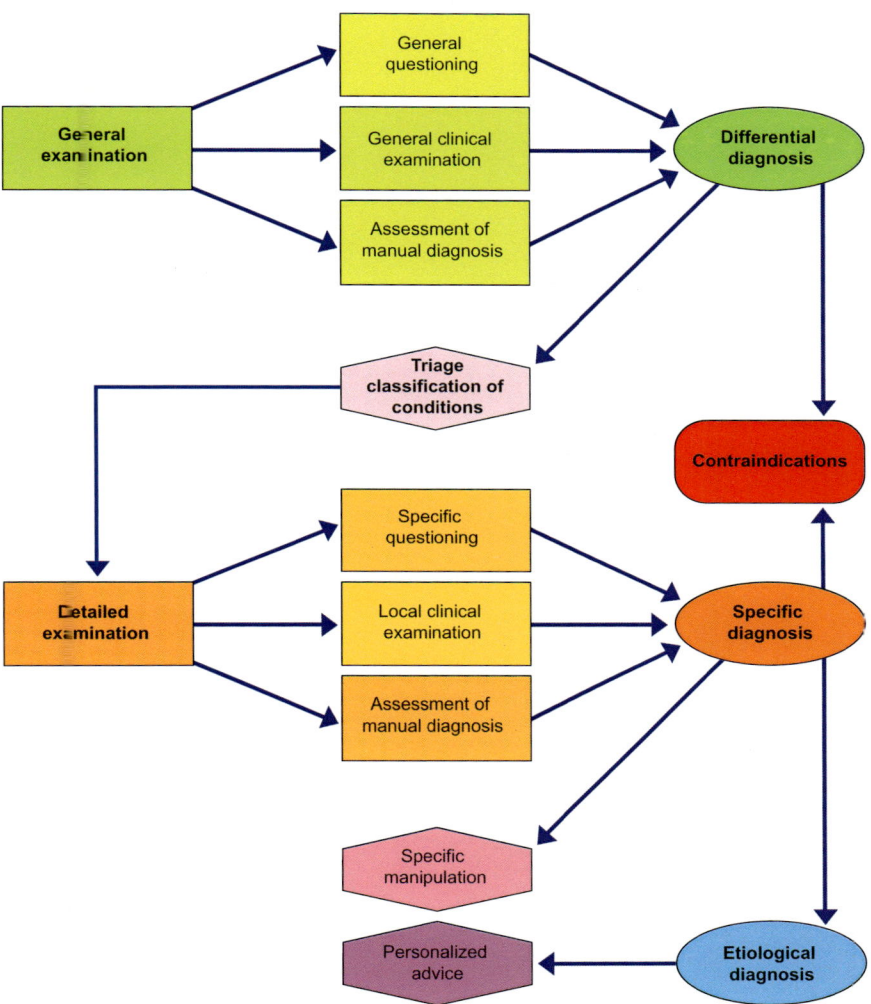

Figure 8.3. General practical organization of an osteopathic diagnosis.

General Diagnosis

Chapter 9

Patient Interview

Common sense is the caretaker of the mind; its duty is to not let doubtful ideas enter or leave.

— DANIEL STERN

Goals of Questioning

The osteopathic consultation is a difficult art. It requires both a rigorous approach to the pathology of the patient as well as the establishment of human contact, tactile and intellectual.

Patient intake and the *questioning* make up the initial visit. Part of their purpose is to initiate a good therapeutic relationship. The trust of the patient is not always acquired immediately. The goal of questioning is to collect relevant information about the patient's complaint. It is necessary to try to evaluate both the condition and the adaptations to it. Questioning is not an exercise in conviviality; it is an essential stage of the clinical examination:

- It provides information that would not be obtained by other methods of investigation. Some targeted questions deal with classical data: personal familial antecedents, surgical interventions, previous hospitalizations, treatments, lifestyle, illnesses, accidents, history of any illness, etc.

- It informs the practitioner about subjective symptoms: pain, treatments that have aggravated or ameliorated the problem, various sensations, etc. These findings are by definition only describable by the patient.
- All of the clinical signs do not necessarily show up during the short period of a consultation. It is often indispensable to ask the patient to make a statement.

The difficulty is not in being exhaustive—all conscientious students have a checklist of questions—but in trying to tailor your verbal approach to the patient and the patient's problem. The technique of conducting a patient interview is not like an interview in journalism, where a list of questions is followed in a systemic manner. The practitioner must learn to be guided somewhat by the patient. The skill is in being able to follow the trail the patient shows us while staying conscious and present. Each situation is different, and we must have a certain mental flexibility to disentangle the patient's narrative.

Communication is one of the keys to successful questioning. It is necessary to be sufficiently directive, but not overly so, and to know how to listen without losing the main train of thought. About half of diagnostic hypotheses can be ascertained through questioning. The other stages of the clinical examination either strengthen or weaken these possibilities and often find other avenues to pursue.

Limits to Questioning

Osteopathic diagnosis is first and foremost tissular. Only the examination and manual decoding of the tissues can determine the location and the nature of the mechanical inadequacy. The patient interview should not prejudice the manual diagnosis. The essence of osteopathic diagnosis is nonverbal. I have often treated patients from other countries with whom I shared no common language; the questioning was obviously quite limited. All the same, through a vigorous clinical examination, I was able to understand what caused the patient to suffer. Only a vigorous clinical examination of the patient allows us to find the main mechanical dysfunction, and examination will never lead us astray.

Similarly, we like to give students the experience of examining patients before questioning them. This exercise is an excellent form of manual training, as it allows students to consider any preconceived notions that could be created from the questioning. This exercise is one of the qualifications to becoming an osteopathic veterinarian.

While it is essential to know medical and surgical symptomatology, in order to develop a clear plan we have to avoid "allopathizing" the questioning. It is not worthwhile asking questions whose answers are of no consequence to the diagnostic conclusion. Reciting a checklist is of no great clinical utility if it is not based on solid symptomatological knowledge. Any unworkable information is of no interest.

Observation, inspection, and the clinical examination are all guides to learning the patient's case history. The choice and personalization of the questions are best determined by the clinical context.

Management of the Questioning

In everyday practice, the questioning may be broken down into two stages:

- a *formal stage*, which generally takes place at the start of a consultation, with the practitioner seated in front of the patient. Often, taking written notes on paper accompanies this initial stage.
- an *informal stage*, which emerges throughout the consultation. Questioning accompanies the findings of the clinical examination as a way of uncovering more precise and more directed symptoms.

Some Rules of Questioning

A well-conducted questioning must follow several rules. It is important to remain alert to any diversionary symptoms in an effort to obtain the most accurate information:

- The practitioner's *attention* is of primary importance; no detail should be neglected. In principle, we do not interrupt the patient. Investigate any points that justify a detail or provide clarification.

    In certain cases, it may be necessary to direct the questioning so as not to be overwhelmed by it. If the narrative becomes vague, you can resort to some direct questions. Asking *how, where,* and *when* is usually more helpful than *why,* which can put the patient on the defensive.

- *Determine the essentials of a detail.* Some patients get bogged down in useless information and secondary considerations. It is not always easy to sort it all out. With this type of patient, pay attention to preconceived ideas and false diagnostic trails.

- Know how to *listen* to the patient. The main principle of questioning is to let the patient relate his story in his own words and to then intervene with questions, prompting him to be more precise about certain details. Listening also shows that you care about the patient himself, his story, and his complaint.

    At times you may need to validate the answers by summarizing them as a way to make certain you understand the motivation behind the consultation as well as the most significant elements of the patient's recollections.

- Know how to *hear* what the patient says. The words she uses and the way she uses them to hide or reveal her thoughts or her story are often charged with feeling. Abstain from judging their value, and retain your objectivity as much as possible.

- Don't let yourself be influenced by personal sympathy or aversion that might affect your judgment of the individual. The patient should always be considered with *respect.* Resist presenting him with your own moral standards by making any reference to so-called "normality." Don't contradict him, except if necessary in the course of pointing out any inconsistencies.

- Adapt yourself to the social and cultural environment of your patient. Ensure that your questions are well understood and adapted to the knowledge and vocabulary of the patient. Likewise, be thoughtful in your choice of words when speaking to the patient about his or her state or pathology. You may find that some terms are best avoided.

Verbal Communication

Choice of Questions

At first, questions should be general. It is necessary to discover why the patient has come for the consultation and the principal symptoms. Ask an open-answer question that gives complete freedom of reply: for example, "What brings you here?" or "What do you think is wrong with you?" After hearing the reply, inquire further: "Is there anything else?' When the subject has finished, you can encourage her to say more by asking: "Tell me about that," or perhaps "What bothers you the most at this moment?" When the patient answers, find the thread of her story and follow it, wherever she goes with it. To obtain more data, you can encourage the narrative with such questions as "And then?" or "What happened next?"

The next step is gathering more precise details through more focused questions. These direct questions should go from *general* to *specific*. For example, "How do you describe your back pain?" "Where do you feel it?" "Show me the location." "Does it stay in one place or does it move around?" "Does it radiate into the thighs? Into the legs?"

Whenever possible, *direct questions* should not be *leading questions*. Try to ask questions that demand a qualitative reply rather than a simple yes or no. If patients are incapable of defining their symptoms without help, assist them by offering multiple-choice questions. For example: "Is your pain continuous, sharp, burning, or shooting?" Each question should have at least two choices.

Ask the questions one at a time to avoid confusion. For example, it might be confusing to ask this kind of question: "Have you had a primary infection, pleurisy, asthma, bronchitis, or pneumonia?"

Use appropriate and comprehensible language. For example, among health professionals *dyspnea* is in common usage, while the layperson would say *breathless*. It is useful to use language familiar to a profession, a country, or a region.

Validate the information you have received. Be certain you clearly understand what the patient has presented. Psychologically, the interview is important for the patient. It allows him to put words to his complaints. Summarizing his narrative ensures you have understood him correctly, and by doing so, the patient will feel heard.

Distrust diagnostic terms that label the patient. Some terms can seem burdensome, and the patient gladly asks for other opinions or diagnoses. I remember a patient who consulted me for sciatica and whose problem was in fact lateral ankle pain due to a commonplace sprain. Her neighbor, who had had sciatica several months before, told her that she had the same thing, and the patient went from one therapist to another for what she called her "sciatica."

Communication Tools

Some people seek help for relatively simple problems, while others suffer from illnesses with complex psychosocial or physiopathological causes. The exact nature of the patient's complaint is not always immediately apparent from the intake form. To better understand the problem, allow each patient to tell his or her own story spontaneously.

If you interrupt the telling prematurely, you risk suppressing the very elements you are seeking. A clinician's role is not entirely passive, however. Listen actively, making a survey of the significant symptoms, emotions, events, and relationships. Then have the patient expand on these points.

Box 9.1. Tools of Verbal Communication

Barbara Bates (1993) and Mark H. Swartz (1991) describe effective methods of eliciting patient information through repetition, clarification, moral support, confrontation, interpretation, and questions that make feelings appear. The behavior of the clinician is important during the course of this process.

- *Facilitation:* Facilitation is a communication technique that is both verbal and nonverbal. It consists of attitudes, acts, or words that encourage the patient to say more about something but without precisely directing him toward a theme. Silence itself is attentive and relaxed, which helps him with recall. Leaning forward to look the patient in the eye to say "hmm," "Go ahead," or perhaps "I'm listening to you," helps him continue his account. Likewise, the practitioner can nod or gesture to continue. Conversely, a facial expression of incomprehension is a nonverbal facilitation explaining that you need supplementary information.

- *Repetition:* Echoing what the patient has said by repeating his words back to him encourages more detailed revelations. Repetition can be useful for bringing facts and feelings to the fore without risk of influencing or interrupting the patient's flow of ideas. Both your tone of voice and word stress are important. Be careful to avoid changing the meaning of words or risk being hurtful by discounting something. For example, the patient might say: "I have such severe sciatica that I haven't worked since 2001." If you repeat "not worked since 2001," you put the emphasis on "not worked" and "2001," which immediately places the patient on the defensive.

- *Clarification:* At times, words are ambiguous, or their associations are not clear. In this case, ask for clarity. For example, "Tell me what you've heard about sciatica," or perhaps "You said that you have experienced the same symptoms as your mother; is that what you wanted to say?"

- *Moral Support:* Moral support shows interest and comprehension. Words of encouragement promote a secure environment in a therapeutic relationship. Support is particularly important after the patient has expressed strong feelings or after he or she suddenly begins to cry. According to Swartz, moral support is based on comfort and empathy.
  - *Comfort:* Comfort indicates to the patient that you have understood her. It can also indicate that you agree with actions she has taken to help herself. Comfort is especially useful when

the patient seem perturbed or scared. It is a very powerful tool, but false comfort can have devastating effects. Comfort should always be based on facts: "I'm very happy that you have shown signs of improvement." "Your condition has improved a lot since our last consultation."

- *Empathy:* When a patient talks to you, she may express with or without words, feelings about which she is embarrassed, ashamed, or reticent. These feelings can be essential to understanding the symptoms and pathology of the patient. Empathy is the capacity to accept the patient's feelings without criticizing them. It is a state of understanding and not just sympathy. To be empathetic is a way of saying "I am here with you"; the patient will feel more secure, and this feeling encourages her to continue. Simple replies like "I understand," "You must have been upset," or even "That must have been very difficult for you" can help the patient relate the experience.

  Empathy can also be nonverbal. For example, offering a handkerchief to a person who is crying or gently placing a hand on her arm or shoulder conveys understanding. A nod is a manifestation of empathy.

- *Confrontation:* Confrontation means drawing a patient's attention to something that she may or may not be conscious of. The confrontation can either be affirmative or slightly demanding. If you observe signs of anger, anxiety, or depression, for example, confrontation could help to bring these feelings to light: "Your hands tremble when you talk about that," "Are you angry?" or "Why aren't you saying anything?"

  Confrontation can also be useful to clarify possible contradictions in the account: "You say that you have no idea what triggers your stomachache, but each time you have one, it seems to me that it follows a period of overwork." As another example, you expect that a patient is about to describe a painful thoracic symptom, and you notice there are tears in her eyes. Say to her kindly, "You have a troubled look." By doing so, you encourage her to express her emotions.

Confrontation should be used with care because in excess it can be considered impolite or overly insistent.

- *Interpretation:* Interpretation goes beyond confrontation. Interpretation is a type of confrontation based on a deduction rather than observation. The clinician interrupts the flow of the patient's story, encouraging her to observe her own role in the problem. In this case you intervene instead of observing. For example: "Apparently nothing has gone right for you these last few times." "You seem tired of all the therapy." "It would seem that your symptoms are more intense after you have had an argument with your wife."

  Note: Be certain to have judged the signs and explanations of your patient correctly before discussing them. In interpreting a patient's words or behavior, you risk going off on the wrong track and disrupting any subsequent communication. When used wisely and deliberately, an interpretation can show support and improve understanding.

- *Questions about Feelings:* Rather than attributing a feeling to her, you could simply ask the patient if she resents something, perhaps her symptoms or a particular event in her life. It is advisable to tell her you are interested in her feelings as well as the clinical facts. Otherwise she may hide them from you, and you can miss out on important signs.

NOTE

Use all these tools cautiously. Used thoughtlessly, they can undermine the interview. A consultation is not a commercial relationship—a therapist isn't selling anything—so remain as truthful as possible, respect the patient, and preserve your authenticity.

Box 9.2. Nonverbal Messages

Nonverbal messages can be placed in several categories:
- *The environment—familiar objects and clothing:* such elements can hold an indirect but often strong message. In a general way,

included in this category are the furniture of an apartment, house, or office and the luxury, modesty, extravagance, or simplicity of its decor. In the course of a consultation, familiar objects and clothing are often discussed. Purses, glasses, cufflinks, jewelry, ornaments, pens, watches, and briefcases all carry messages about taste, refinement, simplicity, vulgarity, social status, education, class of origin, or how the person wants to appear to others. This applies also to perfume, makeup, and, of course, the character, shape, color, and purpose of clothing. Clothing is the expression of the thinking and psychology of how a person dresses.

- *Physical appearance:* height, weight, color of the hair and eyes, complexion, the shape of the face, scents, beauty or lack of it, and tone of voice all influence our first impression when we meet a person. From factors such as facial features and thinness or obesity we immediately deduce, more or less consciously, traits of character, mental attitudes, and behaviors. The viewer is sometimes not able to avoid showing an attitude of sympathy or antipathy, attraction or disinterest. Permanent psychological impressions can instantly arise from the shape of the mouth or eyebrows, the pattern of a smile, or the tone of voice. Whether true or false, it is important to consider how much these perceptions determine our attitudes.

- *Gestures, postures, and expressions:* a large majority of the body movements that we observe in the course of interaction among individuals is totally instinctive. These movements include those of the hands, the limbs, the head, or the entire body. They can be full or barely discernible, although they are precisely identified subconsciously by those who perform them or by the person they apply to.

When the head is moved forward half an inch, it signifies approval, waiting, or inviting. Holding back the torso even as little as half an inch signals disagreement and is recognized by the other person's right brain, even if he or she does not consciously know it. As a consequence, the exchange is altered. Words also come with gestures that help to convince, affirm, or otherwise emphasize a point.

Posture reveals a great deal about the emotional state of the person talking and those listening. Muscular tension expresses disagreement and anger. The head and torso leaning forward shows that someone acknowledges defeat and acquiesces. Crossing the arms often indicates a defensive attitude or refusal to get involved, as does a turned-away stance.

Fatigue and depression can be read by the manner in which the shoulders are held. Trembling, clenched fists, and crossing and uncrossing the legs are examples of involuntary responses that are nevertheless seen and interpreted.

Facial expressions are, of course, the most revealing. A combination of tilting the head and moving the lips, jaws, and eyebrows or fluttering the eyelids can transmit a thousand different messages, causing involuntary responses in speech or posture. Anger, sadness, contentment, fear, dislike, surprise, scorn, defiance, and reproach are quite obviously expressed by our body language independently of whether we decides to speak or not. Likewise, gaze plays a considerable role. Eye contact in dominant primates is a way of affirming dominance, but this is not the case among humans. The listener looks into the eyes of the speaker, especially if she is of higher status, and the speaker often looks elsewhere. But when she wants to stop speaking, she again looks at the listener. Some research goes as far as to analyze the contraction and dilation of the pupils, a very discrete phenomenon but one that is easily and consciously perceived by the other person.

- *Touch:* in an adult, touch as part of the interaction before loving or sexual relations expresses either an intimacy already established or pursuit of intimacy or trust. But it could have a subconscious strategy. A person who wants to end a relationship taps lightly on the other person's shoulder, who stiffens if he does not see things in the same way.

109

- *The distance between two bodies:* at the core of every culture, the distance that separates two speakers holds precise meaning. The space that separates two people having an intimate relationship differs from the space between two friends, two colleagues, or two people talking at a party. On public transportation or in a crammed elevator, contact is only tolerable on two conditions: it is not accompanied by meeting the other person's gaze, and the muscles express a certain tension rather than being relaxed. There is thus a close connection with the notion of an animal's territory, and all sorts of strategies are put in place so that this territory is respected by strangers. Some people go so far as to measure the distance between the armchair for a visitor and their own armchair or desk. Uninvited territorial invasion tends to trigger stereotypical postural reactions.
- *Nonverbal communication* encompasses multiple notions, such as tone, delivery, inflection, the sonorous force, the length of the silences, and the speed with which the words are taken up again when the speaker is quiet. There are also interjections of throat-clearing, lip-smacking, and all the phenomena that modulate delivery. All these elements give indications about the mood of what is said (denial, doubt, sarcasm, surprise, conviction, irony, etc.). The right cerebral hemisphere registers what is heard together with all the nuances, hesitations, or contradictions. These elements, which we as practitioners have to decode, often involve instinctive responses.

Nonverbal Communication

In addition to spoken words, body language is an important form of non-verbal communication (box 9.2) that can round out our perception of the patient. As therapists we should give some weight to what is unspoken between ourselves and the patient. Does the patient avoid looking you in the eye? Are there unexpressed clues that the body is trying to express?

An individual who taps her hand or fist on the table while talking emphasizes that she intends to speak in an intense manner. A person who squirms in his chair and cannot get comfortable is obviously ill at ease. Frowning eyebrows can indicate boredom, disapproval, or sometimes a lack of understanding. A person who drops and returns to the topic of her marriage many times might have ambiguous feelings about it. A hand on the heart affirms sincerity and credibility. Often, people who are rubbed the wrong way may avert their eyes to show their refusal to accept a comment. A patient who doesn't agree with something the practitioner says but doesn't say anything may pick fluff off his clothing.

According to Lucien Israel (1995), "The world of nonverbal communication is immense, at times unable to transcend the cultural barriers between people." Research reveals that nonverbal signals directed toward others or exchanged in the course of our interactions represent sixty-five to ninety percent of interpersonal communication.

In right-handed people, the left brain is thought to represent the analytical and logical hemisphere, while the right brain is more global and analogical in function. Thus in nonverbal exchanges, the right brain plays a bigger role. The left brain is not totally excluded from these exchanges, however, making nonverbal communication somewhat intentional. The most quantitatively significant part of our interactions with others is directed by the right brain. Also, in an exchange between two people, nothing escapes two right brains that communicate in parallel with a conversation by the two left brains.

Discussion about the interpretation of nonverbal exchanges is worthwhile. We can easily measure the importance of the nonverbal part of communication by the difficulty we experience in telephoning someone in a foreign language. Experts say it is without doubt the most arduous linguistic task because it is done without benefit of the usual nonverbal clues. Nonverbal communication is vital to any high-level communication.

Complete interpretation of body language is only possible in the cultural and ethnic context of the patient. Arabs and Asians often speak with lowered eyelids, while in a European or North American this mannerism would be seen as abnormal and could indicate depression or lack of attention.

Keep in mind your own facial expression when facilitating a conversation. An attentive appearance shows interest in what the patient is saying. You can also demonstrate you interest by leaning forward slightly. A hand resting on a patient's shoulder expresses support. The practitioner approaches a patient in a straightforward way in the hope of gaining respect and confidence. Gazing alternately into each of the patient's eyes expresses interest. In this way, the listening is looking at the patient's soul.

Don't forget that nonverbal communication has meaning on both sides. It is useful in gathering diagnostic information, and it allows patients to feel whether or not the therapeutic relationship suits them.

Patient Behavior

The behavior of the patient during a consultation is influenced by personality structure. Blétry and Godeau (1995) set up four tables to distinguish more or less archetypical behaviors demonstrated by patients during a consultation: self-satisfied and talkative; intimidated and quiet; methodically meticulous; and demanding. I will also describe three others common personalities: the seducer; the patient with multiple symptoms; and the anxious patient.

Self-satisfied and talkative patients want to express themselves and share family and professional ties, give an exact account of their last vacation, and talk about leisure plans and general opinions. They often take the initiative and may even interrupt you, seeking your opinion on a certain therapy, examination, or intervention that they think should be applied to their pathology. They often self-diagnose and want you to confirm their analysis. It is difficult to get a word in and to obtain a response to a specific question. The practitioner has to abandon open questions, facilitation, and silence. Each question elicits a lengthy reply, and even the responses to closed questions seem interminable in detail.

It is necessary to try to channel the questioning. A courteous interruption, followed by another direct question, momentarily brings these patients back to the subject of the discussion.

Intimidated and quiet patients can also be difficult. They considers all attempts at communication to be a sort of exhibitionism. This tendency can be linked to distress, a psychological block, or to defiance toward therapy or all forms of medicine, due to mistaken ideas, previous experiences, or perhaps just natural timidity on a topic they consider personal. In this case, the practitioner should attempt to reassure, win over, and relax the patient. Sometimes an occasional digression on subjects unrelated to the consultation can be helpful, and then you can return to more classical questioning. It is generally of little use to ask them open questions, but several replies can be obtained from carefully directed questioning. With certain patients, the physical examination can even be undertaken before having completely carried out the questioning. Physical contact, in this specific context, can serve to establish communication. Silent patients can easily be depressed; this could be the direct result of their mental state.

Methodically meticulous patients are generally classified as having obsessive personalities. They may supply you with a personal résumé or an uncommonly detailed medical history. This document is not useless but it does not replace the classical questioning. Consciously or unconsciously, these patients may have omitted essential points from their exhaustive list. The document provided should be kept on file.

Demanding patients have a tendency to be paranoid to some degree. From the outset they are contrary, critical, hostile, and defiant. Usually they have already consulted numerous doctors and therapists of all kinds. They are convinced of the incompetence, low intelligence, and inadequacy of their former therapists. They complain that these therapists did not listen or understand anything about their disease, while they spent money, wasted time, and made no progress. They will tell you that you are different, otherwise they would not be there, and they are confident that you can resolve their problem. Don't be especially flattered; this state of grace will not last, and the false confidence very quickly reveals a thinly veiled threat: they dare you to be successful. With these patients it is necessary to keep a low profile and act with a certain amount of humility: "I am not better or worse than the others"; "I don't have a magic bullet." Admit that all therapies have their limits, and that if you try to help, in no way can you guarantee the results that they so ardently hope to obtain. You can connect them w th the treatment: "Let's try to find the way to treat you or to make you better together"; "You seem to have such a good understanding of your problems." You can enter into a sort of therapeutic contract with a defined term. In the absence of any improvement in symptoms after one or two consultations, they will be advised to get another opinion.

Seducers are in every respect more difficult than demanding patients. They often fit the profile of hysteria. Fantasies of intimate relations with the therapist and a certain exhibitionist tendency often guide the behavior of these extroverts. As a general rule, they do all they can to please the therapist. Behind the scenes, they often feel a sense of rejection generated by anxiety. Faced with this type of patient, the therapist must always show complete professionalism. Empathy and comfort are reduced to a minimum so as to avoid reactivating their desire. As clinicians, we have to protect ourselves from engaging in relationships that could put our efficacy and self-respect in jeopardy.

Practitioners of both genders can find themselves attracted to their patients. The emotional and physical intimacy of the therapeutic relationship can generate erotic feelings. If we acknowledge these feelings, they can be accepted as normal human reactions. Needless to say, sexual or sentimental relationships with patients are unethical. We have to keep relations with the patient within the strict confines of professional relationships.

It is also necessary to reflect on your own behavior. Are you too warm or cordial? Do you express affection physically? Do you seek affectionate support from a patient? Do you dress seductively? It is best to avoid these inclinations as much as possible.

Patients with multiple symptoms: some individuals seem to have every symptom imaginable. Although it is conceivable that they could manifest multiple organic illnesses, it is more probable that they have simulated serious problems. Hypochondriacs are excessively preoccupied with the health, functioning, and general state of their bodies. Often linked to narcissistic overinvestment, this close self-inspection is disquieting. They fixate on the smallest unusual cenesthesic sensations and greatly magnify their significance. This causes them to repeat their requests for advice and care. At times their entire existence, and even that of their families, is organized in a hypochondriacal way: excessive attention to precautions, diets, ritualized meals, sleep, and bowel movements.

Anxious patients: anxiety is a common and natural reaction to suffering or to the therapy situation. For certain patients, anxiety is the result of all perceptions and reactions, while for others it is an integral part of their disease. Practitioners must be receptive to verbal and nonverbal signs of anxiety. For example, anxious people may sit in a tense way, playing with their fingers or clothing. They often sigh, moisten dry lips, sweat profusely, or tremble. The carotid pulse can reveal a rapid heart rate. Some anxious people remain silent, incapable of speaking freely or of confiding. Others try to hide their feelings with words, carefully avoiding their true problems. If you sense underlying anxiety, you must encourage patients to talk about their feelings.

This catalog of behavioral caricatures does not apply to more routinely encountered patients. There is no standard, no "normal." Each patient is a unique case. The "normal" patient will often be the one you naturally find likeable or with whom you tend share certain tastes or ideas.

Adolescents in crisis, drug addicts, and ailing seniors are not easy patients. In all difficult situations, it is necessary to maintain perspective and to remain focused on our role as a therapist. It can be useful to try to understand how a particular patient annoys us, and how his or her story or behavior resonates with our own personality.

All human relations are based on a sort of theatrical play that is more or less an attempt at seduction. The osteopathic consultation is no exception, and it is useful to remember this.

Unusual Cases

The "very important people," "intellectuals," "scientists," and "celebrities" can at times have some prejudices about our profession. This can cause obstacles to establishing a relationship of trust. The personality of a patient can similarly represent an emotional charge that is overwhelming for the therapist. Be especially careful not to be intimidated or paralyzed by the importance of the person you are consulting with. This applies to treating a Nobel laureate, a head of state, an athlete who has won a world championship, or one who is preparing for the Olympics. It is necessary to center yourself on the fact that you are in front of a human being who is having difficulty, who is soliciting your help, and to whom you will lend your assistance. Specifically, do not think of the social function of the patient, but focus on his or her individual dimension. The main thing is to remain yourself, be true to your values, and not feel threatened in any way, even by the distrust of the patient, so that your diagnostic and therapeutic abilities are not affected.

Professionals, including doctors, surgeons, health practitioners, and colleagues, are sometimes problematic, especially in the initial meeting. The osteopathic art is complex and rests on working with feelings. It is necessary to resist the temptation to provide an intellectual explanation of the application of the theory. In my opinion, the initial questioning should be rather brief, passing quickly to the manual evaluation so as not to become overly biased by the intellect.

It is important that you share your diagnostic pursuit and explain your gestures and your manual findings. This establishes good contact with patients and reassures them of your competence. It also verifies that your approach is rational, that there is nothing magical going on, and that it is founded on common knowledge. This exchange and sharing even out a number of difficulties, including cultural differences. It is essential that patients feel the mechanical connections through their bodies. Nothing secures the trust of disbelievers more than to have them perceive the unusual feelings generated by the mobilization of a part of the body whose mechanics are defective.

Patient Reactions

Silence

In the course of a consultation, silence can make us feel ill at ease. Some people feel obliged to maintain the conversation. This is not always ideal. Silence has a variety of meanings and is sometimes useful.

- In the course of trying to recall past occurrences of their complaint, certain patients need to pause to reassemble their ideas and memories, or simply to reflect on what they are going to describe to you or omit, and to trust what they are going to say. An attentive silence is generally the best response, and at times it can be usefully followed by a brief encouragement to continue. We must observe our patients and especially their nonverbal signs.
- In the course of diagnosis or treatment, difficulty in controlling an emotion can cause patients to be silent. In this case, their expression is often unclear: they could be on the verge of tears, altering their breathing, or retreating within themselves. The practitioner can help by gently confronting them in saying, for example, "You seem to be upset; do you want to talk to me about it?"
- People who experience an organic cerebral stroke, or even some depression, can lose their spontaneous expression. After giving a short reply to a question, they become mute. In these cases it is always useful to direct the questioning toward the exploration of cerebral functions.
- At times silence can result from error on the part of the practitioner or from our insensitivity. Have we asked too many direct questions? Is the rhythm of the questions too intense? Is the patient offended by something? Was something overlooked (an annoying symptom, pain, etc.)? Most often the solution is to be truthful. Ask patients what has come up, or if you have misunderstood something. Allow them to explain their point of view and abbreviate the remaining questioning, leaving it until later.

117

Silence is a useful tool from the point of view of communication with quiet patients. Used gently, it can generate rapport and show support. If we as clinicians remain silent, we must nevertheless remain attentive and maintain direct visual contact. After having respected the patient's silence, we can return to the interview by asking: "What do you think about that?" "It's not easy to talk about that," "You said . . . ?" or "You were going to say . . . ?"

As clinicians we can choose silence when patients are overcome with emotion. This allows us to lower the tension that the account or treatment has brought up, and indicates to patients that it is all right to cry.

While it is necessary to make good use of silence, to resort to it too frequently can be interpreted as scorn or indifference. On the other hand, we must never be silent with talkative individuals; if you let them "take the floor," they will not let the therapist direct the interview at all.

Tears

Tears are an important sign of emotions. They often express sadness and can also reveal distress or frustration. If patients seem to be on the verge of tears, a kind remark or an indication of sympathy can allow them to cry. When they stop crying, offer them a handkerchief and wait for them to become calm. In this context, most patients rapidly feel better and are able to continue the discussion or treatment. In our culture, tears make most people feel ill at ease. As clinicians, we must nevertheless make an effort toward helping patients accept this significant manifestation.

Availability and Listening

When I started in this profession, my friend Jean-Pierre Barral said to me one day, "When someone comes into your office, he or she becomes the most important person in the world during the consultation." This advice captures perfectly the state of mind that must preside over the consultation. We must be "all ears" and "all eyes" for two reasons:

- Mental presence, in both the questioning and the examination, allows you to focus on the patient. Paying close attention, we can sometimes grasp a symptom's brief signal, which reveals something essential in establishing the diagnosis.
- The patient ought to perceive this outright therapeutic attention. Nothing is more disagreeable for a patient than to have the impression that the clinician is hurried, looking at his or her watch, or replying to phone calls.

For some patients, even the act of reading or writing in a file or typing on a computer represents a lack of attention and inadequate listening (Njølstad et al. 1992). If note-taking seems too annoying and interferes with the spontaneity of the interview, it is best to complete notes as faithfully as possible after the interview.

Beyond having our full attention, patients must sense in the therapist solicitude, human warmth, and great comprehension—the keys of good communication and a successful consultation.

The Presence of a Third Party

The presence of a third party can sometimes be useful, and at other times it can hinder the atmosphere of the consultation. Preferably, the interview should be between the therapist and the patient alone. In some cases, however, the presence of a third person is inevitable and can help shed light on the patient's condition. It is necessary always to inquire right away what the relationship is between the patient and the third party without trying to guess. This will help to avoid comic or upsetting situations.

Some patients are completely incapable of reporting their own history due to age, dementia, a language barrier, or other deficiencies. In all these cases, the presence of a third party is desirable and indispensable.

The presence of a spouse can be helpful. He or she can offer details, correct errors, and point out the importance of symptoms that the patient may have minimized. The directive or authoritative side of a spouse or parent can be disagreeable or ill-suited for the consultation.

It is up to the therapist to direct questions specifically to one person or the other to elicit the best information. At times it is necessary to interview the patient alone in order to rekindle the intimacy of the consultation.

Sensitive Topics

In all consultations, approaching certain topics can present unusual difficulty. This is the case with topics that have been taboo or tend to be suppressed, such as alcohol, drugs, sexuality, illegal activities, psychiatry, death and dying, domestic violence, family relations, financial worries, and physical deformities. The evolution of ideas is radically different from one setting to another and from one region to another according to age, across religious beliefs, by ethnic origin, and so on. There can be a wide gap from one patient to another. If the questioning must touch on these subjects, it is necessary to do it with tact. Never asks patients straight away questions such as "How much do you drink?" "Are you a drug user?" "Are you gay?" "Are you impotent?" and "Are you averse to sex?" It is necessary to try to assuage patients' guilt should it arise when dealing with this kind of topic. Assure them:

- We are not judges or police officers; it is possible to understand things without making a value judgment.
- We are conscious of life's difficulties.
- We ourselves are not models of exemplary virtue.

It is necessary to present an atmosphere of kindness so that patients feel encouraged to confide in us what might appear to them to be shameful. Nonverbal communication works well here to show our absence of judgment and to encourage patients to pursue their recollections. It is always necessary to be careful that our *comprehension* does not imply *approval.* In some cases, approval could be a factor in the reinforcement of destructive behavior, such as with alcoholism or a drug habit.

Alcohol and Drugs

Many practitioners have difficulty asking patients about their consumption of alcohol and drugs, whether illicit or prescribed. We don't have to approve of the use of these products, but they can be directly linked to symptomatology. Our investigation aims to gather a maximum of data. It is sometimes necessary to appraise the repercussions of alcoholism on the health of the patient in order to develop an adaptive therapeutic response (box 9.3). After all, liver manipulation has no real usefulness for a patient who regularly overindulges in alcohol.

Sexuality

Questions concerning sexual function and practices can have several applications. Beyond the diagnosis of an unwanted pregnancy or sexually transmitted diseases, certain genital symptoms can relate directly to certain dysfunctions and need to be considered in the broad scheme of things.

Some patients have questions or problems with their sexuality. Given the opportunity, they might be quite willing to talk about it. Even if they don't confide in you during your first meeting, it is wise to have approached the subject, making you a potential listener.

Questions regarding sexual function or practices can evoke moments of forgetfulness. Sexual practices are often only considered in the course of a person's gynecological-obstetrical history or in terms of urogenital symptoms. In approaching this topic, say something like: "Next I would like to ask you several questions about your sexual life." You can then begin with questions about sexual behavior and sexual satisfaction. Focusing on the information that is necessary, some questions should be asked with complete neutrality: "What method of contraception do you use?" If the patient says they don't use it at all, ask: "Have you tried to have a child?" "Do you have pain during intercourse?" "Is your sex life satisfying?" and "Do you feel concerned about HIV/AIDS or STD infection?"

Remember that sexual activity can begin very early. Adolescents often keep their sexual behavior secret from their parents. The practitioner should be careful, in this case, to maintain confidentiality when broaching this subject with an adolescent.

Box 9.3. Screening for Alcoholism and Drug Addiction

Questions regarding alcohol and other toxic chemicals can follow quite naturally those concerning coffee and cigarettes: "How much alcohol do you drink?" or "Tell me about you alcohol consumption" are good introductory questions that can avoid easy yes-or-no answers.

It is imperative to inquire about alcohol consumption in the case of abdominal pain. To do this, ask supplementary questions: "Have you ever had problems with alcohol?" and "When did you have your last drink?" An affirmative reply to the first question and having had an alcoholic drink in the last twenty-four hours indicate possible alcoholism (Cyr and Wartman 1988).

For other concerns, the CAGE questions (cutting down, annoyed by criticism, guilty feelings, and eye-openers), can also be useful in detecting alcoholism (Mayfield et al. 1974):

- "Do you resent the need to cut down your alcohol consumption?"
- "Are you annoyed by the criticism of your alcohol consumption?"
- "Do you have guilty feelings regarding alcohol?"
- "Do you ever drink first thing in the morning to calm your nerves or to overcome dry mouth?"

The questions concerning drug addiction are similar: "Do you take any mind-altering substances?" "What quantity of marijuana do you use?" "Do you take pills to sleep? To lose weight? For pain?" "Have you tried to stop?"

Be aware that alcoholism and drug addictions can begin in childhood or adolescence. Approaching this subject with adolescents is difficult. Start by asking them about friends and family who may consume these substances. "Many young people take drugs nowadays. What is it like at your school? What about your friends?" When patients realize that you aren't going to judge them but are showing an interest in them, they can feel more at ease and tell you how they became drug users.

Mental Illnesses

Considered and treated differently than organic illnesses, mental illnesses are much more the object of deeply rooted prejudices in our society. It is often easier for a patient to talk about something like having diabetes and injecting insulin than to talk about having schizophrenia and taking antipsychotics.

If you want to direct the questioning to previous mental illnesses of patients or their families, address them with open questions: "How did you come to have emotional or mental problems?" or "Have you previously had depression?" Then you can follow with questions about treatment: "Have you previously consulted a psychotherapist or psychiatrist?" or "Has anyone in your family been hospitalized for an emotional or mental problem?"

Many psychiatric patients are high-functioning and are frequently capable of speaking openly about their diagnosis, symptoms, hospitalizations, and course of treatment. Be comfortable enough yourself to inquire about all of it without embarrassment so that you can evaluate the point at which the symptoms can cause suffering.

Even though depression is a common problem, it is often poorly diagnosed and treated. It is good to keep in mind the possibility of depression in all patients who complain of fatigue, vague symptoms, weight loss, insomnia, or unexplained pains. Mood changes are not necessarily the only symptom of depression. To alleviate depression, it is necessary to know the characteristic symptoms and to explore the manifestations. "How was your mood or your spirits last month?" "Do you take interest and pleasure in your everyday activities?" Bates (1993) insists on the importance of evaluating the seriousness of a person's depression. It is as important as thoracic pain, both potentially being lethal.

Serious Illnesses, Death, and the End of Life

Even though incurable patients are rare in an urban practice, we are increasingly asked to help bring comfort to people with serious illnesses under the label of palliative therapy. In communicating with patients dealing with incurable illnesses or with those at the end of their lives, we can be confronted with our own anguish. Patients who know they are dying rarely like to talk much about their illness. It is necessary to listen to them if they want to talk, or to be content with more superficial conversation if they don't. The illness is only one part of the patient's life, and at times, a smile, a joke, a discussion of the surroundings, or a comment on a publicly shared event can offer better support than a serious discussion on pathology and the suffering that it causes.

A good way to communicate is to reflect what the patient says. Incorporate into the conversation terms that the patient uses. If the patient does not use the word *death*, then don't use it at all. Conversely, if the patient uses the word *cancer*, that authorizes you to use it too.

Anamnesis (Patient History)

In an osteopathic consultation, the questioning does not follow the methodology of classical medical questioning. It should be rigorous enough, however, not to leave anything to chance. A classical examination usefully completes taking the patient's history by putting the elements obtained from the interview into perspective. All interviews begin by identifying the patient, learning his or her last name, first name, date of birth, gender, relationship status, and profession.

Reason for the Consultation

One of the goals of questioning is to determine the precise complaint of the patient. When the case is simple, as in whiplash or torticollis, the reason for the consultation is evident. Other times, it is more difficult to discern. Some patients are not even certain what we can do for them and are consulting us on the recommendation of someone close to them, so their request is vague and imprecise. Help them to describe as best they can what brought them to consult you. Other patients come with several dysfunctions, pathologies, and different illnesses, causing confusion. They often hope we have the power to correct everything with our treatments. In this case, help patients chose the most troubling issue. Make them contain their requests and prioritize their complaints. At a convenient time, record the requests in writing in the patient file. We should always keep notes about the reason for the consultation. This written record is essential:

- It identifies the start of the therapeutic relationship, which forms a point of reference that often has great importance in subsequent consultations.
- Between treatments, some patients forget their initial complaint, particularly as more of their symptoms have evolved.
- Some patients have a selective memory: either they avoid discussing what doesn't always work or fit, or they hold back about what has improved since their last appointment.

Only your notes will allow you to objectively verify, point by point, what has improved and what has not changed. Be as precise as possible about how patients perceive the illness or symptoms. Which symptoms are the most disturbing? To what degree does the ailment interfere with their life and functioning? Similarly, consider the written notes.

Signs and Symptoms

The clinician ought to know how to discover and recognize a great variety of signs and symptoms. The word *symptom* refers to what the sick person feels: breathlessness, pain, nausea, diarrhea, constipation, double vision, and vertigo are all symptoms. They are not absolute and are influenced by culture, intelligence, and socioeconomic environment.

The word *sign* applies to an objective finding discovered by the clinician, without reference to the perceptions of the patient. Signs are observable, identifiable, and often quantifiable by different observers. In osteopathy, signs are more numerous than they are in allopathy, since manual examination identifies all loss of tissular and articular mobility as abnormal.

Certain signs are also symptoms. A sick person may describe an episode of bronchial wheezing, making it a symptom. The clinician could also hear wheezing in the auscultation, making it a sign. Semiology uses the terms *clinical sign* or *subjective sign* as synonyms for *symptom* and *sign of the examination* or *objective sign* to designate signs.

A *syndrome* is a group of symptoms and the telltale signs of a dysfunction, joined by one or more anatomical, physiological, or biochemical anomalies. It underlies the failing of an organ or of a group of organs or tissues.

Symptoms help the osteopath understand the complaint, discern the ailment of the patient, and make the differential diagnosis. In terms of understanding the mechanical dysfunction, experience shows that the cause is often far removed from the symptom. While it is important to understand the patient's complaint and to analyze the symptoms, it is not necessary to be blinded by these findings for the rest of the diagnosis.

Previous History

A thorough history-taking is necessary to establish the basis on which patients describe themselves and their symptoms, to evaluate how patients see their past, and also to learn from actual past medical records. The history-taking explores previous illnesses, traumas, wounds, and surgical interventions. The evolution of a patient's general state of health concerns current health, environmental conditions, personal habits, and any ongoing care. The compilation of previous history must be carried out in a methodical way and organized according to age, for example, childhood, adolescence, young adulthood, etc. A degree of tact is required when asking about facts apparently unrelated to the current affliction.

We distinguish between *personal* and *familial* previous histories. This allows us to be precise about the nature of the patient. Classically, the personal history comprises the following:

- general state of health
- previous illnesses
- wounds, injuries
- hospitalizations
- surgeries
- allergies
- vaccinations
- abuse
- diet
- sleep
- current medications

Past events carry different weight depending on the age of the patient and the time of life whey they occurred.

Familial previous histories help to evaluate any risks that predispose a patient to certain illnesses. They are mainly focused on:

- cardiovascular events
- diabetes
- cancer

Treatments and Medications

If a patient is taking medications, it may suggest precautions in taking on therapeutic responsibility. Some symptoms can be created and others hidden by taking certain medications; in this way they can complicate diagnosis. Numerous undesirable effects are linked to medical interventions, and certain symptoms are directly attributable to them. Continuing to take a medication can be the origin of true intoxification of the organism. Some visceral manipulations are contraindicated by medications. Finally, certain treatments, like anticoagulants and corticotherapy over a long period, can present difficulties in the choice of manipulative techniques.

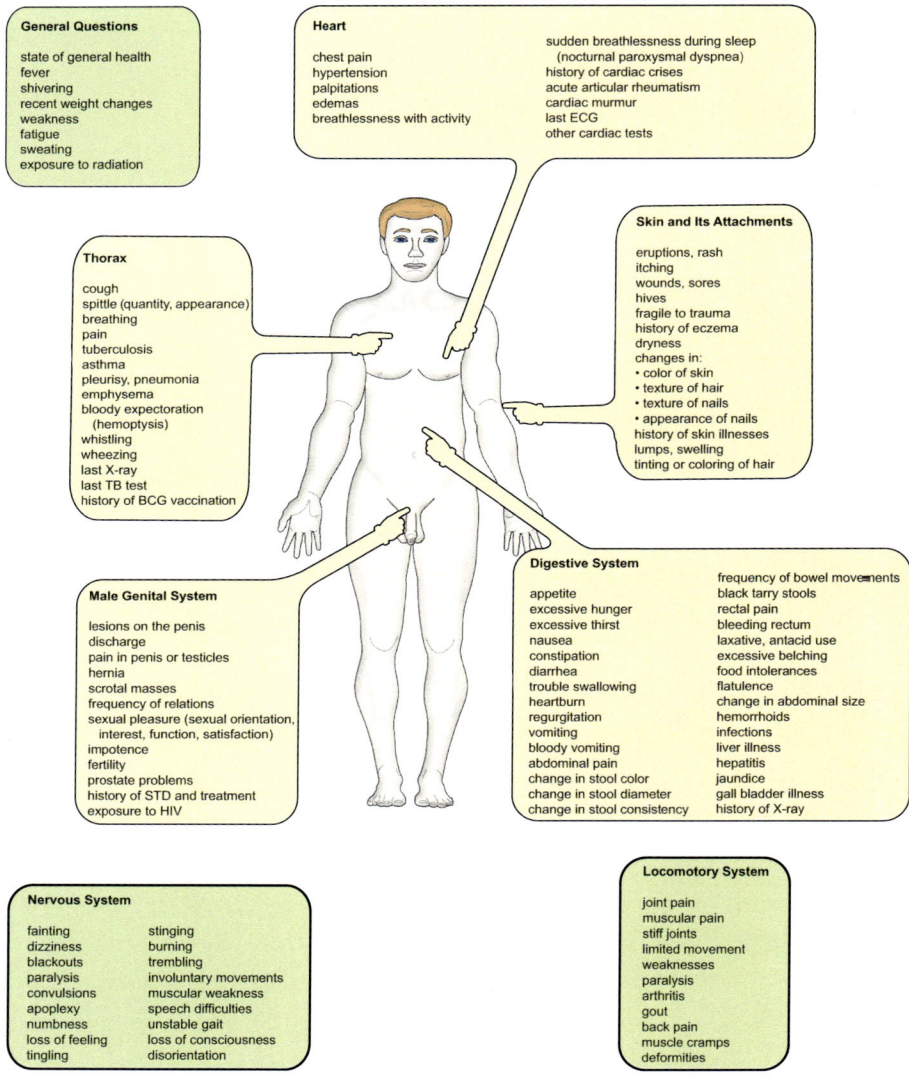

General Questions

state of general health
fever
shivering
recent weight changes
weakness
fatigue
sweating
exposure to radiation

Heart

chest pain
hypertension
palpitations
edemas
breathlessness with activity
sudden breathlessness during sleep
   (nocturnal paroxysmal dyspnea)
history of cardiac crises
acute articular rheumatism
cardiac murmur
last ECG
other cardiac tests

Skin and Its Attachments

eruptions, rash
itching
wounds, sores
hives
fragile to trauma
history of eczema
dryness
changes in:
• color of skin
• texture of hair
• texture of nails
• appearance of nails
history of skin illnesses
lumps, swelling
tinting or coloring of hair

Thorax

cough
spittle (quantity, appearance)
breathing
pain
tuberculosis
asthma
pleurisy, pneumonia
emphysema
bloody expectoration
   (hemoptysis)
whistling
wheezing
last X-ray
last TB test
history of BCG vaccination

Male Genital System

lesions on the penis
discharge
pain in penis or testicles
hernia
scrotal masses
frequency of relations
sexual pleasure (sexual orientation,
   interest, function, satisfaction)
impotence
fertility
prostate problems
history of STD and treatment
exposure to HIV

Digestive System

appetite
excessive hunger
excessive thirst
nausea
constipation
diarrhea
trouble swallowing
heartburn
regurgitation
vomiting
bloody vomiting
abdominal pain
change in stool color
change in stool diameter
change in stool consistency
frequency of bowel movements
black tarry stools
rectal pain
bleeding rectum
laxative, antacid use
excessive belching
food intolerances
flatulence
change in abdominal size
hemorrhoids
infections
liver illness
hepatitis
jaundice
gall bladder illness
history of X-ray

Nervous System

fainting
dizziness
blackouts
paralysis
convulsions
apoplexy
numbness
loss of feeling
tingling
stinging
burning
trembling
involuntary movements
muscular weakness
speech difficulties
unstable gait
loss of consciousness
disorientation

Locomotory System

joint pain
muscular pain
stiff joints
limited movement
weaknesses
paralysis
arthritis
gout
back pain
muscle cramps
deformities

Figure 9.1. Review of the systems.

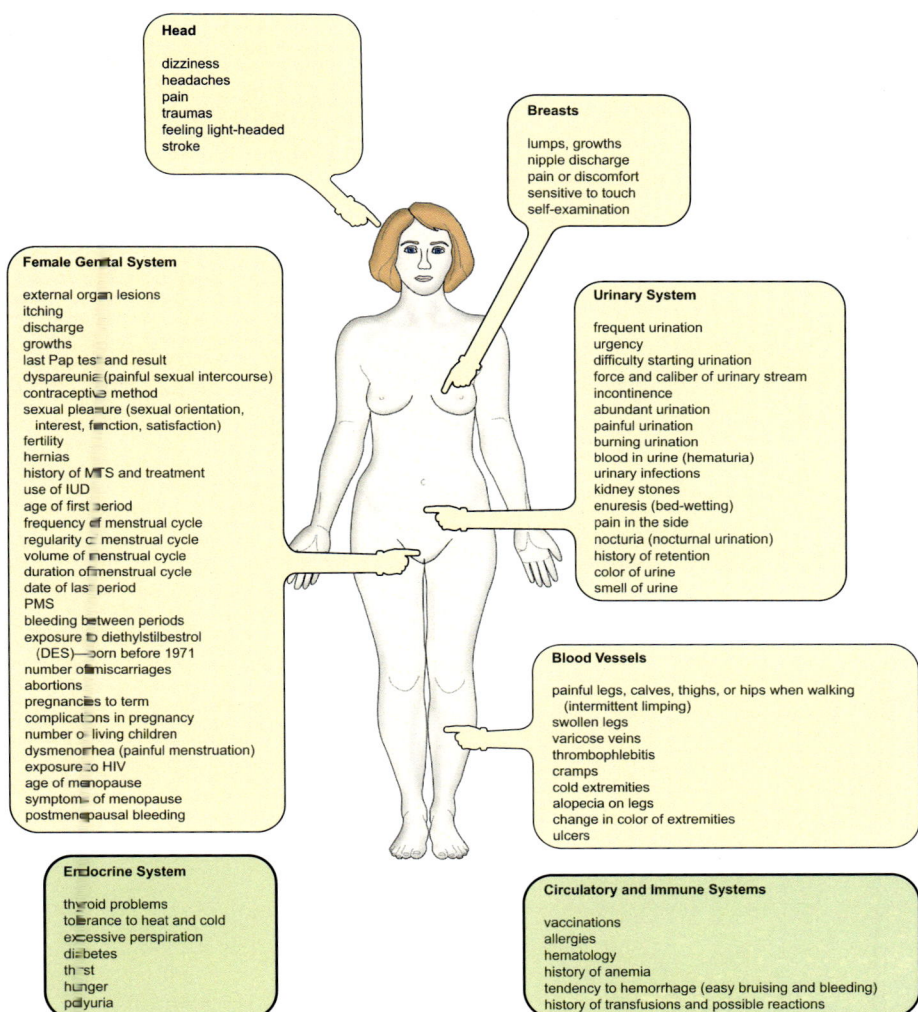

Head

dizziness
headaches
pain
traumas
feeling light-headed
stroke

Breasts

lumps, growths
nipple discharge
pain or discomfort
sensitive to touch
self-examination

Female Genital System

external organ lesions
itching
discharge
growths
last Pap test and result
dyspareunia (painful sexual intercourse)
contraceptive method
sexual pleasure (sexual orientation,
   interest, function, satisfaction)
fertility
hernias
history of MTS and treatment
use of IUD
age of first period
frequency of menstrual cycle
regularity of menstrual cycle
volume of menstrual cycle
duration of menstrual cycle
date of last period
PMS
bleeding between periods
exposure to diethylstilbestrol
   (DES)—born before 1971
number of miscarriages
abortions
pregnancies to term
complications in pregnancy
number of living children
dysmenorrhea (painful menstruation)
exposure to HIV
age of menopause
symptoms of menopause
postmenopausal bleeding

Urinary System

frequent urination
urgency
difficulty starting urination
force and caliber of urinary stream
incontinence
abundant urination
painful urination
burning urination
blood in urine (hematuria)
urinary infections
kidney stones
enuresis (bed-wetting)
pain in the side
nocturia (nocturnal urination)
history of retention
color of urine
smell of urine

Blood Vessels

painful legs, calves, thighs, or hips when walking
   (intermittent limping)
swollen legs
varicose veins
thrombophlebitis
cramps
cold extremities
alopecia on legs
change in color of extremities
ulcers

Endocrine System

thyroid problems
tolerance to heat and cold
excessive perspiration
diabetes
thirst
hunger
polyuria

Circulatory and Immune Systems

vaccinations
allergies
hematology
history of anemia
tendency to hemorrhage (easy bruising and bleeding)
history of transfusions and possible reactions

Figure 9.1. Review of the systems (continued).

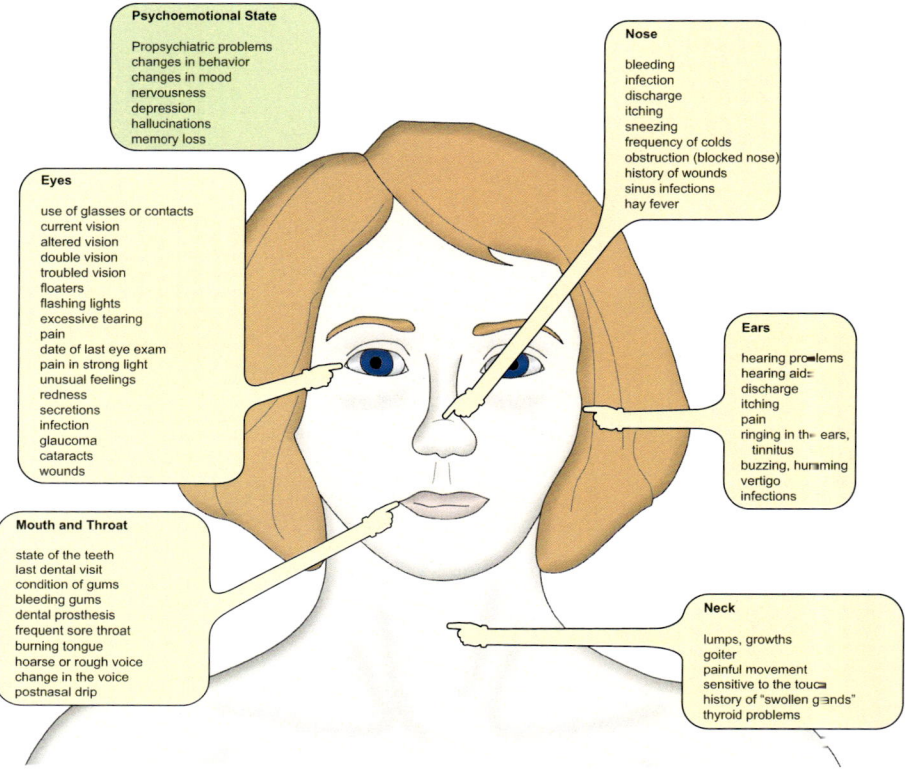

Psychoemotional State

Propsychiatric problems
changes in behavior
changes in mood
nervousness
depression
hallucinations
memory loss

Nose

bleeding
infection
discharge
itching
sneezing
frequency of colds
obstruction (blocked nose)
history of wounds
sinus infections
hay fever

Eyes

use of glasses or contacts
current vision
altered vision
double vision
troubled vision
floaters
flashing lights
excessive tearing
pain
date of last eye exam
pain in strong light
unusual feelings
redness
secretions
infection
glaucoma
cataracts
wounds

Ears

hearing problems
hearing aids
discharge
itching
pain
ringing in the ears,
    tinnitus
buzzing, humming
vertigo
infections

Mouth and Throat

state of the teeth
last dental visit
condition of gums
bleeding gums
dental prosthesis
frequent sore throat
burning tongue
hoarse or rough voice
change in the voice
postnasal drip

Neck

lumps, growths
goiter
painful movement
sensitive to the touch
history of "swollen glands"
thyroid problems

Figure 9.1. Review of the systems (continued).

Review of Systems and Research on Cardinal Symptoms

In classical medicine, the essential goal of the review of systems (fig. 9.1) is to assure the clinician that no major symptom has been overlooked, especially in an area that has not been completely explored as part of the reason for the consultation. This review of systems is often the chance for the therapist to refer back to his or her checklist. It is typical classical medical questioning.

For an osteopath, this stage is not done rigidly in the course of questioning and can easily be integrated at the time of the physical examination. It is easy enough, during palpation and examination, to ask

130

the patient about the function of the elements being observed. These questions arise in connection with organs that are suspect on palpation or found to be fixed in mobility tests. For example, it is logical to ask a patient about previous history and about urinary function when you discover a fixed or ptosed kidney during the examination. With more experience, questioning takes up less time at the start of the consultation, but it follows naturally from there.

If you proceed to a review of systems in the framework of the questioning, it is useful to ask a very general question introducing each system. This focuses patients' attention, allowing them to move from general to specific within each system, and can eventually provide everything you need to know. The more or less detailed character of questions in each field depends, among other things, on patients' age, what is bothering them, their general state of health, and the reason for the consultation. An older patient, running the risk of cardiovascular illnesses, cancer, and prostrate problems, for example, would be asked more detailed questions in fields that would probably not concern a patient of age twenty in apparent good health.

This review of systems is classically done "from head to toe," but other mnemonic or memorized techniques can be used. Explain that you are going to ask them if they have previously experienced specific symptoms, and that they will reply "yes" or "no." When the response is yes, follow-up questions are asked. You do not have to repeat questions that have already been asked, except when supplementary information is needed.

The questions must be clearly understood. For example, a question concerning possible dyspareunia is asked in this way: "Do you happen to have pain during sexual intercourse?" Each of the questions assigned to an organ or a system investigates the specific symptoms that relate to that system.

Summary

The questioning is a subtle and curious mixture. On one hand, it combines cognitive aptitudes and the techniques of the practitioner. On the other hand, it is an encounter of the personalities and feelings of the patient and the therapist. As therapists, we must conduct the interview in the most neutral way possible so that our own problems do not encroach on the patient. We also need to have a sound grasp of signs and symptoms. Without seeming overly technical, we need to be able to bring some method to the interview and the communication. A well-conducted interview ought to rely on the following points:

- *listen:* concentrate the attention of the practitioner on the patient. It is important to hear the patient's *complaint* and to discern the *request.*
- *evaluation:* separate what is pertinent and what isn't *(selection of pertinent information),* the distinction and classification of information by order of significance. It means being *discerning.*
- *questioning:* realize that the probing of significant areas may require more precision. It is necessary to ask questions about cardinal symptoms in the different systems. The mind, using semiological knowledge, helps to round out questions to elaborate. We need to be mindful of *method* and *curiosity.*
- *observation:* proceed to gather and explore the data from nonverbal communication. It involves using our *insight.*
- *understanding:* appreciating disquiet, fear, or apprehension in the patient allows the practitioner to be empathetic. It involves acting with *humanity.*

The questioning should be flexible, spontaneous, and noninquisitive. Used well, it constitutes a powerful diagnostic tool.

Chapter 10

General Evaluation

My object is to make the osteopath a philosopher, and place him on the rock of reason. . . . When you fully comprehend and travel by the laws of reason, confusion will be a stranger in all your combats with disease.

— Andrew Taylor Still

Osteopathy is accomplished from numerous general evaluations in the course of a consultation. It finds the signs and cardinal symptoms that determine the attitude to adopt. A patient may present some risk factors or revealing signs of an organic pathology; only a rigorous estimation of risks allows us to judge the necessity of supplementary advice.

Symptoms

There is a precise method to evaluate a symptom. In principle, we classically consider seven points. The major symptoms should be the object of investigation in terms of:

- the center of localization
- quality
- quantity or severity
- chronology: duration and frequency
- circumstances of appearance

- factors accentuating or extenuating the symptom, for example standing or sitting
- associated manifestations

Patients who consult an osteopath have often already benefited from other clinical support. It is interesting to know about previous treatments and their effects on symptomatology. These elements provide precise diagnostic indications. For example, a vertebral problem not alleviated by nonsteroidal anti-inflammatories can be a sign of a pain related to, or referred from, visceral or neuromeningeal origin.

The results of laboratory examinations also form part of the evaluation. Certain significant negative results aid in the differential diagnosis, for example the absence of some associated symptoms, or those symptoms that are general signs of various diagnoses.

It is necessary to discern the functional discomfort of the patient, which means to evaluate the effects of this ailment or of its symptoms in everyday life. It is also necessary to measure the concerns that the pathology can create, and to appreciate the anxiety, anguish, or depression that can interfere with the patient interview. Pain that affects locomotion, for example, is at times accompanied by the "fear of ending up in a wheelchair" or the fear of premature aging. In other respects, chronic pain and depressive disorder are frequently linked, although it is not necessarily easy to determine which causes which.

The psychoemotional approach to symptoms should also be considered in the interview, especially concerning the impact of unexpected symptoms or ailments. Pathology originating from an emotional shock, mourning, separation, divorce, or a socioprofessional conflict is sometimes clearly seen by patients, but it is rare that they are able to verbalize it spontaneously. In offering them the opportunity to talk, we often gather essential information for establishing a diagnosis. If necessary, we can start the discussion with an open question, for example: "Do you think your present mental state is connected to a specific event?" or "Did you receive difficult news any time before the appearance of your first symptoms?" Partially opening the door in this way is enough for patients to recall, if they want to, difficulties they have encountered.

General State

Evaluation of the general state constitutes a key element in establishing a differential diagnosis. Long-term deficiency in the general state can be considered an exclusive sign of various organic illnesses. Deficiency in the general state can be constituted by varying association of three significant signs: asthenia (weakness), anorexia, and emaciation. Frequent sleep disturbances also shed light on the general state. These signs are described in the following paragraphs.

Emaciation and Anorexia

Emaciation is characterized by a *loss of more than five percent of the subject's usual body weight.* Weight loss is an important symptom with multiple causes. One or several of the following can be considered:

- decrease of food intake (anorexia, dysphagia, vomiting, or insufficient food)
- deficient absorption of nutritive elements by the digestive tract
- increased metabolic requirement and/or loss of nutritive elements in the urine, in stools, or due to cutaneous lesions

Anorexia is defined as a decrease or total loss of appetite. More often a total loss, it can sometimes be selective for certain foods. The questioning is essential because:

- It allows us to establish the evolution of the subject's weight and to make a distinction between a constitutional weight loss and emaciation.
- Asking about eating allows us to evaluate the daily amount of food intake. It is known that a diet of less than 1,500 calories over twenty-four hours leads to weight loss. It is necessary to determine whether

food consumption has decreased during the same time period, if it has stayed the same, or even if it has increased.

The *causes of emaciation* are numerous:

- Misery, old age, isolation, physical handicap, emotional or psychiatric problems, dental extraction, poorly fitting dental prostheses, alcoholism, and drug addiction increase the probability of malnutrition. The signs of malnutrition are at times discrete and nonspecific: weakness, easily becoming fatigued, intolerance to cold, squamous dermatitis, and swelling of the ankles.
- I would also cite gastrointestinal ailments, endocrine pathologies, chronic infections, cancers, cardiac deficiencies, chronic pulmonary or renal problems, depression, and mental anorexia.
- Selective anorexia for meat is classic in cancers of the digestive system.
- Refusal of food is a positive diagnostic element of mental anorexia.
- Emaciation despite normal food intake and normal appetite is seen in hyperphagia, bringing to mind diabetes, hypothyroidism, adrenal deficiency, or intestinal malabsorption.

With the presence of emaciation or anorexia, the interview must find the associated signs:

- fever
- symptoms pointing to a precise organ
- psychological context and lifestyle

Asthenia

In the case of fatigue, it is necessary to eliminate any organic factors and then to think of depression as a way of asking for psychological help. The interview can precisely determine the character of fatigue:

- in the morning on rising or in the evening, or after a day at work
- at work or during holidays
- when active or at rest

136

These findings are characteristic of depressive disorder:

- morning fatigue, lifting at the end of the day
- troubles associated with fatigue such as: loss of interest, initiative, or eagerness; sadness; self-deprecation; and loss of the vital impulse

If fatigue is an accompanying symptom in the depressed and anxious states, it is also present in many organic illnesses. We must consider:

- infections: hepatitis, infectious mononucleosis, HIV, endocarditis, brucellosis, or tuberculosis
- endocrine disorders: hypothyroidism, adrenal deficiency, diabetes, or hypopituitarism
- cardiac deficiency
- chronic pulmonary ailment
- renal or hepatic deficiency
- electrolyte imbalance, as in hypercalcemia
- moderate or severe anemia, or hemopathy
- certain digestive or bronchial cancers
- some nutritional deficiencies
- medications
- toxic withdrawal

NOTE

Muscular weakness is different from fatigue. Muscle weakness is an objective loss of muscular force, which corresponds to a neuroanatomical source.

Chronic Fatigue Syndrome

Chronic fatigue syndrome is a recognized pathology of the nosological order. Even though several viral etiologies have been suspected, none have been proven. We consider it in the absence of a precise organic cause and on the following diagnostic criteria:

- fatigue that:
  - is not alleviated by rest
  - reduces activity by at least 50%
  - lasts for six months or more
- at least five of the following symptoms:
  - fever
  - adenopathy
  - myalgia
  - headaches
  - arthralgia
  - insomnia
  - allergies
  - emaciation
  - abdominal pain
  - psychiatric problems

A diagnosis of chronic fatigue syndrome is only prudent after the exclusion of a known pathology.

Other Components of Evaluation

Appraisal of the general state should be completed by a physical examination:

- weight
- evaluation of adipose tissue
- appraisal of muscle tone
- finding associated signs: adenopathy, hepatomegaly, splenomegaly, tumor mass, objective neurological problems, abnormalities found on palpation of the kidneys or pelvic organs

NOTE

All deficiencies in the general state require caution and should prompt us to systematically seek supplementary advice or a second opinion. Most often, several simple examinations permit us to specify a clinical picture.

- biological examinations:
  - speed of sedimentation
  - C-reactive protein
  - numeration of blood formula
  - blood ionogram
  - hypercalcemia, glycemia
  - serous creatinine
  - electrophoresis of proteins
  - hepatic tests (transaminases, alkaline phosphatases, bilirubin, gamma glutamyl-transpeptidase)
- radiographs: plates of the thorax, front, and profile

Sleep

Clinical Interest in Sleep

Fatigue reflects on more than the general state. The quantity and quality of sleep must also be considered. Sleep takes up a third of our lives: at age sixty, we have slept for twenty years. Indispensable for the recuperation of our physical and psychological faculties, it is essential for good quality of life. These days, however, we don't give it the weight it deserves, and often consider it time lost. Abused by overwork or shift work and altered by drugs that harm health, sleep may no longer play its refreshing role.

Sound sleep enhances the proper functioning of the body and helps maintain it. Sleep problems can contribute to the rise of medical, mental, or psychiatric states, or conversely, sleep problems may originate from them. Digestive, endocrine, respiratory, or neuropsychic dysfunctions can be revealing signs.

Elements of the Physiology of Sleep

To a great extent, the physiology of sleep still remains a mystery. What ends does it serve? There are several hypotheses, but the conclusions are far from clear. We only know for certain that it is vital. Deprived of sleep, an animal's central nervous system becomes disorganized and can no longer maintain body temperature, causing death within several weeks.

A night's sleep consists of the regular alternation of REM sleep and deep or non-REM sleep with long brain wavelengths. The noticeable effects of this alternation has revealed an association between dream recall and REM sleep.

Waking-Sleep-Dream Cycle

Falling Asleep

After a period of being awake, people show precursory signs of sleep: yawning, blinking, and losing awareness of the environment. If people resist going to sleep, the desire to sleep lasts for about fifteen minutes and returns one to two hours later. If people follow the sleep indicators, they go to bed and assume a posture that allows optimal muscular relaxation.

In the course of a day, there are generally two periods when the organism has a natural tendency to fall asleep: the nocturnal period, from midnight to 7 a.m., and the middle of the afternoon, between 2 and 4 p.m.

Deep Sleep with Long Brain Wavelengths

Going to sleep and deep sleep are characterized by closing the eyelids, immobility, progressive slowing of the vegetative functions (respiration and cardiac rate), and decrease in body temperature and muscle tone. Electroencephalography (EEG) allows us to distinguish four stages (N1 to N4), according to the depth of sleep, judged by the presence of long wavelengths of large amplitude. This is called non-REM or deep sleep, and it lasts sixty to seventy-five minutes.

REM Sleep

The subsequent REM sleep phase is sometimes called paradoxical sleep because its signs are muscular atony, rapid EEG waves, rapid eye movement (REM), and irregular respiration. REM sleep has a median duration of fifteen to twenty minutes. It is when dreams happen, which has been verified by dream recall in subjects woken during this phase of sleep.

Cycling

The alternation of deep sleep and REM sleep, called the ultradian rhythm, seems to have a metabolic support function. A cycle of sleep lasts about ninety minutes. After a brief awakening, another cycle starts. In the course of one night, three to five cycles of sleep can follow one another, according to the duration of sleep. The presence of short awakenings at the end of the cycles, up to a total of twelve to fifteen minutes, is completely normal. Most of the time, on rising in the morning, the person does not remember those wakeful periods. Some aged individuals remember only those wakeful periods and thus believe they have not closed their eyes during the night.

Duration of Sleep

In an adult male, the physiological duration of sleep ranges from three to twelve hours, according to the individual. Each person needs a sleep time that is appropriate for that individual. The mean duration of sleep is eight hours, but there are "big" sleepers and "little" sleepers, each with different needs. Some people need ten hours of sleep each night, while others are content with four to five hours.

The physical environment (temperature and light), social environment (stress), and food all influence the duration of sleep. Heredity is significant. There are families of short, medium, and long sleepers. The tendency to sleep more or less, starting early or late, is inherited from our parents, like height and hair color. The influence of the environment and education modulates this inheritance.

Sleep is unique. Each person has to know their own sleep requirements in order to be rested and in good form. It is also necessary to know the effects of lack of sleep and to be able to manage the limits of recuperation.

Physiological Effects of Sleep

All the main physiological systems are influenced by sleep. For example, decreases in arterial pressure and cardiac rhythm occur during the course of sleep. This explains why certain disorders of cardiac rhythm can occur at night. Respiratory function is similarly modified; breathing frequency and output vary with the phases of sleep. During sleep, the ventilatory response to hypercapnia is suppressed. These modifications of respiratory function can be part of the pathogenesis of sleep apnea or of sudden infant death syndrome (SIDS).

Endocrine function also varies in the course of sleep. Generally there is an increase of the secretion of prolactin. In young people, deep sleep is accompanied by a peak in the secretion of growth hormone (GH). Sleep also has an effect on the secretion of luteinizing hormone (LH). During puberty, there is an increase in the secretion of LH. In adult women, however, there is a decrease of the secretion of LH during the follicular phase of the menstrual cycle. Falling asleep and deep sleep are associated with inhibition of the thyroid stimulating hormone (TSH) and of adrenocorticotropic hormone axis (ACTH-cortisol), which is independent of the circadian rhythms of the two sleep phases.

Sleep is also associated with changes in thermoregulation. There is a decrease of the threshold of hypothalamic neurons that attenuate heat and cold responses.

Clinical Evaluation of Sleep

Sleep is a good indicator of the state of people's health and relationship with their surroundings. Ask patients how many hours of sleep they usually need to feel that they are in good form; then ask how many hours they actually sleep.

Insomnia is often the mark of intense cerebral activity. Hypersomnia is a telltale sign of depression. Ask patients if they snore, and if their snoring annoys others in the household. Finally, ask if they feel drowsy during the day and have headaches on waking.

142

General Physiopathology

Many people lack sleep during the work week, which makes them sleep longer on the weekend or on vacation. At times this sleep recuperation is insufficient, and drowsiness sets in. Being deprived of sleep, even in the course of a single night, can create a sleep deficit that grows until sufficient sleep can be obtained. Aside from sleeping, no other means can cure a sleep deficit.

Certain sleep disorders can be the cause of daytime sleepiness. The consequences can be serious: falling asleep while driving or at work, reduced school or work performance, psychological disorders, or relationship, family, or social difficulties.

Sleep apnea affects close to five percent of the population. It is defined by stoppages of respiration during sleep, and it has cardiovascular consequences if left untreated. As with restless leg syndrome, bruxism, or somnambulism, the causes of sleep apnea are not clearly understood.

Furthermore, certain cardiovascular or respiratory disorders can be aggravated in the course of sleep, during the periods when our organism is functioning differently than when we are awake.

Insomnia

There are more than eighty indexed sleep disorders. The most common is insomnia, regularly affecting close to fifteen percent of the population. Most of us suffer from at one time or another. Clinical experience shows that most cases of insomnia are *by origin* a disorder of arousal—in effect, very strong stimulations of the alertness system that prevent sleep. Fundamental research on the mechanisms of sleep confirms that what happens during an alert period conditions falling asleep and the quality of sleep that night.

Insomnia is often perceived as an injustice, but it is not abnormal. A usually short sleeper who has an exceptionally long night isn't disturbed, even though it is analogous to insomnia. It occurs unnoticed because it is tolerated better.

Insomnia in which an individual has difficulty falling asleep often translates as mental activity frequently revisiting the events of the day. Insomnia in the middle of the night interrupts the complete sleep cycle and can be a source of mental hyperactivity. Insomnia is quite common in many anxious, nervous, psychasthenic, or hypochondriac subjects. They can display true anxiety about going to bed, often involving rituals or an abusive consumption of hypnogenic medications.

Some who experience insomnia prefer to get up and free themselves with a positive or gratifying activity (reading, watching television, reflection, work, etc.), in this way profiting from their insomnia and benefiting from a quiet moment when everyone else is asleep.

Respiratory Disorders Linked to Sleep

Respiratory disorders related to sleep are linked to partial or total obstruction of the upper air passages, responsible for clinical problems from snoring to obstructive sleep apnea. These problems have in common *snoring* and *diurnal somnolence*. Besides a decline in attention that increases the risk of accidents, these disorders expose the patient to complications in the form of arterial hypertension and cardiorespiratory deficiency.

Snoring

Snoring afflicts about fifteen percent of the population. It is twice as common in men as in women. Sixty percent of men and forty percent of women snore after age sixty.

During sleep, respiration undergoes two phenomena: it produces a modification of the excitability of the respiratory center (central phenomenon) and a decrease of muscle tone in the upper air passages (peripheral phenomenon). The simplest and loudest of these breathing variations is snoring. A sound is produced on inspiration, either by vibration of the soft palate or by vibration of the base of the tongue. In contrast, expiration is silent or only faintly noisy. Accentuated muscular hypotonicity with aging explains the age-related increase in this problem. There are two main forms of snoring:

- *simple snoring.* There are no other reverberations that disturb the sleeper, with minor diurnal somnolence.
- *snoring with a clinical resounding noise.* Here we find fatigue, headaches on waking, diurnal somnolence, and arterial hypertension. Snoring can be accompanied by respiratory anomalies or by sleep apnea.

Treatment varies according to the actions taken: weight loss, decreased alcohol consumption, decreased tobacco consumption, and decreased use of benzodiazepines (which lower the muscular tonus); abandoning sleeping on the back; and maintenance of the permeability of the nasal fossae. There may be a rhinopharyngeal cause, such as a deviated septum or hypertrophy of the tonsils.

Sleep Apnea

This syndrome essentially affects men between age forty-five and sixty-five, and it especially affects snorers. Sleep apnea occurs immediately after falling asleep and is characterized by respiratory stops lasting about forty seconds, with resumptions of the respiratory rhythm always coinciding with waking. The repetition of apneas, often more than five per hour, involves a reduction and disorganization of sleep, diurnal somnolence, and systematic alveolar and pulmonary hypoventilation, transitory at first and later permanent.

The usual classical treatment is positive pressure: a nasal mask that the patient wears to deliver air under constant pressure. This system allows the suppression of apneas and assures opening of the upper air passages. This therapy reorganizes sleep, ends diurnal somnolence, and prevents any development toward an insufficient cardiac episode.

Hypersomnia

Hypersomnia is defined by sleep lasting more than twelve hours. This can be idiopathic, psychiatric, or posttraumatic. Some patients can sleep up to twenty hours per day. This problem relates to hyperactivity of the nonarousal system. Hypersomniacs are distinguished by diurnal somnolence.

145

Narcolepsy

Narcolepsy is a disorder of the control system governing REM sleep. It manifests as irrepressible bouts of daytime sleep. Cataplexy is a sudden and transient episode of loss of muscle tone, often triggered by emotions. It is a rare disease but frequently affects people who have narcolepsy. This disorder may be linked to a particular gene group, HLA-DR2 and HLA-DQ1.

Fever

Definitions

Despite environmental variations, the human body normally stays at a constant temperature. Temperature regulation provides equilibrium between the loss and production of heat by the various tissues, notably the muscles and the liver. Fever is defined as elevation of core temperature above 99.5 degrees Fahrenheit. It results from modifications in the thermoregulatory center, which is situated in the anterior hypothalamus.

There are individual variations in temperature. A person may also feel a fever even before the core temperature rises above the usual values for a given individual. A state of moderate fever, between 99.5 and 100.8 degrees, is called febrile.

Fever can be accompanied by shivering. This is a succession of muscular shakes, lasting five to ten seconds, starting at the jaw and intensifying during inspiration.

REMARKS

Fever due to a release of pyrogenic substances is distinct from hyperthermia, which corresponds to a fault in the elimination of heat. It can be seen during exercise, in an extremely hot environment, or with some medications that inhibit transpiration. For example, a negative side effect of antipsychotic drugs can cause the core temperature to reach 107.5 degrees.

Hypothalamic Control of Temperature

Human metabolism produces more heat than it needs in order to maintain a core temperature of 98.6 degrees in neutral ambient temperature. Body temperature is controlled by the hypothalamus. The neurons of the preoptic region of the hypothalamus receive two types of information:

- The first, driven by the peripheral nerves, relays the degree of external heat.
- The second indicates the temperature of the circulating blood.

A very richly vascularized region of the hypothalamus, called the organum vasculosum laminae terminalis (OVLT), can liberate the metabolites of arachidonic acid, among which prostaglandin E2 is the most powerful inductor of fever known. These metabolites modify the adjustment of the thermoregulatory center, and many signals are sent to the efferent neurons.

- Thus the sympathetic fibers innervating the peripheral vessels cause vasoconstriction to avoid the loss of heat.
- Similarly, some messages are sent to the cerebral cortex, initiating changes in behavior such as seeking out a warm environment, clothing, or a special position.

The combination of these two phenomena can increase the body temperature by 3.5 to 5.5 degrees. If adjustment of the hypothalamus asks for more heat, involuntary muscular contractions, generated by shivering, arise to increase heat production.

Conservation of heat and the increase of heat production are monitored by the blood temperature flooding the neurons of the anterior hypothalamus, allowing it to reach a new point of equilibrium.

Variations of Temperature

In practice, measurement of core temperature should be made in ideal conditions in order to limit the influence of factors that can cause it to

147

vary, including emotions or stress, physical exercise, digestion, or sudden changes in ambient temperature. In addition to these factors, there are some physiological variations in temperature:

- In the course of the nycthemeron (twenty-four consecutive hours): vesperal temperature is higher by one to two degrees than temperature taken in the morning.
- During the menstrual cycle: temperature in the second part of the cycle (after ovulation) is higher by about one degree than in the first part.

NOTE

All increases in temperature do not imply a fever. Bouts of heat called hot flashes along with perspiration can also occur in menopause.

Physiopathology

Pyrogens

Substances that bring on a fever are called pyrogens. They can be of exogenous or endogenous origin. *Exogenous pyrogens* come from the environment. They include microorganisms and their byproducts or toxins. *Endogenous pyrogens* are products of an illness, generally in response to an infection or inflammation. Hidden at the local or general scale, they reach the circulation and act at the level of the hypothalamic thermostat. The most important pyrogens are the *interleukins* and *interferon.* The endogenous pyrogens are also called *cytokines.* This term has been adopted because these substances are produced any number of inflamed cells. Cytokines consist of polypeptides produced by a wide variety of cells: monocytes, macrophages, lymphocytes, endothelial cells, hepatocytes, epithelial cells, keratinocytes, fibroblasts, and others.

The body possesses its own antipyrogens. These are arginine vasopressin, the hormone melatonin, and corticosteroids. All are able to modifying the capacity of endogenous pyrogens to stimulate prostaglandin production.

NOTE

Fever is not synonymous with infection. It can be tied to:

- a thromboembolic dysfunction: phlebitis, myocardial infarction, pulmonary embolism, etc.
- an inflammatory illness: diffuse erythematous lupus, ankylosed periarthritis, purpura, etc.
- a hematologic disorder: acute leukemia, profound hematoma
- a parasitic or fungal infection: malaria, amebiasis, etc.

Consequences of Fever

Positive Consequences

Fever has been with us for hundreds of thousands of years, spanning animal evolution. Elevated temperatures stimulate the activity of polynucleotides and lymphocytes. They also alter the growth and virulence of many microorganisms. Fever thus increases the capacity to fight infection. Generally, it is preferable to have this natural defense mechanism.

Negative Consequences

Beyond occasional discomfort, the energetic cost of fever for the patient is considerable. For each two-degree elevation of body temperature, oxygen consumption increases by thirteen percent, measured by caloric expenditure. This increase in metabolism can test the patient's cardiac functions or limit cerebral vascularization. Fever speeds up muscular catabolism and favors weight loss. It reduces the level of alertness and can be the origin of episodes of confusion or obtundation (reduced mental capacity). Children are subject to convulsions.

According to Harrison (1995), in a pregnant woman, a simple fever of one hundred degrees or greater during the first trimester doubles the risk of spinal bifida in the fetus.

Semiology of Fever

The level of response (acute, progressive, or insidious) and the evolution of fever (continuous, remittent, intermittent, recurring, cyclical, undulating, or disarticulated) offer interesting information to the clinician, who must prepare a precise pathological diagnosis. This data can also assist us in determining the stage of a pathology.

Sensations of cold, goose bumps, and chills accompany a climbing temperature, while a sensation of heat and sweating accompany a falling one. Body temperature naturally rises during the day and falls during the night. When fever disturbs this variation, night sweats occur. Discomfort, headaches, and muscular and articular pains are often seen with a fever. It is important to control diuresis, consciousness, and respiration.

It is necessary to recognize the signs of poor tolerance to fever, which constitutes the need for emergency medical help, especially in an infant. Poorly tolerated fevers can be observed at any age, but especially in infants and young children or in the elderly. The principle risk s the possibility of heart failure, or convulsions in a child.

Much significance is placed on the pulse rate. It is estimated that at 100.5 degrees, the pulse rises to 90; at 102 degrees, to 100; and at 104 degrees, to 110. Dissociation between pulse and temperature, meaning a slower pulse with elevated temperature, indicates infectious ailments such as typhoid fever, malaria, or meningitis. Conversely, an excessively rapid pulse is an index of potential gravity, notably in a person with a cardiac prosthesis.

There can be prolonged fevers of inexplicable origins, which sometimes cause considerable diagnostic problems for specialists.

NOTE

Afebrile infectious states can arise, in particular if the patient is being treated with steroids, has taken aspirin, is aged, or suffers from renal insufficiency. The decline of interleukins during renal insufficiency explains the weak febrile reaction of insufficient kidneys.

Practical Advice

The source of many diagnostic traps, fever is an element of nonnegligible gravity. Generally it contraindicates our intervention, even if it is conceivable that a slightly elevated temperature may not be a formal contraindication. It is imperative that the exact cause of the fever be determined and that a specific treatment of *disease* be applied.

I strongly recommend that you have an auricular thermometer in your consultation kit or briefcase. Taking temperature is quick and precise, and it allows us to avoid many pitfalls, especially with infants and children.

Adenopathies

Adenopathies must be systematically searched for as soon as the practitioner suspects a general pathological process. The existence of general signs, such as asthenia, weight loss, fever, night sweats, and pruritis, must lead us to palpate lymph node areas. Sometimes, a swollen lymph node is discovered by chance during a clinical examination.

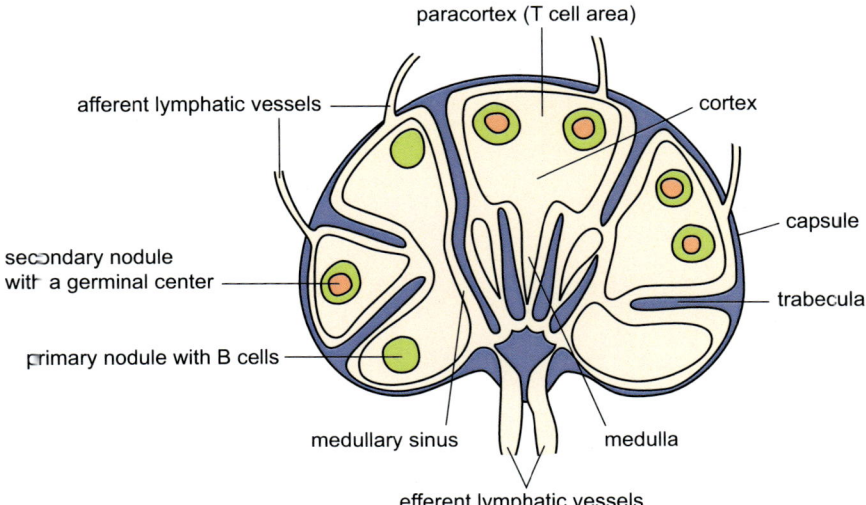

Figure 10.1a. Structure of a lymph node.

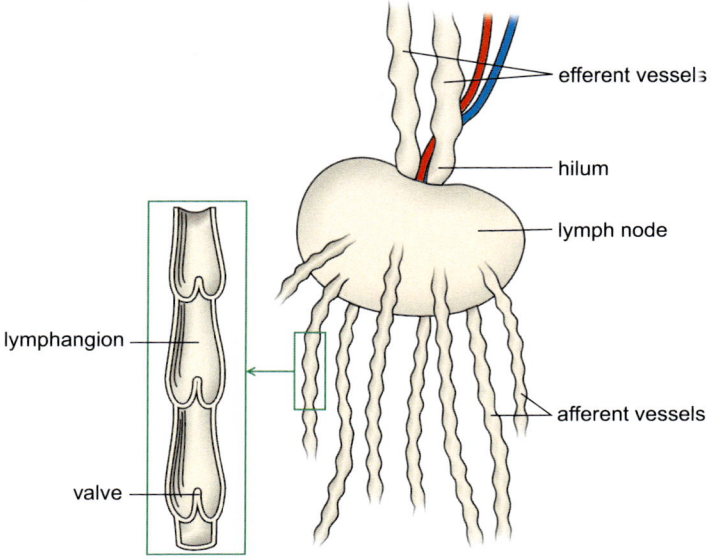

Figure 10.1b. Structure of a lymph node.

Characteristics of Adenopathies

Lymph nodes are easily recognized (figs. 10.1a and b). They are small masses the size of a lentil or a pea, normally painless and mobile under the skin. They are often nonpathological. Five parameters should be investigated:

- mobility
- form
- dimensions
- consistency
- sensitivity

It is also necessary to investigate whether a suspect lymph node is isolated or in a group. When it was discovered, how it became apparent, and the speed of its development are fundamental points to ascertain in the patient interview.

A positive diagnosis of superficial adenopathy is founded on palpation of hypertrophic lymph nodes. A diameter of more than three-eighths of an inch is considered pathological. In some areas, such as the inguinal region, a lymph node over three-quarters of an inch is considered pathological, while the presence of a lymph node of less than three-eighths of an inch in the subclavian area can be alarming.

Lymph Node Areas
Cervical Area

It is necessary to carry out a palpation circuit (fig. 10.2), allowing you to discover lymph nodes in these regions:

- submental
- submandibular
- mastoid
- malar
- parotid

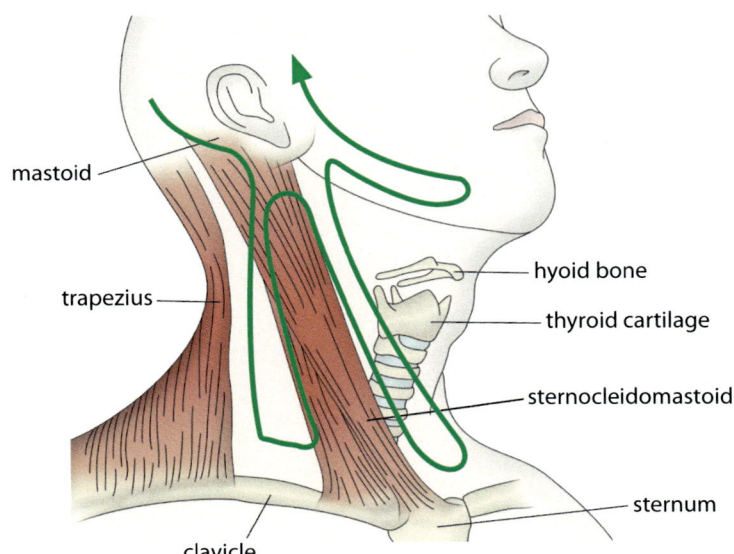

Figure 10.2. Palpation of lymph nodes in the head and neck.

- retromandibular
- jugulo-carotid, the length of the vascular axes
- spinal
- occipital
- subclavian (fig. 10.3)

Axillary Area

The axillary lymph nodes can be palpated in the seated or lying position (fig. 10.4). In the seated position, the patient can place a hand on your shoulder. In the lying position, it is necessary to hold the arm in abduction while grasping the wrist of the patient. Exploration of the axillary area is made from upper to lower areas, against the thoracic wall, by executing small rotations from the ends of the fingers, curled back slightly. The axillary group consists of anterior, posterior, central, lateral, and brachial lymph nodes.

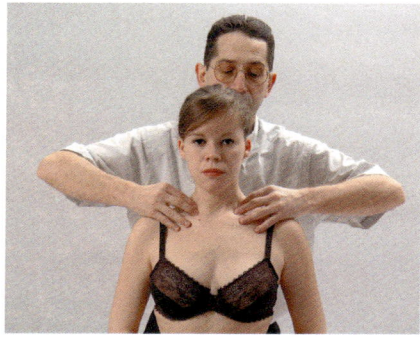

Figure 10.3. Searching for supraclavian adenopathies.

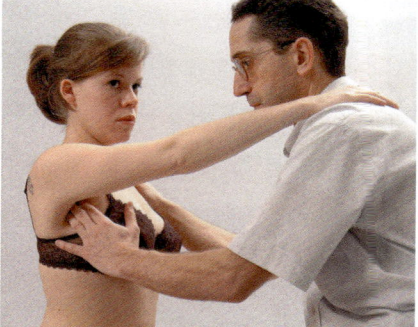

Figure 10.4. Searching for axillary adenopathies.

Supraepitrochlear Area

The subject has a bent elbow, and the examiner palpates the groove situated between the biceps and triceps, one inch above the epitrochlea (fig. 10.5).

Inguinal Area

The lymph nodes here are found in the femoral triangle, with the patient lying down (fig. 10.6). The superficial inguinal lymph nodes consist of two chains. The horizontal chain is palpated just below the inferior border of the inguinal ligament, and the vertical chain runs the length of the great saphenous vein.

Popliteal Area

The lymph nodes of the popliteal crease are found by passively bending the knee (fig. 10.7). The hands surround each side of the knee, while the fingers of both hands find the lymph nodes. It is necessary to thoroughly investigate the height of the popliteal fossa.

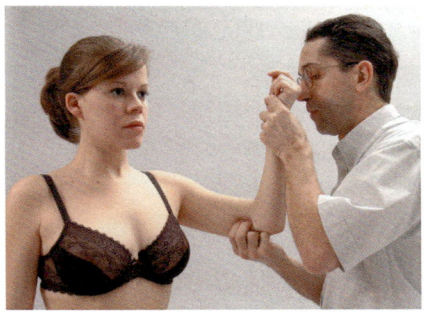

Figure 10.5. Searching for epitrochlear adenopathies.

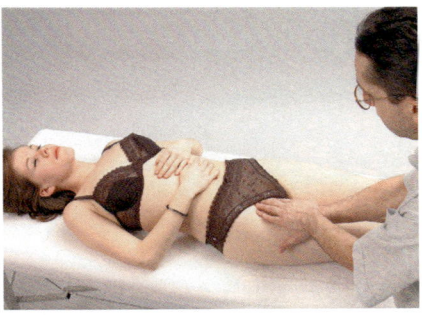

Figure 10.6. Searching for inguinal adenopathies.

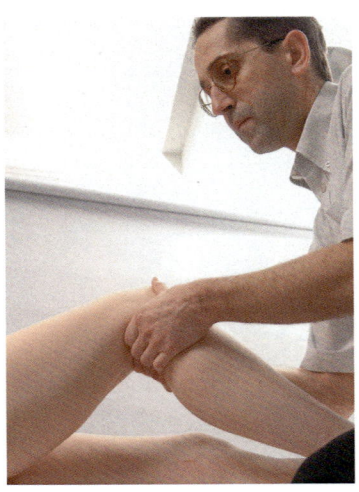

Figure 10.7. Searching for popliteal adenopathies.

155

Drainage Therapy

We must look for a lesion in the drainage route of the lymph node we are concerned with:

- Cervical areas drain the cutaneous area of the face, the scalp, the otolaryngological area, and the thyroid (Fig. 10.8).
- The subclavian areas drain the mediastinum. The lymphatic flow of the subdiaphragmatic viscera converges with the thoracic canal. This explains the elective localization of superficial adenopathies corresponding to the hollow subclavian angle (Virchow's node).
- The axillary areas drain the upper limbs, the thoracic wall, and the mammary glands.
- The inguinal and retrocrural areas (fig. 10.9) drain the lower limbs, the external genital organs, and the anal border.

REMARKS

Certain adenopathies are especially indicative:

- Epitrochlear adenopathies are found in cases of sarcoidosis and syphilis.
- Occipital adenopathy is observed in cases of infectious mononucleosis, syphilis, and rubella.

Extranodal Damage

In cases of adenopathy, we must be particularly attentive to detect possible extranodal damage. It is necessary to find in particular:

- hepatomegaly
- splenomegaly
- hypertrophic tonsils
- a thymic mass, palpable in the sternal notch

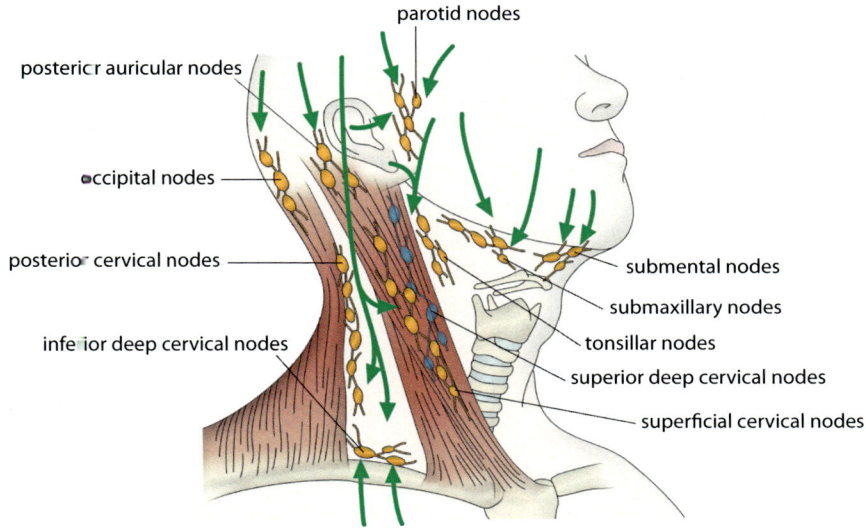

Figure 10.8. Lymph nodes of the neck and corresponding drainage.

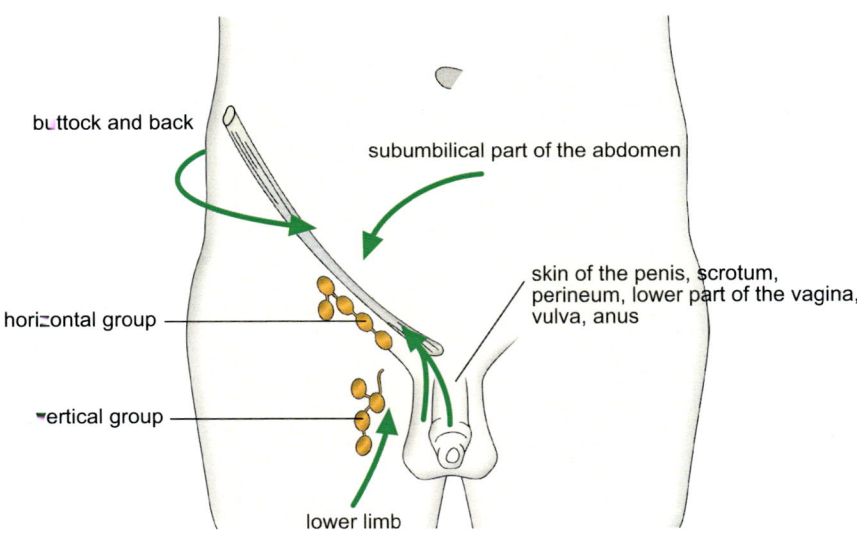

Figure 10.9. Drainage area of the inguinal lymph nodes.

Diagnostic Procedure

Several questions can be asked when the osteopath is confronted with an adenopathy.

- Does it concern a lymph node or not?
- Is the injury or damage to the lymphatic system localized or generalized?
- Is it a case of primary damage (lymphoproliferative disease) or a secondary one (infection, inflammatory disease, cancer, etc.) of the lymphatic system?
- Is the pathology implicated as benign or malignant?

Differential Diagnosis of an Adenopathy

Occasionally we must use imaging, notably ultrasonography, to concisely identify a lymph node. In all areas, it is possible to confuse a lymph node with:

- a neuroma
- a lipoma
- a fibroma

At the cervical level, it is possible to confuse a lymph node with:

- a large salivary gland: parotid, submaxillary, or sublingual
- a cyst: dermoid, branchial, or thyroglossal
- an aneurism of the carotid glomus
- a tumor: thyroid or muscular
- an abscess of soft tissues
- a cervical rib

In the inguinal area, it is possible to confuse a lymph node with:

- a hidradenitis (suppuration of an apocrine sweat gland)
- a cold abscess
- a hernia

- a twisted cyst
- an arterial aneurism or a venous ectasia

Lone or Grouped Adenopathies

Schematically, a sensitive, red, hot, mobile, and soft adenopathy or a bundle of painful lymph nodes suggest an infectious pathology that may emanate from the drainage region. It can involve a bite, a wound, infected stitches, a sexually transmitted disease, or a reaction to an inoculation.

A chronic cervical adenopathy that is a bit inflamed could be caused by a tonsillar or dental injury, and at times by tuberculosis.

A voluminous adenopathy, hard, painless, and adhering or infiltrating, should highly suspected of malignancy. It could involve a lymphoproliferative disease (Hodgkin's disease, lymphoma, leukemia, etc.), cancer, or myeloproliferative disease.

Polyadenopathy

In an acute context, with fever or in a febrile state in a young subject, we must think of infectious mononucleosis, HIV infection, toxoplasmosis, cytomegalovirus infection, brucellosis, or syphilis. In a more chronic context, it might be prurigo, a systemic disease (lupus, polyarthritis, or sarcoidosis), a lymphoproliferative disease, cancerous metastases, or leukemia. The existence of associated splenomegaly indicates the generalization of lymphatic damage, especially in the case of a viral infection, mycobacteriosis, lupus, sarcoidosis, and lymphoproliferative diseases.

Pain on Absorption of Alcohol

Lymph node pain stemming from alcohol absorption was once considered specific to Hodgkin's disease. In reality, this mysterious symptom has also been observed in tuberculosis, septic lymphangitis, sarcoidosis, some cancers, and non-Hodgkin's lymphomas.

Edemas

Definition and Physiopathology

Edema is an accumulation of fluid in the extracellular tissues. It can be due to an increase of plasmatic ultrafiltration across capillary walls or perhaps to a decrease of lymphatic resorption of liquids from interstitial spaces.

- The increase of filtration is favored by:
  - increase of hydrostatic pressure; this is why edemas predominate in lower areas of the body.
  - lowering of oncotic intracapillary pressure; for example, in the case of hypoproteinemia
  - increase of extravascular protein concentration in the case of inflammation, allergy, or lymphatic edema
- The decrease of venous resorption is linked either to anomalies of the venule wall (chronic venous deficiency), to an obstruction of the main venous trunk (iliofemoral thrombophlebitis), or to an increase in venous return pressure, as in congestive right-heart failure.
- The decrease in lymphatic resorption can be due to congenital anomalies of lymphatic drainage (congenital lymphedema), digestive anomalies (exudative enteropathy), or the branching or obstruction of the main drainage ducts (lymphoma, ganglionic dissection).

Semiology

The most objective sign is *weight gain*. All weight increases without polyphagia indicate the existence of edemas. It is necessary to distinguish a true edema from the false edemas encountered in myxedema or lymphedemas and linked to lymphatic stasis.

The fingerprint test is a very good clinical sign of edema. A finger pressed onto an edema leaves an imprint, which disappears more or less rapidly as the liquid refills the indentation. For a fingerprint to be clinically observable, the increase in interstitial liquid volume will be on the order of ten to fifteen percent.

Once diagnosis is confirmed, we must ascertain the acute or chronic character of the edema. The gravity of an edema depends on many factors, such as its location and its extent:

- If the edema is localized, its significance varies depending on its location. For example, if it is located in a lower limb, it indicates the possibility of phlebitis. At the level of the face, it could be an angioedema.
- If the edema is diffuse, it is generally not immediately clinically evident. The body can retain water that increases body weight by almost seven pounds without the edema being visible. An edema affecting both lower limbs must be considered a diffuse edema.

In principle, edema predominates in the lower parts of the body: the lower limbs at night, and the lumbar region if the patient is bedridden. If it is generalized, it can affect the eyelids, the face, and the hands.

If the edema is painful, its inflammatory character can be studied: redness, heat, or loss of ability to mobilize a limb.

Etiology

The etiologies of edema are numerous and multiple (fig. 10.10). For the lower limbs, they are dominated by cardiac deficiency, decompensated hepatic cirrhosis, nephritic diseases, and profound phlebitis. Edemas can reveal an organic pathology. The practitioner must examine carefully:

- the thyroid: look for hypothyroidism or hyperthyroidism
- the heart: right-heart or total cardiac deficiency or failure
- the liver: search for signs of hepatocellular deficiency or portal hypertension
- the kidneys: proteinuria or renal deficiency

	Acute Edemas	Chronic Edemas
Localized Edemas	osseous tumors Paget's disease muscular sarcoma arthritis (septic or inflammatory) ruptured tendon angioedema (allergy) urticaria wasp stings Lyme disease phlebitis lymphangitis cankerous fascitis (gaseous gangrene) erysipelas periarthritis	vascular causes congenital lymphedema lymphatic congestion algodystrophy neurological edemas: cerebrovascular accident (thalamic syndrome), tumor
Diffuse Edemas	allergies (alimentary, medicinal, or other) urticaria glomerulonephritis treatment by interleukin (vascular hyperpermeability) vasculitis hypovolemic shock cyclical edemas ovarian hyperstimulation toxemia in pregnancy angioedema	medications vena cava syndrome cardiac deficiency portal hypertension hypoproteinemia: hepatic, digestive, or renal scleroderma endocrinopathy: hypothyroidism, hyperthyroidism, insulin-dependent diabetes, hypokalemia

Figure 10.10. Edema etiologies (after Blétry et al. 1995).

Venous or Lymphatic Edema

The classical treatises of semiology describe in great detail the clinical nuances distinguishing a venous edema from a lymphatic edema of the lower limbs. According to Blétry (1995), the subtleties of an examination are unfortunately often overshadowed by these defaults. In practice, we say that an edema is of lymphatic origin if there is an evident cause of lymphatic stasis, or when there is a venous obstruction.

Thrombophlebitis is swelling (inflammation) of a vein caused by a blood clot. Homans's sign is a sign of deep vein thrombosis (DVT). A positive sign is present when there is pain in the calf or popliteal region with the examiner's abrupt dorsiflexion of the patient's foot at the ankle while the knee is flexed to ninety degrees. However, this sign has poor reliability because it is often positive in individuals without DVT. A positive Homans's sign does not positively diagnose DVT—it has a poor positive predictive value—and a negative

Homans's sign does not rule out the DVT diagnosis (it has a poor negative predictive value).

Diagnosis of thrombophlebitis of the lower limbs cannot be clinically affirmed. *Any suspicion, in all cases, must be confirmed by Doppler sonography, conducted on an emergency basis.*

Pain

Diagnostic Interest in Pain

Pain is one of the principal motivations for consultation. Classical semiology precisely covers this complaint: in effect, the intensity, locale, radiation, duration, and alleviating or aggravating factors allow us to identify the pain. Throughout life and across cultures and ages, however, the feeling and expression of pain varies. In practice, the traditional semiology is rather outdated because pain does not always present its signature. Some characters, however, are somewhat reliable:

- pain with exertion indicates angina pectoris, constrictive and distressing
- agonizing pain from a branch of the trigeminal nerve
- the stabbing pain of a perforated ulcer
- the pain of the right hypochondrium blocking inspiration and spreading from the hepatobiliary system to the shoulder, etc.

But the list ends quickly. The specificity of colic, pelvic, thoracic, or articular pain is impossible to establish.

All pain has two components: one precise, analytical, and descriptive; the other emotional, translating the suffering. Patients who talk about their pain gradually make it more analytical and less emotional. Listening to patients talking about it actually soothes it. Any pain specialist will confirm this. It is therefore useful to let patients express their own physiopathic conceptions, with descriptions such as "the beak of a parrot spiraling up my spine," or of the calcaneus, "driving a nail into my heel."

Diagnostic Value of Pain

Recall that osteopathic diagnosis strives to distinguish effects and causes. It must consider the pain but not be blinded by it. In general, pain is lying, a false friend that must not influence our manual diagnosis. Often it leads new practitioners astray if they let themselves be taken in by the painful side, just as the needle of a compass is attracted to the north. The osteopathic investigation should be guided by adequate clinical analysis. Richard (1987) gives the following general rule:

- When the pain phenomenon (referred pain) is located to the side of the restriction of mobility, it concerns a recent case.
- When the pain phenomenon is on the opposite side and free, it involves a rather older case.

Pain, therefore, is due to a functional overexertion of a compensation. Considering this simple example, we can easily understand that pain is not the best element to use to construct an osteopathic diagnosis.

The Age of Painful Phenomena

There are two types of pain: acute and chronic. They are not differentiated by their intensity but by their age. Pain does not have the same significance if it comes on suddenly, driving the patient quickly to a consultation, as pain that developed gradually and insidiously without the patient being able to date it precisely. Acute pain can involve medical or surgical emergencies. This is notably the case for posttraumatic pain and pain linked to an infection or acute inflammatory process, or to an acute visceral pathology. Chronic pain is pain that persists for several weeks or months. It usually indicates a degenerative inflammatory or neoplastic pathology.

Acute Pain

Acute pain has a sudden onset that alerts the organism to the existence of a trauma, a burn, a visceral lesion, or a developing pathology. It is often accompanied by a feeling of anxiety. The interview and clinical examination should be able eliminate a medical or surgical emergency. If supplementary examinations seem advisable, it is best for the patient to consider the situation an emergency until there is more information.

Chronic Pain

Pain is said to be chronic when it has persisted for at least six months. It has lost its alarming character and can be secondary to:

- an uncontrolled evolving pathology, such as cancer or osteoporotic vertebral compression
- a sequela of an illness considered healed, for example pain after a bout of shingles
- a definite lesion, such as a neural lesion
- a benign functional pathology, like a migraine or colitis

Chronic unmastered pain is sometimes labeled as psychogenic. All the same, depressive disorder can take on the mask of pain without a physical source. Whatever the cause, when pain tends to persist, multiple physical, psychological, and behavioral repercussions are added, which complicate the diagnosis. For neurophysiologists, this evolution of symptomatology constitutes the transition from *pain symptom* to *pain illness.*

Types of Chronic Pain

For the same pathology, chronic pain can have diverse semiological expressions. In differential diagnosis, it is necessary to distinguish spontaneous and provoked pain, diurnal and nocturnal pain, fulgurating pain, etc.

Inflammatory Pain

Inflammatory pain happens typically at rest. It is not alleviated by a comfortable position; it appears during the second part of the night and is followed by notable stiffness in the morning.

Mechanical Pain

Mechanical pain occurs after exertion. It decreases with rest and when comfortable. If stiffness is present in the morning, it is short-lived, lasting only several minutes.

Neoplastic Pain

Cancer pain is very complex. Nevertheless, any type of pain may be of cancerous origin. During the evolution of a given malignant tumor, the causes of pain are diverse. The problems presented by pain in the terminal phase are often beyond the reach of our abilities.

Neurological Pain

Neurological pain presents difficult diagnostic problems. This kind of pain varies with locale and the nature of the lesion. We distinguish:

- deafferentation pain due to loss of sensory input into the central nervous system, as occurs with avulsion of the brachial plexus or other types of lesions of peripheral nerves, or due to pathology of the central nervous system. This pain is spontaneous, unrelenting, and resistant to analgesics, even morphine. Patients feel a strange disagreeable feeling that they describe as burning, stabbing, prickly, crushing, or like an electrical discharge. This kind of pain is relieved or aggravated by stimulations that are not normally painful: a movement, effort, or a simple tactile stimulation. The best example is trigeminal neuralgia.
- hypersensitive nociceptive pain is due to painful hyperstimulation. The pain message originates from peripheral lesions, such as inflammatory processes, traumatic or ischemic lesions, or visceral distention. In a general way, there is cellular destruction bordering on locoregional metabolic disturbances.

The somatic examination must assess the neurological damage. It is necessary first to find a motor deficit: problems of tonus or contracture in the painful area. Sometimes we can ascertain the most complex

166

problems as a dystonic mental state, trembling, or even vasomotor or nutritional problems contributing in sympathetic participation.

Psychological Pain

Psychological pain is generated by the somatization of various conflicts. We discover them:

- when there is masked depression: physical pain is accompanied by signs of depressive disorder.
- sleep and libido problems, anxiety, irritability, and loss of interest in activities
- when there is hysterical neurosis or anxious neurosis of the hypochondriacal type
- when certain delirious or schizophrenic psychiatric states are seen in their initial stage

Listening to the patient's description of pain and its accompanying signs together with the clinical examination can orient you toward a psychological cause. But diagnostic certainty cannot be attained only by the absence of abnormalities that are expected to cause certain clinical manifestations. The classification of pain in this category must be made carefully and moderately. Pay attention to the information received and to diagnostic traps: the analgesic action of antidepressants, especially tricyclics, is a pharmacological reality. Their efficacy does not remove the existence of underlying depression.

Subacute Pain

Certain authors distinguish a third type of pain: subacute pain, which encompasses persistent or recurring pain, similar to pain that appears gradually. Very often, one or more suspect diagnoses have been made, and the patient comes for another point of view or another therapeutic response. The medical history is often long and involves many therapeutic failures. In these situations, it is necessary to return the investigation to the beginning and to trace the diagnostic path to its origin. The more complicated a case appears, the more necessary it is to return to an *elaborate clinical reflection.*

In reconstructing the clinical history of the illness, the practitioner should question patients again with know-how and using psychology. They may be reticent to reply yet again to questions they have been asked many times before, which may seem to them to be of no interest. The clinical examination must be very thorough to address all the elements that could have been missed in previous investigations. Finally, the osteopathic examination should be complete and thorough to discover every mechanical dysfunction and to try to bring to light the pathology of the complaint.

Projected Pain

Pain called "projected" is pain felt at a distance from the affected zone. It can be of two types: *transient pain* and *referred pain.*

Transient Pain

Transient pain expresses itself in the cutaneous region of a visceral lesion, or even in the dermatome, depending on the nervous structure affected. For example, compression of the nervous trunk or a spinal nerve expresses itself in the corresponding cutaneous region. A pleuropulmonary injury can seriously affect the thoracic wall with regard to the zone injured and evoke back pain. It is necessary, however, to distrust certain oddities. Some nervous structures have little to do with pathology, and their innervation regions are not well known. For example, in the case of some canal diseases:

- Subscapular nerve disease causes pain that is easily confused with muscular or osseous pain of the scapular region.
- Pudendal canal disease presents with perineal neuralgia.
- Compression of the lateral cutaneous nerve of the thigh under the iliac spine shows up as paresthetic meralgia.
- Compression of the digital nerves causes pain in the lateral aspects of the finger articulations.

■ Tarsal tunnel disease causes burning plantar and other surfaces.

The pitfall is to improperly deduce a lesional mechanism based on topographical data. Sciatica is readily attributed to a herniation, but it can depend on a truncal injury of the sciatic nerve in the lower pelvis, or even a compression under the piriformis muscle. In all three cases, the pain topography is identical, but the modes of relieving the pain will be different, and the therapeutic responses will be diametric.

Viscera and the structures that protect them do not always correspond to the same metameric level of innervation. The lungs are under the influence of nerves issuing from T1 and T2, but the pleura are innervated by different intercostal nerves. Thus a pneumopathology of the inferior lobe presents different lower costal pain than irritation of the pleura.

Referred Pain

Referred pain is the most misleading form of projected pain. There is little relationship between the anatomical location of the lesion and the locale where the pain is expressed. This is explained by the notion of convergence and projection (fig. 10.11):

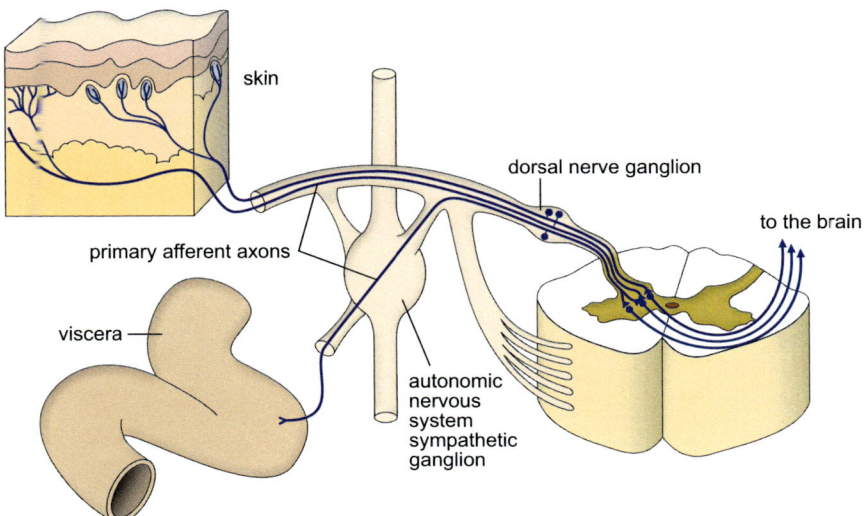

Figure 10.11. Convergence and projection of pain.

- *convergence:* two afferent neurons from two distinct anatomical regions converge toward the same medullary segment or myelomere because of their embryological origin. The innervation of the myocardium comes from metameres T1 to T5, and the upper limb is innervated by the brachial plexus issuing from metameres C5 to T1.
- *projection:* an error in integration of the nociceptive message releases pain in a different region but at the same metameric level, translating as "confusion" between the two regions.

This is why, classically, the heart expresses pain in the region of the left brachial plexus, and more specifically in the region of the ulnar nerve (C8 to T1). The liver and gallbladder, connected to the afferent path of the phrenic nerve, produce pain in the area of C4, corresponding to the right scapular region. Most facial or cranial pain comprises transient or referred pain, for example pain of a supratentorial origin in the region of the second cervical spinal nerve (fig. 10.12). Thus with meningitis, there is no pain in the meninges, but referred pain is expressed as headaches in the region of the trigeminal nerve or the C2 nerve.

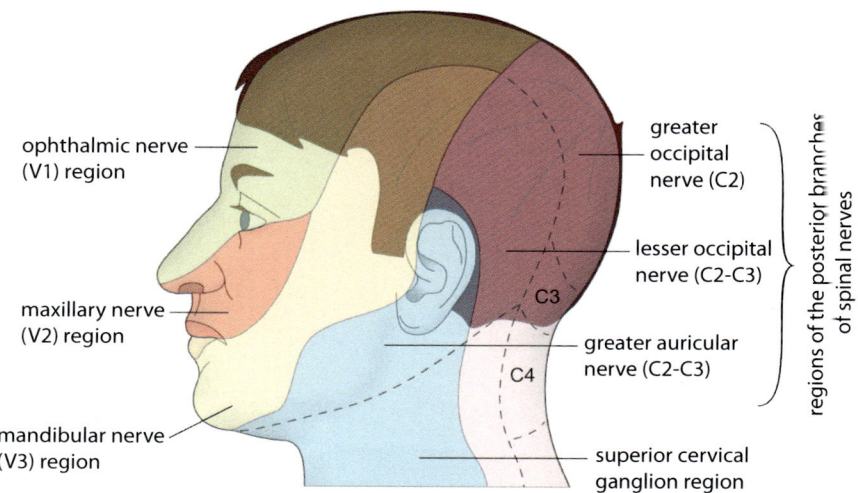

Figure 10.12. Innervation of the head.

Individual Experience of Pain

The anatomical organization and physiology of the receptors of the cerebral centers is identical in all organisms, but each person reacts in a different way when overcome with pain. The individuality of pain is fundamental. Each of us raises or lowers our pain threshold according to whether we focus on pain or are inattentive to it due to mental or physical activity. People who feel better enjoy life more, look better, understand better, make better judgments, and have more sensitivity. They are generally also more sensitive to pain.

By contrast, "mental poverty" is often accompanied by reduced sensitivity. Some schizophrenics are capable of tolerating pain and even inflicting frightening self-mutilation without appearing to suffer. Other personal, geographic, ethnic, historical, philosophical, and religious factors are part of the variation in sensitivity to pain. When evaluating pain, we must always take these factors into account.

Moaning and Suffering

Moaning

Moaning does not reflect on the seriousness of pain. It translates as a cry for help, rescue, and consolation. It is a true expression of the body in sound. Moaning expresses the experience of the patient and brings about the therapeutic meeting.

Suffering

According to Paul Ricoeur (1994), the term *pain* is for effects felt as localized in the organs, certain parts of the body, or the whole body. The term *suffering* refers to the open effects of patients' relationship to themselves, connection with themselves, connection with others, and their connection to meaning and questioning. Pure pain is uniquely physical, while suffering is purely psychic. But there are connections between the two notions, and one rarely exists without the other. Still, according to Ricoeur, the phenomena linked to suffering can start on two axes:

1. *The self-other axis:* suffering jointly involves an alteration of the connection to self and to others:

- People who suffer appear intensified by the feeling of being cut to the quick ("I suffer, therefore I am").
- Connection to others is modified; there is separation and isolation in suffering.

In the first stage, suffering seems unique. In the second stage, suffering is incommunicable: no one can understand it or help. In the third stage, even more intensely, others can be seen as enemies or as the cause of suffering, wounding the sufferer. At the highest degree of virulence, the feeling of being chosen to suffer can appear: suffering is lived as a personal curse. Questions of "why?" "why me?" and "why my child?" arise; this is the hell of suffering.

2. *The acting-suffering axis:* suffering causes a decrease in the power to act. There are four levels of incapacity: in the ability to say, to do, to describe, and for self-appraisal.

- Suffering induces an *inability to speak,* often expressed in an elective way at the level of mimicry, tears, or shouting. It takes the path of a complaint, request, or cry for help to someone else. From there, it shows itself with pain, which often remains enclosed in silence in the organs.
- Next comes an *inability to act.* Common to pain and suffering, it creates a discrepancy between wanting to do something and being able to do it. *To suffer* also means "to endure." A minimal degree of action is incorporated in passive suffering.
- The third level is characterized by the *lack of narrative function* to establish personal identity. For people to understand themselves means they must be capable of relating to themselves with both acceptable and intelligible stories. Suffering makes communication difficult, and breaks can occur in the thread of a story.

- Finally, suffering confronts people as an *inability to appraise themselves*. Being able to appraise themselves is tied to the possibility of regarding things as a function of judgments of good and bad. Suffering thrusts low self-esteem and guilt onto the individual. For example, sometimes a suffering individual has been heard to say, "I should really be punished for something."

Questioning about Suffering

The question inevitably arises as to what the sense of suffering is. According to the Greek philosophers, suffering "teaches." But what does it teach? We can only try to answer that with respect for those who are suffering. Suffering may exist without this answer, but it never goes without questions like "Why me?" "Why is this happening?" and "How long will this go on?"

Pain Glossary

The definitions in quotation marks are from the International Association for the Study of Pain (IASP). The annotations that follow without quotation marks are not part of the IASP definitions but originate, for the most part, from Zetlaoui (1994) and clarify certain points.

allodynia: "Pain caused by a stimulus that normally does not provoke a painful sensation. In allodynia, the (pain) threshold is lowered."

analgesia: "Absence of pain to a normally painful stimulation." The abolition of sensitivity to pain is made without suppression of other sensory modalities (heat, cold, or touch).

analgesic: A pharmaceutical substance that acts on pain, having essentially a central action (example: morphine).

anesthesia: 1. Absence of pain to a normally painful stimulation. This word is most often used in the same sense as *analgesia*. 2. A set of medical techniques used to lessen and abolish painful sensation. Anesthesia can be general (with the use of a hypnotic), locoregional (only addressing one anatomical region), or local.

antalgic: Pharmaceutical substance that acts on pain, having essentially a peripheral action (example: paracetamol).

causalgia: "painful syndrome combining a continuous pain with a type of burn, an allodynia, or a hyperpathy after a traumatic nervous lesion, often associated with a vasomotor and sudoral dysfunction and with trophic problems of secondary appearance." It involves chronic pain.

central pain: "Pain associated with a lesion in the central nervous system." It always concerns chronic pain.

dysesthesia: "Abnormal and disagreeable provoked sensation. A dysesthesia is not always but often painful."

endorphins: Substances released by the organism whose pharmacological effects are similar to those of morphine.

hyperalgesia: "Exaggerated response to a stimulus normally recognized as painful. The threshold of stimulation is not lowered."

hyperesthesia: "Exaggerated sensitivity felt as painful with a stimulation, itself usually recognized as not painful. The term *hyperesthesia* defines both the lowering of the pain threshold and the exaggerated response to a normally recognized stimulus. As for hypoesthesia, the stimulus and its site of application should be precise. Hyperesthesia encompasses both allogynia and hyperalgesia."

hyperpathia: "Painful syndrome characterized by an exaggerated response to a stimulus that is repetitive, but also from which the threshold is increased. Hyperpathia can be associated with a hyperesthesia, a hyperalgesia, or a dysesthesia. Frequently there is a problem of localization and identification of stimuli. The pain associated with a spreading and retentive feeling."

hypoalgesia: "Decrease of the painful sensation provoked or evoked by a stimulus normally recognized as painful. In hypoalgesia, the pain threshold is elevated, and the response is decreased."

hypoesthesia: "Decrease of the sensitivity to a stimulus, with the exception made of specific sensory systems (vision, auditory, etc.). The stimulus and its applied location should be specified."

level of pain tolerance: "The higher the level of pain that an individual is disposed to or capable of tolerating." It involves a subjective parameter, like a pain threshold.

neuralgia: "Pain seated in the distribution region of one or several nerves. It does not necessarily concern a recurring pain."

neuritis: "Inflammation of one or several nerves. This term should not be used when an inflammatory process is present."

neuropathy: "Problems of functioning or pathological modification of a nerve. For a nerve, the term *mononeuropathy* is used; for several nerves, *multiple mononeuropathies*. The term *neuropathy* is reserved for symmetrical and bilateral injuries."

nociceptive stimulus: "A stimulus is known as nociceptive when it is capable of provoking a tissular lesion."

nociceptor: "A preferentially sensitive receptor to a nociceptive stimulus, or which would be if it prolonged itself."

pain: "Sensorial or emotional disagreeable experience, associated with an actual or potential tissular lesion, or described in terms of evoking such a lesion." It always involves a subjective sensation that is difficult to quantify. This definition allows us to account for strongly psychogenetic pain.

painful anesthesia: "Pain felt in a zone or a region of anesthesia."

pain threshold: "The weakest painful experience that a subject can recognize. The notion of a weak intensity of a stimulus that a subject perceives as pain."

paresthesia: "Spontaneous abnormal sensation. A paresthesia is not always and even rarely painful."

somatotopy: "Cellular distribution of the interior of a nerve center in correspondence with precise anatomical localizations."

sympathetic reflex dystrophy (algoneurodystrophy): "Continuous pain of a burning type, present in an extremity, accompanied by a sympathetic hyperactivity, secondary to an injury without a lesion of the nervous trunk." The difference from causalgia is in the identifiable absence of a lesion in the nervous trunk.

Excess Weight and Obesity

Nourishment is one of the most influential factors affecting health and illness. Body weight is an indicator of the state of general health. Malnutrition and weight loss are rare in industrial societies. On the other hand, excess weight and obesity represent basic nutritional problems. Obesity is a risk factor for many diseases.

Weight gain results from quantitative changes, either at the tissular level or at the level of liquids in the organism. The definition of ideal weight in adults remains debatable, but it is based on the relationship of weight to height (fig. 10.13). The data presented vary with gender and bone structure.

Measuring Weight

Weight gain is produced when calorie intake exceeds calorie expenditure at a given time. Typically it appears as an increase in the volume of corporal fat (adipose tissue). When water retention is weak, it is invisible. It has to be several pounds before it appears as edema.

NOTE

All weight gain that happens without increased appetite or nutritional intake must be examined for the existence of edemas or an endocrine pathology.

Body Mass Index

Several indices have been created, but the Quetelet index, better known as the body mass index (BMI), is used internationally. It expresses the connection between body weight measured in kilograms to the square of height measured in meters:

BMI = weight ÷ height^2 (kg/m^2)

BMI correlates well with the quantity of adipose mass and depends very little on height or gender. Obesity is defined as an excess of adipose

Age Height	20–29	30–39	40–49	50–59	60–69
4 foot 11	83–109	92–118	98–125	105–112	114–140
5 feet	86–115	95–124	104–130	111–139	119–148
5 foot 1	93–123	101–130	110–139	117–148	126–156
5 foot 2	94–125	103–136	112–143	121–154	130–163
5 foot 3	99–129	107–138	116–147	125–156	134–167
5 foot 4	101–133	111–144	120–153	129–162	138–170
5 foot 5	103–135	113–146	122–155	131–164	140–173
5 foot 6	106–139	115–148	126–159	135–168	144–179
5 foot 7	108–146	119–154	128–163	137–174	148–183
5 foot 8	112–147	121–158	132–167	143–178	152–189
5 foot 9	114–151	125–162	136–173	147–182	156–195
5 foot 10	118–155	129–166	140–177	149–188	160–199
5 foot 11	121–161	135–172	146–183	157–194	168–208
6 feet	128–171	142–184	153–195	166–208	177–219
6 foot 1	133–177	146–188	157–201	168–212	181–225
6 foot 2	137–181	148–194	161–205	174–218	187–231
6 foot 3	141–185	152–198	165–211	178–224	191–237
6 foot 4	143–189	156–204	169–217	182–230	195–241

Figure 10.13. Weight range as a function of height and age.

tissue. In current practice, this index allows us to determine whether individuals have a body weight appropriate to their height. Be careful to note that it involves generalizations; it is not necessary to establish a "norm" with patients.

- "Normal" is a BMI between 20 and 25.
- An individual is considered to be carrying excess weight if BMI is between 25 and 30.

- Obesity is a BMI above 30 in men and above 29 in women; morbidly obese is a BMI over 40.
- Emaciation is having a BMI less than 20.

Figure 10.14 shows some flexibility in the BMI scheme, and it indicates the norms of BMI as a function of age.

Age	Optimal BMI (kg/m2)
19–24	19–24
25–34	20–25
35–44	21–26
45–54	22–27
55–64	23–28
65 and over	24–29

Figure 10.14. Optimal body mass index (BMI) as a function of age.

Distribution of Adipose Tissue

The distribution of adipose tissue is important because the risks of different complications depend on it. The work of Jean Vague (1955) allows us to distinguish three types of obesity:

- android fat distribution
- gynoid fat distribution
- visceral obesity, a more recent discovery, with or without excess weight

Between the two extreme forms of android and gynoid obesity, there is a range of intermediary states.

Android Obesity

Android obesity (fig. 10.15) gives the body the shape of an apple. It is seen more commonly in men. The fat concentrates in the upper part of the body: the abdomen above the umbilicus, the thorax, the shoulders, the hollows above the clavicles, the neck, and in a characteristic manner, the nape of the neck. To compensate, adipose tissue appears decreased at the level of the buttocks and thighs. We often

178

note a florid face (erythrosis), and in women pilosity increases (hypertrichosis). This resembles the serious damage of hypercortisolism (Cushing's syndrome), but unlike hypercortisolism, we see neither cutaneous hypotrophy, nor characteristic weals, nor amyotrophy. Android obesity increases the risks of diabetes, hyperlipidemia, arterial hypertension, and atherosclerosis.

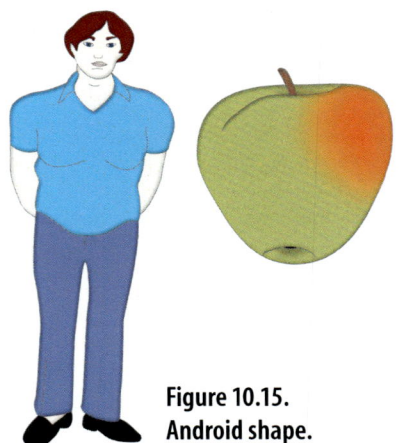

Figure 10.15. Android shape.

Gynoid Obesity

Gynoid obesity (fig. 10.16) shows a pear-shaped body. It is more common in women but not out of the ordinary for men. The fat concentrates in the lower part of the body: the abdomen below the umbilicus, the thighs, and the buttocks, like an exaggeration of the common feminine jodhpurs look. Metabolic risks are not major in gynoid obesity, but nevertheless the health picture is complicated by venous deficiency in the lower limbs,

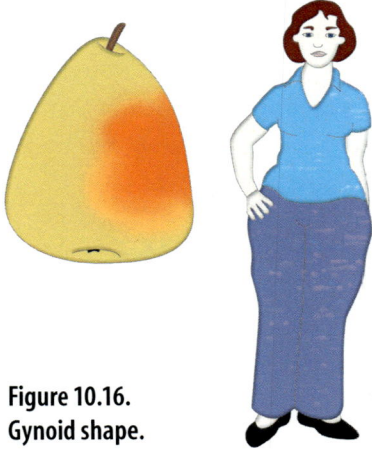

Figure 10.16. Gynoid shape.

articular degradation in the form of gonarthritis or hip arthritis, or even vertebral lumbago with lumbar hyperlordosis.

The causes of fat distribution remain unclear and are the subject of much research. Starting with the android form, we examine:

- genetic factors
- environmental factors (stress, alcoholism, smoking, sedentary lifestyle)

- endocrine factors (elevation of sympathetic tonus, hypersecretion of cortisol, hyperinsulinism, decrease of testosterone in men, decrease of progesterone in women)

The influence of sexual hormones on the distribution of fat could explain why the risk of metabolic diseases is comparatively higher in men than in premenopausal women.

Visceral Obesity

Visceral obesity corresponds to an increase of intra-abdominal, peritoneal, and visceral fat. Via the portal system, its metabolic work steadily maintains drainage to the liver, with free fatty acids released by the intra-abdominal adipose tissue. Usually, increased visceral adipose mass is accompanied by an android fat distribution, but it can occur in isolation when found in the absence of excess weight. Visceral obesity without excess weight is missed by the classical medical approach and seems especially able to benefit from our mechanical approach.

PRACTICAL ADVICE

The intervention of several health practitioners is often necessary before obese or overweight patients will accept the need to go on a diet. Patients are often sensitive to the idea that their weight could be responsible for their pain. We can simply explain that excess weight generates pain by increasing stress on articulations and discs, which also creates real tissular distentions and favors cardiovascular diseases.

Clinical Consequences

Several studies have shown a relationship between mortality and weight. Obesity and excess weight considerably increase the risks of morbidity and mortality (fig. 10.17). The principal clinical consequences concern arterial hypertension, diabetes, dyslipidemia, coronary heart disease, cerebrovascular accidents, gallstones, arthrosis, degenerative articular illnesses, respiratory problems, and certain cancers. The lowest mortality observed is in an ideal BMI range of 23

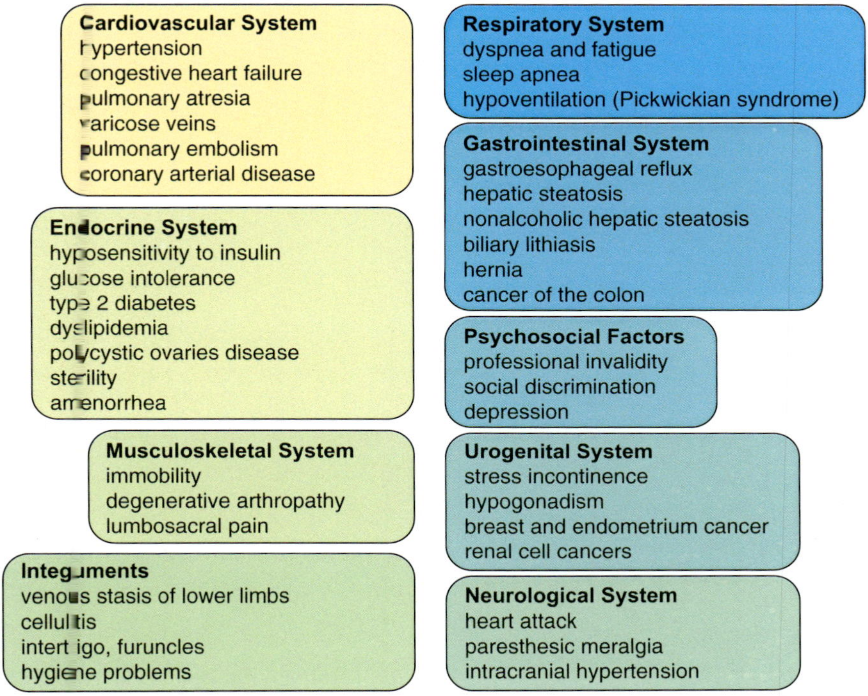

Cardiovascular System
Hypertension
congestive heart failure
pulmonary atresia
varicose veins
pulmonary embolism
coronary arterial disease

Respiratory System
dyspnea and fatigue
sleep apnea
hypoventilation (Pickwickian syndrome)

Endocrine System
hyposensitivity to insulin
glucose intolerance
type 2 diabetes
dyslipidemia
polycystic ovaries disease
sterility
amenorrhea

Gastrointestinal System
gastroesophageal reflux
hepatic steatosis
nonalcoholic hepatic steatosis
biliary lithiasis
hernia
cancer of the colon

Psychosocial Factors
professional invalidity
social discrimination
depression

Musculoskeletal System
immobility
degenerative arthropathy
lumbosacral pain

Urogenital System
stress incontinence
hypogonadism
breast and endometrium cancer
renal cell cancers

Integuments
venous stasis of lower limbs
cellulitis
intertrigo, furuncles
hygiene problems

Neurological System
heart attack
paresthesic meralgia
intracranial hypertension

Figure 10.17. Symptoms and diseases linked to obesity (after Swartz 1991).

to 25. Above or below this ideal zone, the risk of mortality essentially increases by:

- cancers, when BMI is 18 to 23
- cardiovascular disease, when BMI is over 25
  - mild risk between 25 and 30
  - moderate risk between 30 and 40
  - high or elevated risk—four times greater—over 40

Arterial State

The arterial system is an area where osteopathy and allopathy can come together with good agreement. For osteopathy, the cardiovascular system in general and arteries in particular are of the utmost conceptual and therapeutic significance. For allopathic doctors, early detection of cardiovascular diseases is a daily task. Cardiovascular pathologies are very common, can remain quiescent for a rather long time, and their symptoms are sometimes mistaken. In the presence of cardiovascular risk factors, evaluation of the condition of the arteries should be systematic.

Pulse

Generalities

The absence or decrease of a pulse is the most important gauge of an arterial problem. Palpation of an arterial pulse can provide information on the *heart rate,* the *aspect of the pulse,* and the pulse's *amplitude.* The radial, brachial, femoral, popliteal, pedal, and posterior tibial pulses are the peripheral points of a systematic examination of the arterial tree. The peripheral arterial pulse is generally taken comparatively on the right and on the left. It concerns principally comparing the *timing* and the *force* of the pulses. The amplitude of the pulse is graded on the following scale:

0 absent
1 decreased
2 normal
3 increased
4 bounding

Auscultation of the carotid arteries and *palpation of the abdominal aorta* are also important. Without doubt, the carotid pulse provides the greatest potential for analysis of different parameters that orient to a certain degree toward diseases of the heart or large truncal arteries. Data from the carotid pulse can lead us to suspect heart disease or diseases of the large truncal arteries. An arteriopathy generally corresponds to an overall disease of the peripheral arterial tree.

Peripheral Pulses

Radial Pulse

Radial pulses are evaluated by grasping both of the patient's wrists and palpating the pulses with the index, middle, and ring fingers of each hand (fig. 10.18). Recall that at the wrist, the radial pulse is situated on the anterior aspect of the radius, immediately outside the radial flexion muscle of the carpi.

Brachial Pulse

The brachial pulse can be palpated using the pad of the thumb (fig. 10.19). The brachial artery is situated inside of the tendinomuscular junction of the brachial biceps.

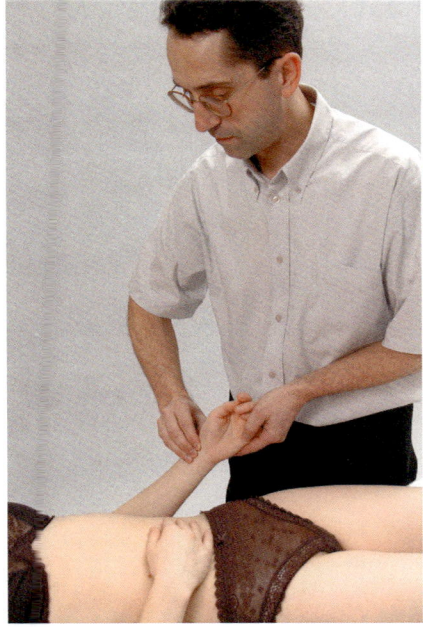

Figure 10.18. Radial pulse palpation technique.

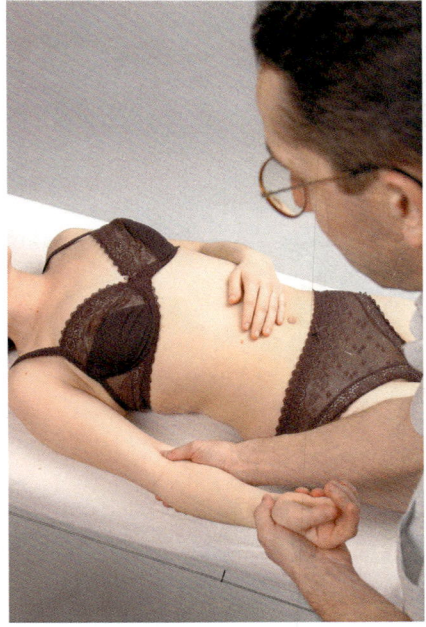

Figure 10.19. Brachial pulse palpation technique.

Femoral Pulse

The femoral pulse is found just below the inguinal ligament at the root of the thigh (fig. 10.20). The femoral artery descends vertically along the line midway between the anterior superior iliac spine and the pubic tubercle.

If one of the femoral pulses is diminished or absent, it is necessary to search for a murmur with auscultation, with the stethoscope placed on the femoral artery (fig. 10.21). The presence of a femoral murmur may be interpreted as a pathology of an aortic or iliac center.

Popliteal Artery

The popliteal pulse is slightly difficult to take. It is best to evaluate each artery separately. The patient is supine with the knees bent. Place your thumbs on the patellae and the bulk of the medius, the ring fingers of

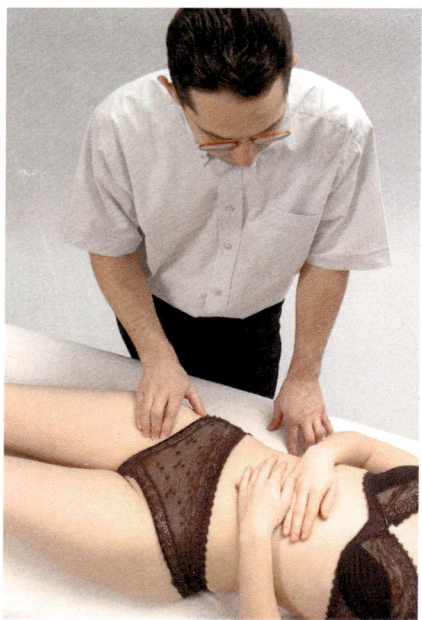

Figure 10.20. Femoral pulse palpation technique.

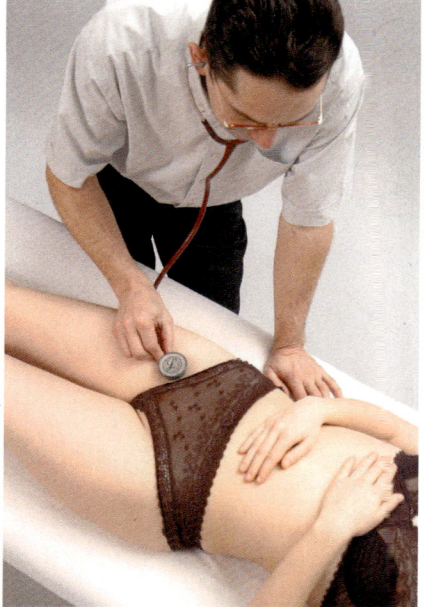

Figure 10.21. Auscultation of the femoral artery.

both hands in the popliteal fossa (fig. 10.22). The artery is situated slightly more inside of the tendon of the biceps femoris. Fairly firm pressure is usually necessary to feel the pulse.

Peda Pulse

The two pedal pulses are checked simultaneously with the pads of the index, middle, and ring fingers (fig. 10.23). For convenience, it is

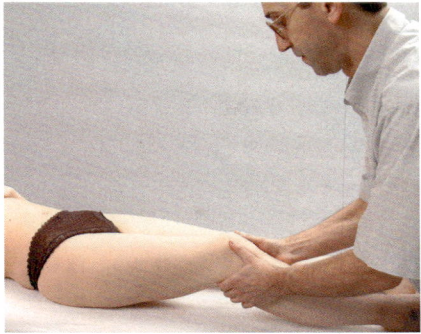

Figure 10.22. Popliteal artery palpation technique.

possible to do it with the hands crossed. The pedal or dorsal pulse of the foot approximately follows the extreme edge of the extensor tendon for the big toe.

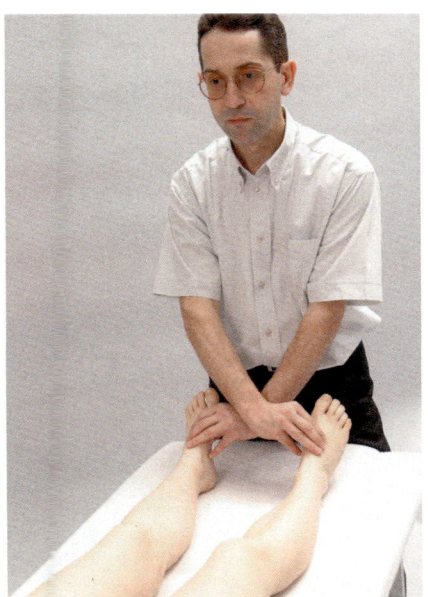

Figure 10.23. Pedal arteries palpation technique.

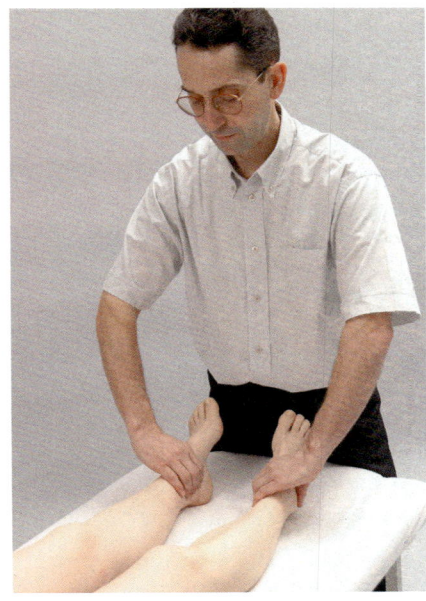

Figure 10.24. Posterior tibial arteries palpation technique.

Posterior Tibial Pulse

The two sides can be evaluated simultaneously. The posterior tibial artery may be palpated just in front of the internal malleolus, between the tendon of the posterior tibial muscle and that of the long flexor of the toes (fig. 10.24). In patients over age sixty, the absence of this pulse is a very strong sign of occlusive peripheral arterial pathology.

Synchronicity of the Radial and Femoral Pulses

By placing one hand on the femoral artery and the other on the radial artery, it is possible to determine the chronology of the pulse, one in relation to the other. This technique must be carried out for each side. Normally, the radial and the femoral pulses are felt simultaneously, or rather, the femoral pulse very slightly precedes the radial pulse. Any slowing of the femoral pulse on the homolateral radial pulse suggests a stenosis of the aorta, in particular if the subject has hypertension.

Vascular Murmurs

Generalities

The auscultatory murmur is due to a turbulence in the blood flow, downstream of an obstacle or a narrowing of the arterial aperture. Auscultation should be comparative.

Carotid Arteries

Auscultation of the carotid is accomplished by placing the stethoscope on the carotid artery of the supine patient (fig. 10.25). The head of the patient ought to be slightly elevated with a pillow or the headrest of the table and slightly turned away from the

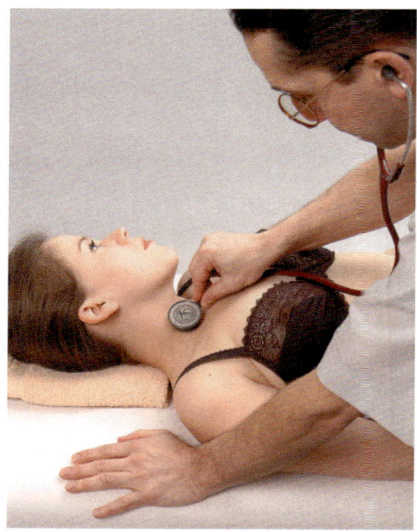

Figure 10.25. Auscultation of the carotid arteries.

artery being examined. After examination of one carotid, the other must be auscultated. It is preferable to ask the patient to stop breathing during auscultation. Normally no sound is heard. After auscultation of the carotid arteries, we proceed with their palpation.

NOTE

The presence of a carotid murmur is an important clinical sign. It could indicate arthrosclerosis of the artery itself, or it could result from transference of an intense murmur originating in the heart or the large vessels at the base of the heart.

Abdominal Aorta

Examination of the abdominal aorta is accomplished by delicately palpating the depth of the medial part of the epigastric and umbilical regions (fig. 10.26). The presence of a pulsating mass with a tendency to expand laterally implies an aneurism of the abdominal aorta. This diagnosis must be made with extreme care in thin people, whose aortic pulsations can normally and easily be felt. An ultrasound exam provides a slightly pricey but risk-free means to alleviate any doubt.

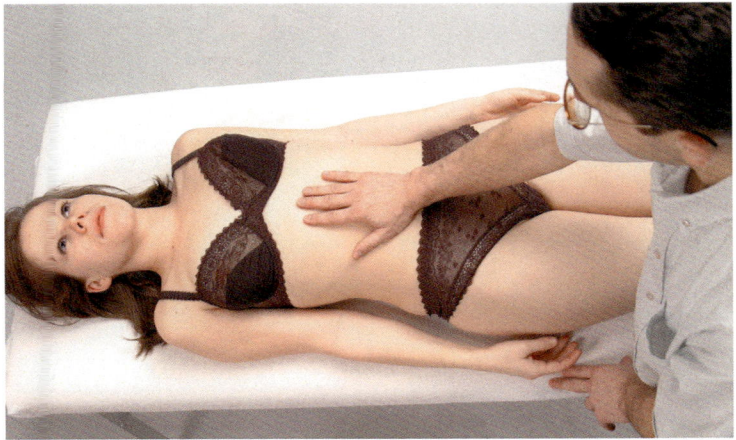

Figure 10.26. Palpation of the abdominal aorta.

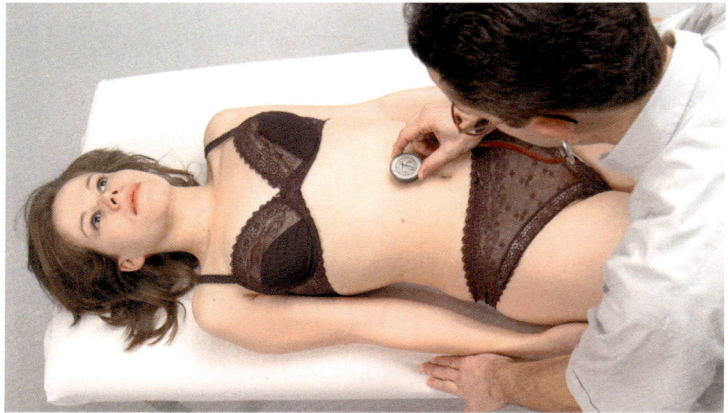

Figure 10.27. Abdominal aorta auscultation technique.

An aneurism of the abdominal aorta is also interpreted by a vascular abdominal murmur, sometimes accompanied by a femoral murmur and a diminished femoral pulse. The patient is supine. Place the stethoscope on the midline about two inches above the umbilicus and carefully listen for an aortic murmur (fig. 10.27). An aneurism of the abdominal aorta is an affliction that kills: eighty percent of abdominal aorta ruptures are fatal. Many of these deaths could be avoided if the patient had known of the anomaly. Signs of detecting an abdominal aortic aneurism:

- pulsating mass
- pulsating laterally
- abdominal murmur
- absence of a femoral pulse

Renal Arteries

Auscultation of the renal arteries is carried out by placing the stethoscope about an inch above the umbilical level, on a horizontal line just over an inch long that is situated about an inch lateral from the medial line (fig. 10.28). A renal arterial murmur can be the only clinical sign of stenosis in a renal artery.

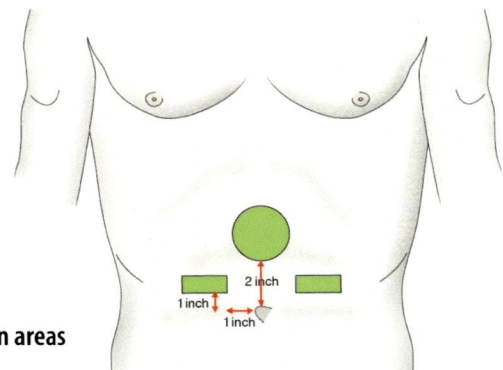

Figure 10.28. Auscultation areas for abdominal murmurs.

Arterial Pressure

Arterial pressure, usually called *blood pressure,* is an important parameter of diagnosis of many afflictions.

Measurement

Blood pressure is measured by a *sphygmomanometer* or a *tensiometer.* Generally, measurement is made on the arms of a supine patient (fig. 10.29). Position the tension cuff around the arm and inflate it until the systolic pressure is high, thus compromising the humeral artery. This state is marked by the disappearance of the radial pulse. Using the valve, slowly deflate the cuff until the pressure is slightly below the systolic pressure. The peak of each wave of pressure then briefly opens the arterial aperture. It results in:

- the reappearance of the radial pulse (palpatory criterion)
- the production of a murmur in the humeral artery, perceptible with a stethoscope at the bend of the elbow, caused by blood turbulence in the narrowly open vessels (auscultatory criterion). This murmur is also called Korotkoff sounds.
- an oscillation of the needle of the manometer (oscillometric criterion)
- the perception by the patient of wave pulsations in the arm (subjective criterion)

189

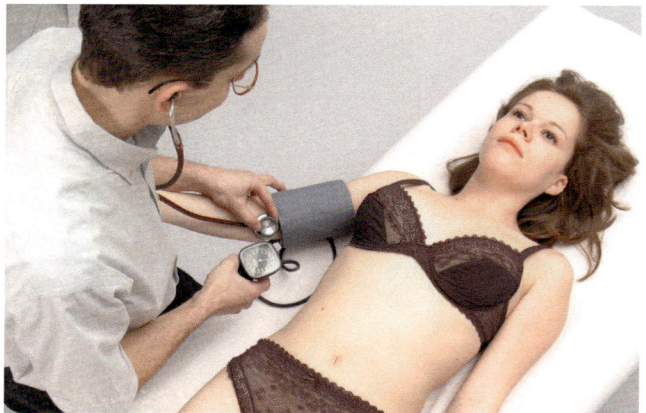

Figure 10.29. Measuring blood pressure.

Read on the manometer the pressure for which these criteria appear; this is the *systolic pressure*. When the pressure in the cuff falls below the diastolic pressure, the murmur at the level of the humeral artery disappears. The sensations of pulsation cease, as do the oscillations on the manometer. The manometer pressure at this moment indicates the *diastolic pressure* (fig. 10.30).

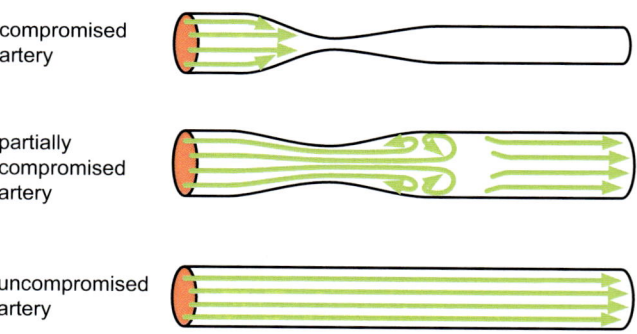

compromised artery

partially compromised artery

uncompromised artery

Figure 10.30. Blood flow in an artery (after Hayek 1953).

Note

The size of the cuff is important to determine blood pressure precisely. The cuff should have a width about twenty percent larger than the diameter of the limb. Using a cuff that is too small for the size of the arm gives a higher blood pressure reading than it actually is. It is necessary to have a large cuff for obese patients and a pediatric one for children. It is recommended that the cuff be adjusted well around the arm, with the lower edge situated just over an inch above the flexion crease of the elbow Place the inflatable part of the cuff so that it meets the artery.

To obtain an exact measurement, the cuff should be at the level of the heart. The patient's arm must be extended to avoid an increase of registered pressure caused by isometric exertion. Excessive stethoscope pressure on the artery does not impact the systolic pressure, but artificially lowers the diastolic pressure.

In an adult, systolic arterial pressure is normal up to 140 mmHg, and up to 85 mmHg for diastolic pressure. The sensitivity limit of any sphygmomanometer is about plus or minus 3 mmHg; arterial pressure must not be restrained beyond 5 mmHg, a number closer to that indicated by the manometer.

Arterial Hypertension

Arterial hypertension, or hypertension, is a major public health problem in developed countries. It is a common but silent affliction and a source of grave complications if it is not treated.

Hypertension is called "the silent killer" because, in most cases, it creates no worrying symptoms. Without treatment, hypertension works the heart excessively and damages the blood vessels. The risks then are blindness, angina pectoris, myocardial infarction, or even heart failure. That is why it is important to verify arterial tension in our patients, especially in those who have not had routine medical examinations or those who have cardiovascular risk factors.

Checking blood pressure with a cuff is a simple examination. Medically, hypertension is defined as when diastolic pressure is greater than

90 mmHg or systolic pressure is over 160 mmHg. Diagnosis of hypertension does not rely on a single blood pressure measurement, however. As soon as hypertension is suspected, arterial pressure must be measured at least twice, at two different examinations, and should be measured while walking. More and more, diagnosis is made by recording blood pressure measurements over twelve or twenty-four hours.

Most hypertensive patients do not directly present symptoms linked to elevated blood pressure. It is only detected by systematic routine examinations. If any symptoms are present, they could be due to:

- elevation of blood pressure itself
- vascular consequences of hypertension
- the causal disease, in the case of a secondary hypertension

Although classically considered a sign of elevated blood pressure, headaches are only observed when there is severe hypertension. They are most often located in the occipital region, present when alert, and disappear after several hours. At times, hypertension produces dizziness, palpitations, abnormal fatigability, or weakness.

The symptoms of vascular damage are numerous: epistaxis, hematuria, vision problems from retinal injury, syncope, giddiness and dizziness linked to a transitory cerebral ischemia or even angina pectoris, and dyspnea related to a cardiac deficiency. Secondary pain at the aortic dissection or at a fissured aneurism is much rarer (fig. 10.31).

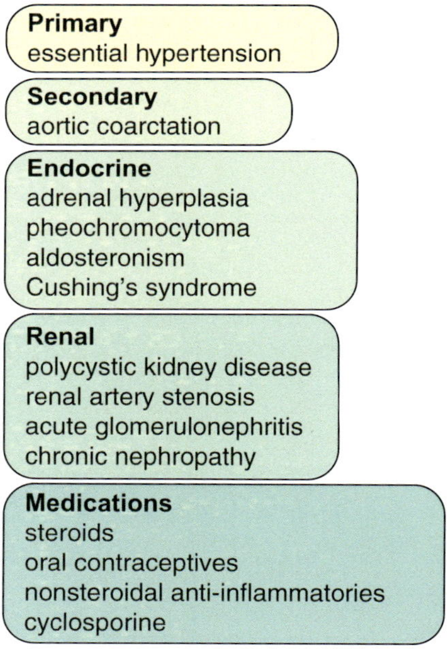

Primary
essential hypertension

Secondary
aortic coarctation

Endocrine
adrenal hyperplasia
pheochromocytoma
aldosteronism
Cushing's syndrome

Renal
polycystic kidney disease
renal artery stenosis
acute glomerulonephritis
chronic nephropathy

Medications
steroids
oral contraceptives
nonsteroidal anti-inflammatories
cyclosporine

Figure 10.31. Etiologies of hypertension (Epstein et al. 2000).

192

Arterial Hypotension

Certain patients have very low blood pressure. Hypotension is diagnosed by its repercussions and by a decrease of cerebral or renal functions more than by an arbitrary blood pressure number. Some patients have orthostatic hypotension, which is manifested clinically by dizziness when they stand up rapidly. Shock is characterized by systolic pressure below 100 mmHg.

Other Pathologies

In certain circumstances, measurement of blood pressure can find rarer vascular pathologies.

Coarctation of the Aorta

If blood pressure is elevated in both arms, measuring blood pressure in both lower limbs is important to check for coarctation of the aorta. Lower systolic pressure in a lower limb—at least 20 mmHg lower than in the upper limb—indicates coarctation of the aorta. Decreased or missing femoral pulses should also be examined. Recall that there could also be a delay in the femoral pulse compared with the radial pulse.

Aortic Stenosis

In the case of aortic stenosis, blood pressure in each arm is different—at least 20 mmHg higher on the right than on the left. The pulse is also fuller on the right than on the left. These anomalies are due to hemodynamic disturbances.

Chapter 11

Posture and Morphological Examination

A young practitioner must analyze and study his patients as if they were his best books.

— ANDREW TAYLOR STILL

Posture and Balance

Observing posture is an important element of osteopathic semiology, particularly in all chronic ailments. Distorted posture is generally accompanied by the pain of recurring dysfunctions. Analysis of posture allows us to discern the fascial tensions that are generated by the skeleton.

Studying posture is also a way of verifying the success of a treatment. A change in posture signifies a profound transformation of the mechanics of the patient.

Definitions

Posture is defined as the maintenance and organization of connections among various body segments. Any stationary body position can be considered posture. Posture can be observed according to two aspects of the various body segments:

- their *relative position*, meaning in relation to each other
- their *absolute position*, meaning in relation to the body's axes and to theoretical positions

The body is able to remain in horizontal equilibrium as long as its center of gravity is within its support base. Failing this, the body topples over. The *stability* of a body is much better when its support base is large and its center of gravity low.

Ideal Posture

Attention to appearance and posture that is pleasing to the eye is important in our societies. The importance of posture esthetics is not focused on today. "Stand up straight" and "straighten your back" are old-fashioned parental orders not often heard today. "Stand at attention," "stick our your chest," and "pull in your stomach" are military orders, undoubtedly as old as the existence of armies. All are expressions of the search for a standard posture that is acceptable in the given context.

When soldiers are given the "attention" command, they stand upright with the little finger on the side of the thigh. Even anatomists have adopted this position, with supination of the forearm, as the reference position in anatomy.

All these commands are based on a postural ideal. Usually these encouragements and corrections are lost on children with poor posture. Posture is not a question of will: we don't hold ourselves the way we want to, but rather the way we can.

The criteria for evaluating posture are not fixed. There are no postural "rules." Ideal posture can be defined as posture that respects both the *managerial rules* and the *comfort of the individual*. Ideally, good posture should only require a minimum of energy to maintain. Furthermore, it must neither generate nor favor the appearance of somatic pain.

Lumbar hyperlordosis can predispose an individual to lower back pain. Shearing at the lumbosacral junction and its consequences on the iliolumbar ligaments, when walking and in the upright position, constitute the mechanical argument for this observation.

Poor ergonomics at work can have a negative impact on some articular segments and can cause destabilized posture. For example, people who work eight hours a day on a laptop computer can complain of neck pain, headaches, or vertigo and see their troubles disappear on the weekend or on holidays. This pattern confirms the link between postural symptoms and professional activity.

Structure and Balance

It is clinically necessary to distinguish what comes from the structure of the body and what comes from the *balance* of the body. Balance is the static and dynamic balancing of a given body structure. In the standing position, the human body is relatively unstable because it represents an elevated structure balancing itself on a small base of support.

The shape of an individual forms his or her *figure*. It is recognizable even from afar. This figure arises from physical and psychoemotional factors. Biotypology shows that several body shapes exist. Independently of shape, however, the different body segments should balance themselves in the various spatial planes. Morphostatic examination shows us the balance and the curves of the individual, while a postural examination analyses the position of the body as a whole in relation to its surroundings.

Equilibrium in the Sagittal Plane

In the ideal standing posture, a plumb line drawn from above along the line of symmetry of the body must pass from top to bottom:

- through a point slightly posterior to the apex of the coronal suture
- through the external auditory canal
- through the vertebral body of most of the cervical vertebrae
- through the scapulohumeral articulation
- slightly behind the flexion-extension axis of the hips
- slightly in front of the flexion-extension axis of the knee
- slightly in front of the external malleoli

197

In the upright position, the gravity line—the plumb line of the body—passes through:

- the crown of the head (vertex)
- the odontoid apophysis of C2
- the vertebral body of L3

This line projects into the ground, equidistant between the feet. The scapular and gluteal mass planes are aligned. In adults, the lumbar curvature should be 1.5 to 2.5 inches, or about three finger widths, while the cervical curvature should be about 2.5 to 3 inches, or about four finger widths (fig. 11.1).

Symmetry in the Coronal Plane

In perfectly symmetrical posture, a plumb line from above along the symmetrical line of the body (fig. 11.2) should pass through:

- the inion
- the medial line of the spinal vertebrae
- the sacrum
- the medial part of the coccyx
- a point midway between the two internal malleoli

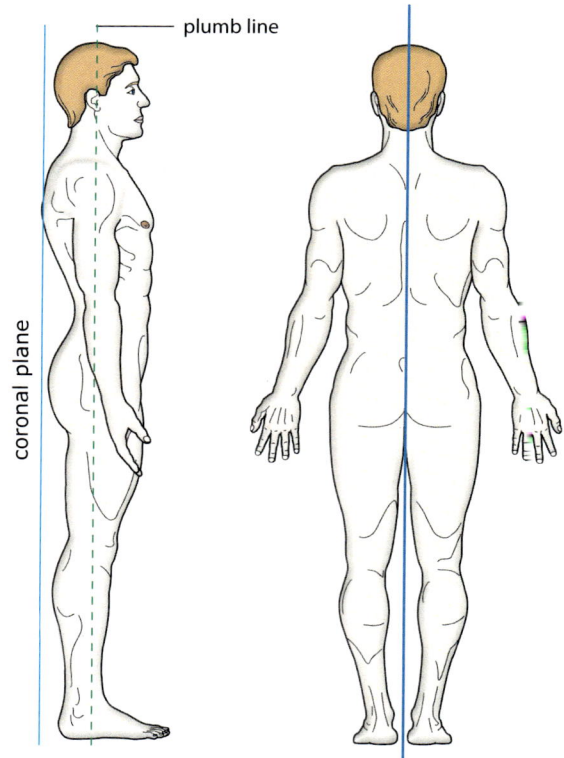

plumb line

coronal plane

Figure 11.1. Equilibrium in the sagittal plane.

Figure 11.2. Symmetry in the coronal plane.

198

A slight dorsal scoliotic posture, with left concavity, is generally considered tolerable.

Balance in the Transverse Plane

Seen from above, the patient should appear neither twisted at the level of the spine nor rotated to one side or the other (fig. 11.3). Neither of the gluteal muscle masses nor the shoulders should be ahead or behind in relation to the other.

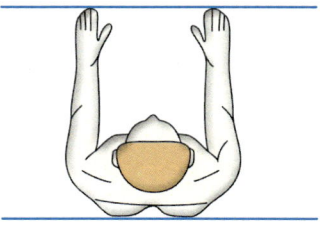

Normal

Figure 11.3. Balance in the transverse plane.

This is how a "normal" stance is defined. Less than ten percent of the population conform to these criteria.

Global Postural Mechanics

Considered in a simplistic way, posture is the geometric result of stacking bones and articulations, maintained and controlled through a muscular system battling the effects of gravity. In reality, posture is the sum of several factors. It is more than the neuromuscular adjustments of the musculoskeletal system. The muscular system plays an important role in the overall balance of the individual, but it should not be considered the only "soft" element that plays a part in posture.

Tissular Organization of Posture

All the tissues of the body—fasciae, ligaments, intermuscular partitions, skin, visceral envelopes, organs, and meninges—participate in the elaboration of posture. Even intracavity pressures contribute to it. All these elements are *generators of passive forces*, which affect posture and corporal structure. For their part, the muscles are not only *generators of active forces*; they also generate passive forces, giving them viscoelastic properties. Body structure is subject to a balance between forces of compression and forces of tension:

199

- tension of the soft elements assures *cohesion* of the system
- compression of the hard elements confers *solidity* to the system

This functional complementary relationship creates a state of restrained equilibrium in which the internal forces balance out. The bones, compressed by gravity, are in balance with the myofascial network tension. The result is a self-governing system in which balance is relatively independent of gravity. When this system loses its balance of forces, it finds itself more subjected to gravity. For example, following soft tissue changes, the spine behaves like a stack of vertebrae subject to gravity. The transfer of forces occurs directly from bone to bone, and instabilities set in.

Combined Forces

Posture is maintained by a combination of passive tensions generated by connective tissues. Intermittent muscular actions rebalance the structural whole. When a ligamentous system is held in an articular position, the body can bear weight on the anterior ligaments of the hip. To discharge the ligaments of their tension, the anterior muscles of the hip periodically contract.

Generally, without any muscular activity, the body oscillates for short periods. General balance is guaranteed as long as the body's center of gravity projects itself in the base of support, delimited by the support of the feet. These oscillations are harmoniously distributed around the ideal projection point, toward the geometric center of the base of support (fig. 11.4). If the oscillations are too large, certain muscle groups contract to prevent the posture from becoming unstable and help bring the body to a position of equilibrium.

Overall, the effects of gravity are mainly encountered by the osseous structures, relying on the ligaments and all connective tissues.

Positioning of the Contents of the Trunk

Classically opposed to the appendicular system of the limbs, the head and trunk form the body's axial system. It contains the vital elements

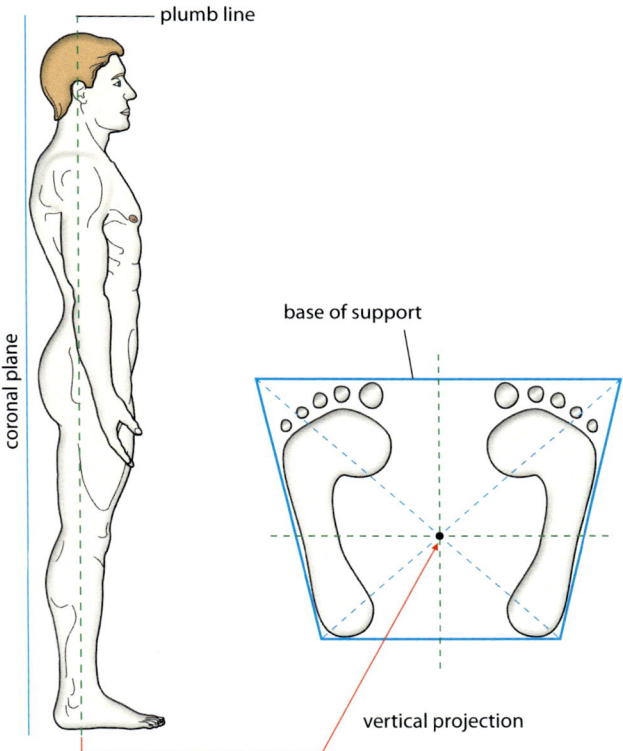

plumb line

coronal plane

base of support

vertical projection

Figure 11.4. Ideal projection point of the center of gravity within the base of support.

that ensure priority functions like respiration, circulation, and digestion. Placed at the core of the vertebral skeleton, the central nervous system is also an element of the highest importance.

The different pressures ruling the thoracic, abdominopelvic, and cephalospinal cavities determine the degree of prestressing in the body. Human beings thus possess a mechanical, almost pneumatic, bearing. The mechanical organization of the trunk contents strongly influences posture and the general form. *Pressure* and *tension* are the two major parameters of this organization. *Each time pressure changes, tension is modified, and vice versa.* The diaphragm and its muscular pressure mobilize three-dimensional compartments by varying thoracic and abdominal pressure. It changes the tension of the abdomen wall and the thorax. It also modifies the degree of longitudinal tension of the mediastinal elements.

For its overall balance, the body tries to align the various centers of gravity that are linked within it. Any change in tension or pressure in the trunk alters the shape of the trunk and thus the position of its center of gravity. The body modifies its postural scheme accordingly to rebalance the whole.

The internal organization of the viscera and the neural axis is accomplished along precise axes, true chains of mechanical influence between the compartment and the contents.

Regulating Posture

Work carried out during the past century allows us to consider the postural system as a structural whole, regulated by multiple components with complementary functions. Our modern holistic vision compels me to add to this traditional conceptualization the connections between the compartments and the contents of the body. It is impossible to deny the interactions between compartments and contents. Without them, posture is reduced to a simple interplay of neuromusculoskeletal sensors and effectors. Visceral elements and neuromeningeal structures are the leading players in postural adaptation, as shown in the SPECT scans that I did with Jean-Pierre Barral when seeking to confirm this.

Requirements

The organism cannot maintain a posture or create movements that would endanger the integrity of certain structures or the maintenance of vital functions. Consequently:

- The mobility and stability of the body are of secondary importance.
- Protecting the body's contents is of primary importance.

Posture has a list of complex responsibilities:

- monitoring the vital functions of the body (respiration, circulation, etc.)
- monitoring the protection of vital elements and the body's contents (vessels, nerves, central nervous system, vital organs, etc.)
- countering the effects of gravity and maintaining an established position
- maintaining balance and opposition to external forces
- accommodating forces and internal mechanical constraints
- accommodating the individual's psychological, emotional, and motor potentials
- balancing the individual in movement

Regulatory System

To achieve neurophysiological prowess, the organism has to integrate information from different sources (fig. 11.5):

- *Exteroceptors* provide information about the situation of the body in connection to its environment. The main afferents involved in postural regulation are vision, the vestibular afferents, and plantar sensitivity.
- *Proprioceptors* provide information about the position of different parts of the body in connection to the whole, in a static position or in the course of movement.
- *Interoceptors* continuously monitor the body's vital elements (viscera, organs, vessels, nerves, central nervous system, etc.).
- *Higher centers* receive the data from the different information sources. They integrate the information and determine the best postural response—one that corresponds to the psychomotor possibilities of the individual and at the same time fits with the external conditions and internal rules of the body.

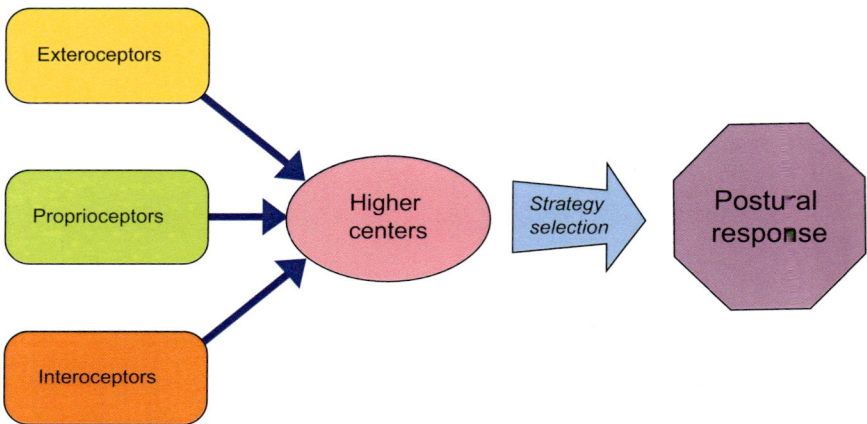

Figure 11.5. Principles of posture regulation.

Psychoemotional Parameters

Regulation of posture is also attributed to psychic states. Posture is one of the visible expressions of our way of being. Biotypology studies the somatopsychic connections that link the human form with psychic tendencies. Balance and postural responses are an integral part of these somatopsychic links. An individual's state of mind, will, and aspects of his or her personality and emotional makeup are all determined by postural response (see Chapter 12). An extroverted personality does not have the same resources as an introverted one. Given identical mechanical conditions, their respective postures are very different.

Postural Decompensation

In disrupted posture, decompensation occurs in two stages.

Management

Management is the first principle to be lost. In order of priorities, the organism maintains at all costs a position that assures the rules of postural regulation, even if it takes a lot of energy to do so. This stage of *posture that is costly in energy terms* can generate fatigue, but it is rare that patients seek consultations at this time.

Comfort

Comfort is the second characteristic to be lost. This is when posture begins to cause annoyances and pain. At this stage, *uncomfortable posture* rapidly becomes a *painful posture*. The pain can be acute, as with a sudden spinal fixation, or can become chronic. This is when the vast majority of patients seek consultations.

Protective Posture

Even painless postures illustrate how posture accommodates the vital contents of the body. Each time an significant anatomical element is affected by inflammation or irritation or is at risk from excessive mechanical demands, posture modifies itself for maximum protection.

In the case of sciatica, the sciatic nerve responds to inflammation and restriction in the boney framework and sends nociceptive and proprioceptive messages to the higher centers. Certain muscle groups are activated to create a painless posture, with contractions that attempt to immobilize defective articular segments and prevent the addition of new constraints on the nerve. In this case, somatic posture modifies itself to protect the neural contents.

A meningeal irritation can affect postural compensations. In the case of meningitis or meningeal hemorrhage, stiffness at the nape of the neck is a cardinal sign for diagnosis. This pain is the consequence of hypertonicity of spinal muscles in the cervical region. This muscle tension prevents all spinal flexion, which in turn leads to tension in the dura mater and adds to restrictions of the cerebrospinal meninges.

The same process is triggered by a visceral irritation. In the case of appendicitis, the body assumes a painless posture comprising flexion of the right hip and right lateral flexion of the lumbar column, carried out by the irrepressible contraction of the psoas. The *muscular defense,* a true hypertonicity of the abdominal muscles, sometimes contributes to the postural scheme.

Thus we see that posture results from more than just the effects of gravity on the stacked skeleton. Other forces influence the cohesion of the compartments and their contents. Hyperactivity of certain muscle groups is often a safe response of the *compartment* in the context of pathology, or of a threat to the *contents*. Seen from this perspective, some muscular contractures should not immediately be overcome, from a therapeutic viewpoint.

Morphostatic Examination

Morphostatic examination screens out mechanical disorders affecting the patient. It provides valuable information and must not be neglected. All disturbances of body harmony generally reveal abnormal fascial tension. The morphostatic examination also allows us to use this tension to gauge the results of treatment.

For instructional purposes, I have separated the routine general examination and the detailed examination of the patient. The routine general examination can be quick, and an experienced practitioner can do it with a glance. The detailed examination clearly demonstrates the methodology of observing posture. It allows us to be systematic and methodical in our approach.

Application

Determining the Directing Eye

In order to avoid any errors caused by parallel vision during the examination, it is necessary to have perfect coordination of the hands and eyes. It is important to determine your directing eye (fig. 11.6):

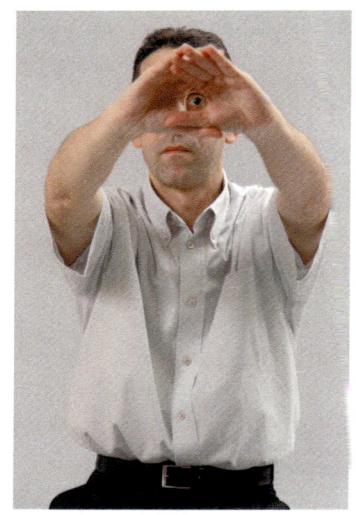

- With both eyes open, pick a distant object as a target.
- Extend your arms and form a small circle by joining the thumb and index

Figure 11.6. Determining the directing eye.

finger of both hands. Reduce the circle bit by bit until you are just able to see the target object.

- Alternately close your right eye and then your left eye. Normally the object disappears from your field of vision in one eye but not the other. The eye that allows you to see the object in the circle is your dominant eye.

Placement

As a general rule, palpation of reference points is done in combination with visual observation. Try to appreciate the following points:

- The hands and the eyes must be at the same height, on the same plane of reference.
- To examine asymmetry, it is important for your directing eye to be placed midway between the two anatomical parts that you are observing or have palpated.
- When the patient is tall, place yourself to the right of the table if your dominant eye is the right eye; place yourself to the left of the table if your dominant eye is the left.

Examination in the Coronal Plane

Examination from Behind

Routine General Examination

Stand behind the patient and observe any noticeable abnormalities (fig. 11.7). Then consider the gravity line: is weight distributed equally on both feet? Has the trunk shifted to one side, loading one leg more than the other? Observe the carriage of the head, the height of the shoulders, and the level of the iliac crests.

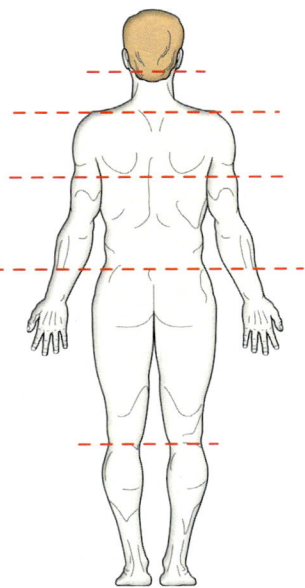

Figure 11.7. Examination from behind.

207

Detailed Examination
Balance of the Head in the Coronal Plane
- Palpate the inion. Is it located on the medial line?
- With a finger under each earlobe, compare their heights; do the same at the level of the mastoid process.
- Are the neck and the head tilted?
- With one finger on the inion and the other at the level of the gluteal cleft, are they aligned vertically?
- Note any lateral deviation of the head and any rotations of the neck.
- All asymmetries can be compensations for the lower body or can sometimes result from a sensory problem. For example, a patient with an auditory problem may have a tendency to rotate the head.

Height of the Shoulders
- Place a finger of each hand on the right and left trapezius muscles. Are they at the same level?
- Shift two fingers laterally onto the two acromion processes. Are they at the same height? Note: be especially mindful of any contraction or retraction of the shoulders that can create an apparent difference of height.
- Place your thumbs on the inferior angle of the scapulae at about T7; compare the level of the angles.
- Shift your thumbs to the spines of the scapula and gauge their distance from the midline.
- Place your palms flat on the posterior surface and your fingers on the superior border of the scapulae, and find the actual rotation of the scapulae.

Any asymmetry can cause a spinal asymmetry or a chronic dysfunction of the shoulder.

The Static Spine
- Observe all apparent rotation of the vertebral column suggested by an enlargement on one side.

- Ask the patient to bend forward. Slide the palms of your hands on the posterior costal angles. You may find an actual hump, indicative of the convexity of a scoliotic structure.
- Find all asymmetry of the vertebrae. Place a finger on the spinous process of T1 and slide it down, along the line of spinous processes, one vertebra after another. Determine if asymmetries or irregularities exist: lateral deviation of the spinous process in relation to the midline; depression or prominence of a spinous process; opening or closing of interspinous spaces.
- Are there smooth vertebral zones? Are there any breaks in the harmony of the spinal curve?
- Observe the symmetry of the space between the arms and the trunk (a parallelogram with four equidistant sides). Any difference between the spaces is frequently due to a spinal asymmetry. Does the more acute angle coincide with the concavity of scoliotic inflexion?

The Static Pelvis

- Crouch down so that you eyes are at the height of the patient's pelvis. Place your index fingers on the iliac crests at the level of the back dimples, and the pad of your thumbs on the posterior superior iliac spines (PSIS).
  - Is there a difference in height of the iliac crests? Is it coherent with the overlying segment?
  - Is there a difference in height of the PSISs? Is it coherent with the height of the iliac crests?
  - Is there a difference in depth between the two PSISs?
- Note any differences in volume or gluteal and spinal muscle tone. Compare the heights of the gluteal sulci.

Balance of the Lower Limbs

- Note all knock-kneed (valgus) or bowlegged (varus) twisting of the knees. Is the dysfunction bilateral or unilateral?
- Observe the flexion creases of the knee in the popliteal crease. Are they situated at the same height?

209

- Note any differences of volume and tension levels of the calves and thighs. In the case of a discrepancy in leg length, find out if it results from a sports injury, a work injury, or an older cause.
- Follow the course of the Achilles tendons to their insertions. Are they arched or stretched?
- Observe the balance of the heels. Is there a tendency toward internal or external pronation? Is it more marked on one side or the other?

Examination from the Front

Routine General Examination

Observe the distribution of weight, the carriage of the head, the height of the shoulders, and the placement of the feet (fig. 11.8). Note thoracic asymmetries and the centering of the umbilicus. You can also find the horizontal alignment of:

- the pupillary line
- the mamillary line
- the radial styloid process line
- the pectoral girdle
- the pelvic girdle

Detailed Examination

Observe:

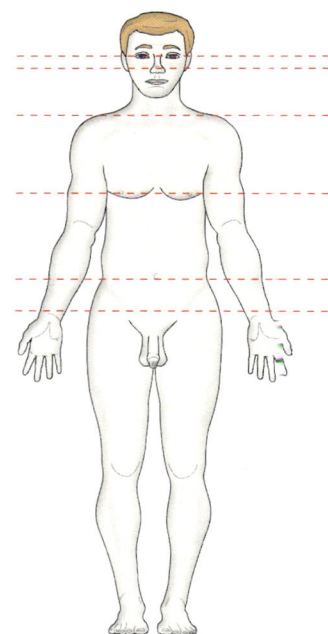

- the symmetry of the neck in relation to the head and face
- the respiratory pattern. Is it superficial? Is the movement more pronounced in the upper thorax, the lower thorax, or the abdomen?
- thoracic symmetry. Is it coherent with observations from behind?
- the outline of retracted or bulging abdominal muscles
- the symmetry of the abdomen

Figure 11.8. Examination from the front.

210

- the position of the patellae in relation to the knees and to associated tension of the quadriceps. Deficiency of the vastus medialis can pull the patella laterally.
- rotation of the lower limb, which is indicated by foot position. Is the direction of the foot the same as that of the patella? Rotation of the limb can have a femoral or tibial origin.
- the parameters of inversion or eversion of the foot. Are the arches collapsed? Slide your fingers between the summit of the arch and the floor to determine if there are differences in height.

Disturbances in the Coronal Plane

Girdle Imbalances

Postural imbalances are most obvious at the level of the pelvic and pectoral girdles.

Tilted Shoulders

In the absence of a grid for visual reference, this imbalance shows up very easily at the level of the wrists. Determining the heights of the radial styloid processes in the standing position is a good clinical indicator of tilted shoulders (fig. 11.9).

Spatial Position of the Pelvis

Only observation of the middle part of the iliac crest, at the level of the back dimples, allows us to visualize the spatial position of the pelvis. Due to the large number of ilium rotation imbalances, the classical anterior and posterior references are often discordant.

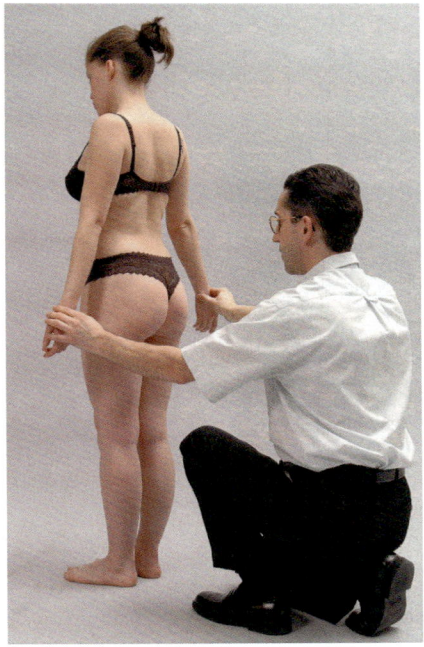

Figure 11.9. Evaluation of the height of the radial styloid processes.

According to studies of posture, three fundamental notions emerge from the morphostatic examination in the coronal plane:

- Imbalance in the pectoral girdle is often linked to laterality (fig. 11.10):
  - For a right-handed person, the left shoulder is generally higher.
  - For a left-handed person, the right shoulder is higher.
  - Exceptions often correspond to disorders of laterality: a left-handed person who was forced to switch, or masked ambidextrousness.
- When the shoulders and the pelvis tilt in the same direction, the first sensory faculty affected is vision. We must therefore check the eyes, corrective lenses, and craniosacral mechanics. Imbalance of the shoulders suggests an inverse pelvis that may also affect plantar positioning. It is necessary to investigate the feet and lower limbs. Examining shoe wear can confirm imbalances.
- Frequently, neuromuscular deficiency or circulatory disorders are discovered in the upper limb on the side of the lower shoulder generally the side of laterality.

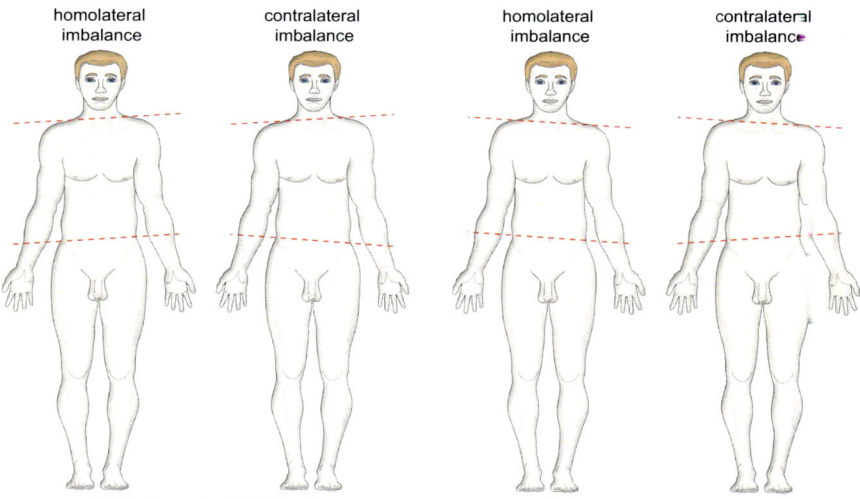

Figure 11.10. Left-handed and right-handed subjects.

Scoliotic Posture

In this posture, the spine or a segment of the spine is inclined to the right or the left. At times, a compensatory curve overlies or underlies the deviation. Any conclusion as to the underlying cause of this posture is informed by knowing whether it comes from true scoliosis or simply from scoliotic posture. *Scoliotic posture* is a lateral deviation of the spine that disappears on lying down. More clinically, there is no hump, and no rotated vertebrae are observable by imaging. *Scoliosis* is a permanent lateral deviation of the spine. It results from a progressive displacement of vertebrae in relation to one another. Observed in the anatomical position, it is organized in the three spatial planes. Because of the vertebral rotation, the patient presents a hump, corresponding to protrusion of the ribs on the convex side of the spinal curve. It is highlighted by forward flexion of the trunk (fig. 11.11).

The evolutionary potential of scoliosis mainly depends on its angular value and the patient's osseous age. Osseous age is evaluated by the Risser sign, which is an evaluation of ossification of the iliac crest (fig. 11.12). It requires a radiological test of osseous maturity, as shown in a frontal X-ray of the pelvis. Risser grades 1 through 5 correspond to increasing age in puberty. The more the osseous age has progressed, the weaker the evolutionary risk of scoliosis.

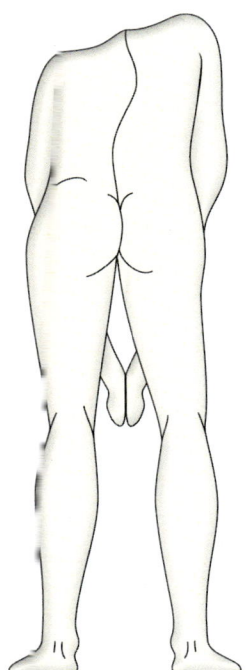

Figure 11.11. Scoliotic hump.

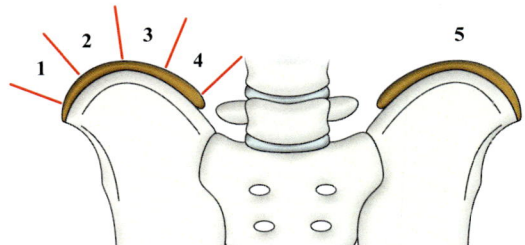

Figure 11.12. Grades of the Risser sign.

Examination in the Sagittal Plane

Examination of the Profile

Because of the absence of natural symmetry, it is more difficult to evaluate equilibrium in the sagittal plane. Even if normal posture can theoretically be defined according to the gravity line, there are a certain number of reasonably efficient postures. With this in mind, the important point to evaluate in profile is primarily the load line. If the body has a tendency to lean forward, the posterior muscles will require increasing energy expenditure to maintain the erect posture. This is accompanied by fatigued or tired posture as well as tissular changes necessary to adapt to this excessive demand.

Routine General Examination

Evaluate the general posture in relation to an imaginary vertical line passing through the external ear canal. Ideally, it should pass through the acromion process, the greater trochanter, and slightly in front of the lateral malleolus. Note any modifications of the head in the anterior and posterior plane; any exaggeration or diminishing of spinal curvature; the flexion of the hip; and flexion or hyperextension of the knee. It is especially important to observe four principal parameters (fig. 11.13):

- the scapular plane
- the plane of the gluteal masses
- cervical curvature
- lumbar curvature

Only figure A is considered "normal" or balanced. There are four principal static disorders:

- B: scapular and gluteal mass planes aligned but with the addition of curvature
- C: posterior scapular plane
- D: anterior scapular plane
- E: scapular and gluteal mass planes aligned but with diminished curvature

214

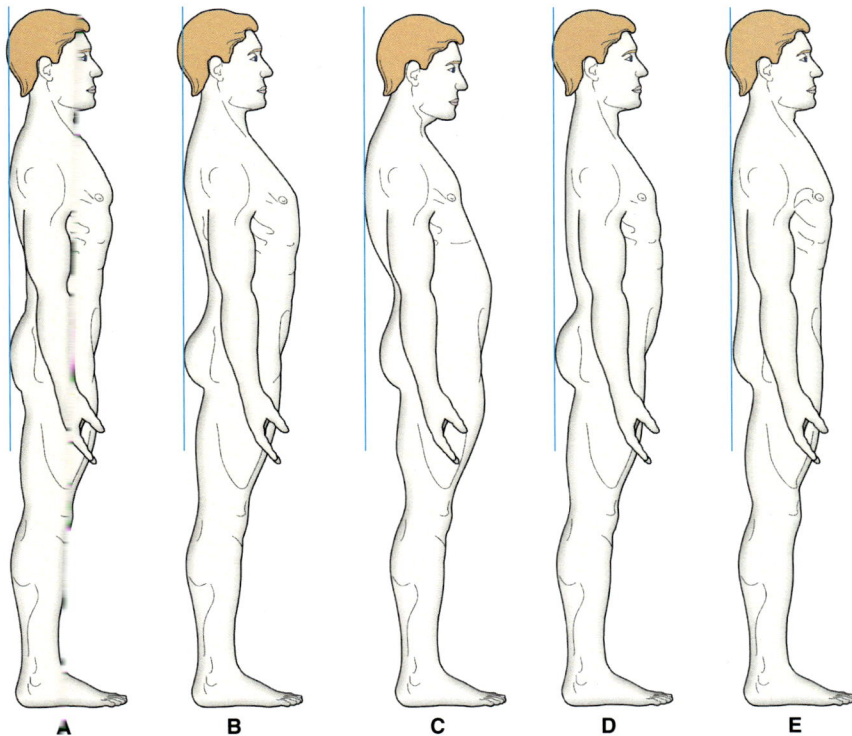

Figure 11.13. Imbalances in the sagittal plane.
A Normal subject
B Planes aligned, with increased curves
C Posterior scapular plane
D Flat back, anterior scapular plane
E Planes aligned with diminished curves

Detailed Examination

Observe:

- cervical posture. Is the head projected forward?
- scapular posture. Is the base of the shoulder in retroposition or anteposition?
- Is spinal curvature increased or diminished? Lumbar hyperlordosis adds to the risk of lumbar pain. Increased thoracic kyphosis can lead to added cervical lordosis, often generating tension and fatigue in the neck and shoulders.

- the tonicity of abdominal muscles and the anterior contour of the trunk. A voluminous abdomen is an important biomechanical element that can orient the diagnosis toward the visceral sphere.
- the pelvifemoral angle. Are the hips in extension or in light flexion? In flexion, is the pelvis relatively anteverted? This can be due to a capsular or ligamentous retraction of the hip, a shortened or overly stretched psoas muscle, or even a significant extension of the lower lumbar column.
- the angulation of the knees. Are they positioned in complete extension or in slight flexion? Is slight flexion of the knees attributable to flexion of the hips or to the position of the lumbar spine? If this is not the case, flexion of the knee is most likely due to a restriction of the joint itself. A shortening of the hamstrings is generally not enough to limit the extension of the knee without also limiting hip flexion.

Sometimes a combined flexion of the hips and knees is observed, as in the case of spondylosyndesis. The patient is trying to lessen the tension caused by the lumbosacral junction.

Lumbar Lordosis

At times overly pronounced and at another times too flattened, what can be said about this notorious curvature? It has numerous variations:

- *Simple lordosis* exhibits an increase of the limited curve in the lumbar region.
- *High lordosis* is defined as an increase of the curve and its migration toward the thoracic region. At times it carries along with it half to two-thirds of the thoracic column in posterior concave curvature. The apex of this curve also migrates higher up, to about the thoracolumbar junction.

Observation of lumbar lordosis informs us about the causative tensions exerted on the lumbar spine by the adjacent elements. Any disturbance of the pelvis, the coxofemoral unit, the angularity of the skeleton of the lower limbs, or muscle tone can reverberate on lumbar lordosis.

The T11, T12, L1, and L2 zone is most commonly dragged anteriorly by the fibers of the pillars of the diaphragm (the crus) and by the psoas muscles. The strong reactivity these muscles have to irritations and toxicities should lead us to suspect visceral involvement.

Disturbances in the Sagittal Plane

Disturbances of balance in the sagittal plane fall into two large categories: the *anterior scheme* and the *posterior scheme,* especially well studied by John Wernham (1985). Besides these opposing schemes, there exist several varying intermediaries.

Anterior Scheme

This is the most common postural attitude. The whole body leans forward, shifting itself toward the front in relation to the plumb line (fig. 11.14). The weight of the body is mainly supported by the forefoot. The knees are in hyperextension, at times very hyperextended. The hips are flexed, and the pelvis is forward. Cervical curvature is accentuated. Significant constraints exert pressure on the lumbosacral hinge, the lumbosacral articulations, the T11–T12 region, and on the cervicothoracic junction. In terms of the myofascial chains, the body is in posterior suspension. Tension in the muscles and their aponeuroses are involved in these suspension affects:

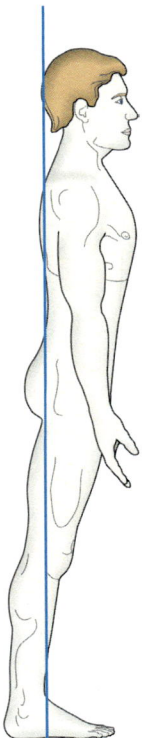

- the flexors of the toes, in particular that of the hallux
- the lateral fibulae and the posterior tibiae
- the soleus
- the hamstrings
- the pelvis-trochanter hinge
- the erector spinae

Figure 11.14. Anterior scheme (after Wernham 1985).

217

There is disequilibrium in the thoracoabdominal pressures: the diaphragm is hypertonic in the lowered position (inspiration), while the abdominal wall is relaxed, appearing hypotonic. In fact, the abdominal organs have a tendency to be ptosed, and the organs of the lower pelvis, such as the bladder, are easily irritated. Because of the weakness of the abdominal muscles, there is increased risk of abdominal hernia.

Posterior Scheme

The whole body leans backward, and equilibrium is maintained by the thrust of the pelvis and the hips toward the front of the plumb line (fig. 11.15). The weight of the body rests heavily on the heels and the arches, which are commonly collapsed. There is flexion of the knees, extension of the hips, and retroversion of the pelvis. Lumbar lordosis is increased, becoming especially pronounced at the mid-thoracic region just above it. Significant constraints come to bear on the sacroiliac joints and on the cervicothoracic junction. Thoracic kyphosis is increased in its cranial portion, and compression occurs at the costochondral-sternal articulations. The cervical column is straight, and the craniospinal junction is in extension. In terms of myofascial chains, the body is in anterior suspension. The implicated muscular tension involved in this suspension affects:

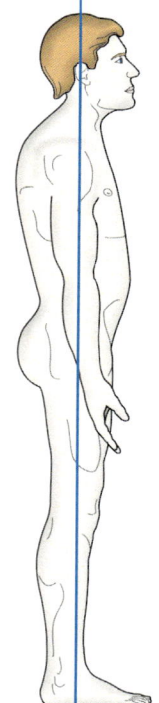

- the extensors of the toes, especially that of the hallux
- the anterior tibiae
- the quadriceps
- the adductors
- the iliopsoas
- the anterior-medial muscle chain: the large right muscles of the abdomen and the muscles above and below the hyoid bone

Figure 11.15. Posterior scheme (after Wernham 1985).

218

Imbalance in parietal thoracoabdominal tension arises. The diaphragm is hypertonic in the upper position (expiration), and the thoracic cavity is retracted, which favors respiratory, cardial, and pericardial dysfunctions and injuries. The strong tension on the anterior abdominal wall can increase intra-abdominal pressure. This factor, coupled with retroversion of the pelvis, compounded by weakening of the perineum, favors ptoses and prolapses of pelvic organs. These conditions can contribute to fluid stasis and congestion. Pelvic congestion with its cohort of urogenital pain, circulatory problems of the lower limbs, and constipation can follow.

Variant Forms of Balance

Posterior Translation Posture

- head projected forward
- increased cervical lordosis
- increased thoracic kyphosis
- diminished lumbar lordosis
- retroverted pelvis
- hip and knee in hyperextension (fig. 11.16)

Flat Back Posture

- head projected forward
- cervical lordosis slightly increased
- high thoracic kyphosis slightly increased, flattening at the mid-thoracic and lower thoracic levels
- flattened lumbar lordosis
- retroverted pelvis
- hip and knee in extension (fig. 11.17)

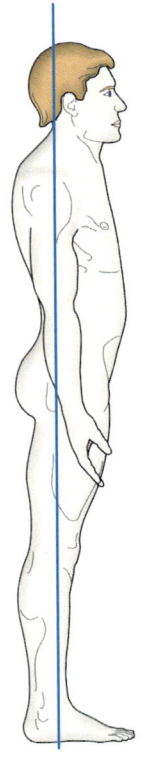

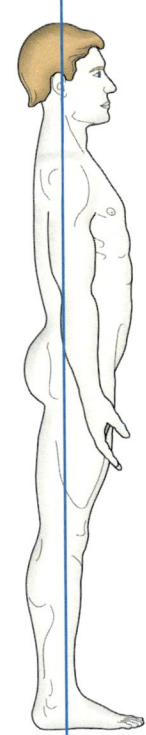

Figure 11.16. Posterior translation posture.

Figure 11.17. Flat back posture.

219

Military Posture

The military posture (fig. 11.18) has been created by a positional exercise: "Stick out your chest; pull in your stomach."

- slight posterior inclination of the head
- physiological cervical and thoracic curves
- chest bulging and elevated, creating an anterior deviation of the cervical column and a posterior deviation of the thoracic column in relation to the plumb line
- increased lumbar lordosis
- anteverted pelvis
- knee in extension
- ankle in plantar flexion

Kypholordotic Posture

- head projected forward
- increased cervical lordosis
- increased thoracic kyphosis
- scapulae in abduction
- increased lumbar lordosis
- anteverted pelvis
- slight flexion of the hip
- tendency to hyperextend the knee
- tendency toward plantar flexion of the ankles in relation to the angulation of the lower limbs
- protruding stomach (fig. 11.19)

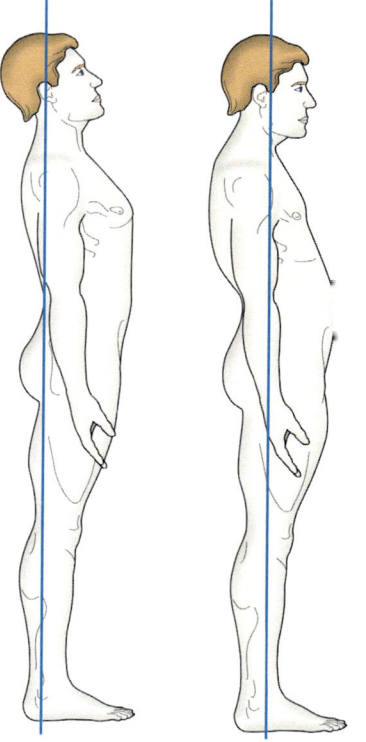

**Figure 11.18.
Military posture.**

**Figure 11.19
Kypholordot c
posture.**

220

Classically, static disorders in the anterior-posterior sense are directly attributed to mechanical problems of the foot and lower limb. They can also be consequences of deformities of the back of the foot or of a lax stride.

Another source of disturbance can be attributed to mastication. Ill-fitting false teeth can alter the position of the head and chest.

The spinal dura mater can also generate constraints all along the spinal axis and increase the curves in the sagittal plane. Finally, certain visceral tensions can reflect back along the central tendon and also create an imbalance in the sagittal plane.

Examination in the Transverse Plane

Examination from Above

This is the study of rotations of the shoulders and of the pelvis. A clear view from above is not easy to accomplish; we have to be content with an approximation of posterior or anterior views from above.

Ask the patient to stand with his or her back against a wall to give you a reference point. It is then easier to see where the shoulders or pelvis are not in contact with the wall. Note the tendencies of the anterior and posterior pelvis and of the anterior and posterior scapulae.

Postural Disturbances in the Transverse Plane

Rotations of the pelvis can occur in the same direction as in the shoulders, or in the opposite direction.

Globally Rotated Posture

The whole body can be rotated right or left (fig. 11.20). This can be initiated by a rotation departing from the ankles and reflected back on the overlying segments.

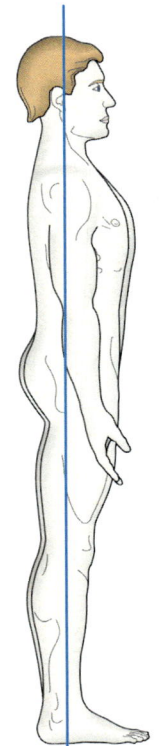

**Figure 11.20.
Rotated posture.**

221

Lateral alignment appears totally different in the right and left sagittal view. In the case of scoliosis, rotation of the thorax is found in the direction of the convexity of the scoliosis.

Posture of Opposingly Rotated Girdles

The observed deformation shows torsion in the pelvic or pectoral girdles, in opposite directions. Rotation of the pectoral girdle is strongly influenced by laterality (fig. 11.21). An injury to organs beneath the diaphragm, such as the liver, frequently generates torsion of the girdles. Commonly, the scapula is posterior on the same side as the injured or dysfunctional organ while the pelvis is anterior.

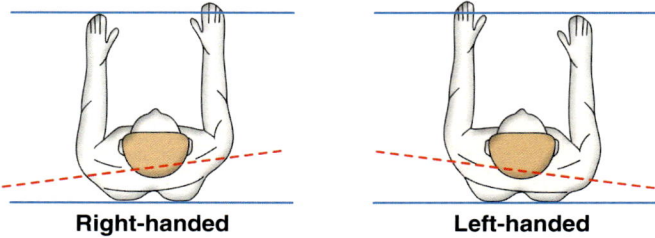

Right-handed   **Left-handed**

Figure 11.21. Imbalances in the transverse plane.

In cases of postural disturbance, the questioning must try to determine precisely the type and level of physical activity to recommend with regard to the maladapted posture. Also, search for any physical abnormalities that could be bound to a particular posture (hemivertebra, transitional anomaly, osteoporosis, etc.). Analysis of postural imbalances is generally carried out before the examination of mobility and palpation of the tissues. It provides valuable indications of the areas where the body is under strain. It shows the myofascial chains implicated, and indicates the patient's adaptability. For example, in the anterior scheme, a vertebral somatic dysfunction in extension will be very difficult to compensate for, while a dysfunction in flexion will be more easily tolerated. It is the opposite for a posterior scheme. This can somewhat explain how the same type of dysfunction sometimes causes virtually no symptoms and other times elicits a hyperalgesic response.

Gait Analysis

It is interesting to observe how posture can change in the course of walking. Observation is made with the patient in their underwear and bare feet. Look at the gait from the front, the back, and the sides. Study the length of the strides, the balancing of the arms, the heel strike, the development of the stride, the inclination of the pelvis, and the adaptation of the shoulders. Note all abnormalities of gait, even the minimal ones. After all, significant pathological injuries are not common in our consultations. Especially note whether the gait is affected by an opposite rotation of the pelvic or pectoral girdles, and if the strides are symmetrical.

Examining Shoes

Pathologies aside, the shoe is a very good reflection of the foot's dynamic carriage and its repercussions for posture (fig. 11.22). When required, examining shoes can provide interesting information. Five principal points are observed:

- *Heel wear.* Normally the foot is placed on the ground on the posterior-lateral side of the heel. This part wears down to a certain extent. A lateral wear pattern translates as someone who has a varus heel, while a pronounced posterior or medial wear pattern is a sign of being pigeon-toed (valgus) at the front of the foot.

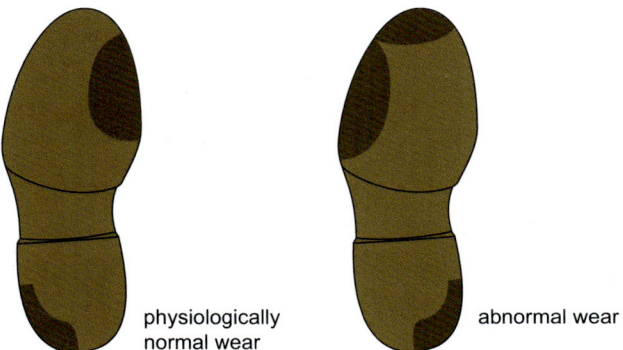

physiologically
normal wear

abnormal wear

Figure 11.22. Sole wear.

223

- *Anterior heel wear.* Normally, the stride ends on the big toe. Thus the anterior-posterior part of the anterior heel is more lightly used. Excessive wear on this anterior-medial part indicates pronation of the forefoot. A wear pattern of the lateral or anterior part of the anterior sole can be observed on a forefoot in supination or an ankylosis of the first metatarsophalangeal articulation.
- *Deformity of the upper* (fig. 11.23). A medially deformed upper on a shoe, especially if it is widened, indicates a pigeon-toed stance. A laterally deformed upper can indicate a varus (bow-leggedness), or a shoe that is too short. In all cases, it is necessary to point out that the shoe itself is not the problem.
- *Wear at the anterior end of the sole.* This is often a sign of a steppage gait. It is necessary to eliminate other causes: shoes that are too long, too heavy, or poorly used; walking on all fours; braking on a bike or scooter; or the use of a skateboard.
- *Creases on the dorsal side.* Normally, propulsion of the foot is principally assured by the hallux. The shoe thus presents transverse creases on its dorsal side. If there is reduced mobility of the metatarsophalangeal articulation of the hallux, propulsion of the foot is made possible by the four other toes. The shoe then presents abnormal oblique creases on its dorsal surface.

Finally, it is important to verify the symmetry of wear on both shoes. More pronounced wear on one shoe should draw your attention to that foot. Abnormal wear that displays a symmetrical pattern on both shoes reveals an imbalance affecting the global posture of the subject.

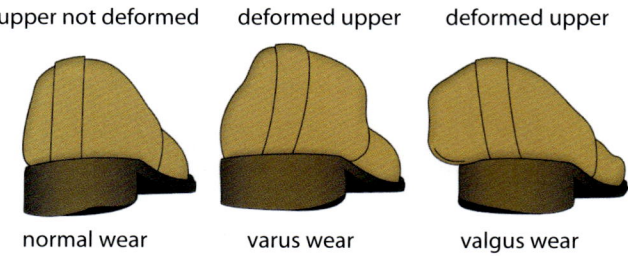

upper not deformed   deformed upper   deformed upper

normal wear   varus wear   valgus wear

Figure 11.23. Deformation of the upper.

Chapter 12

The Nature of the Individual

The normal state of man is to be original.

— ANTON CHEKHOV

Evaluation of the totality and specificity of a patient is a broad undertaking. The contributions of biotypology and clinical psychology are considerable enrichments to the osteopathic art. The difficulty is in finding, among all the approaches that exist, the elements that directly concern our diagnostic approach. The goal is to find the elements of observation that clarify and provide structure to the examination of the patient in its global context. Sometimes it will not be possible to find a dominant lesion, the possible end result of combining approaches.

Biotypology

Generalities

Nicola Pende (1955) defines the individual as a somatopsychic entity who sees, reacts, suffers, and thinks in his or her own unique manner. People obey the laws of a particular morphopsychophysiological heredity and are influenced by external social, environmental, and cosmic modifying agents. This medical approach to a living unity of tissues, fluids, and consciousness is opposed to the generalizations of classical medicine.

The functioning of an individual can be understood on several levels. Biotypology constitutes the basis of the clinical presentation in its totality. It allows us, using multiple approaches, to understand and perceive certain aspects of the functioning of an individual. These diverse approaches bring to light the links unifying structure and function, such as their anatomical or physiological expression. For example, we can consider embryological development and its influence on hormonal balance or on the neurovegetative system. Biotypological explanations likewise allow us to decode the connections existing between personality and physical form.

In the elaboration of a diagnosis, biotypology data aids in determining the strengths and weaknesses of patients, discerning their total functioning and anticipating the foreseeable evolution of their state.

Finally, biotypology guides us toward the most useful therapeutic tool for the specifics of patients by considering their most probable reactions.

Definitions

Biotypology is founded on static and dynamic observations of individuals.

Constitution

Constitution is defined as the physical and psychic structure of the individual. Both inherited and acquired, it consists of static morphological elements and depends on a reactional dynamic, itself regulated by the neuroendocrine system. Constitution is predetermined by a development plan from the genetic code and is influenced by individual variations. On an individual basis, environment plays the same role as personal capacities for action, reaction, and adaptation to life.

Constitution influences the development and course of an illness; it illustrates the notion of *field. The human organism is composed of cells organized into tissues and solid organs, collaborating with the dynamic unity of the body.* Pende (1955) compares this organization to nations' political constitutions, which elaborate on the laws that jointly regulate the collaboration of different groups in a nation for the benefit of the whole.

Temperament

Temperament is defined as the sum of physiological (especially neuro-vegetative), emotional, and reactive dispositions that correspond to constitutional and biotypological traits. In a way, temperament connotes biological factors of the personality. Since Galen and his doctrine of four temperaments (impulsive, choleric, melancholic, and lymphatic), numerous typologies have taken into account the morphological or physiological aspects of different individuals.

Concept of Biotypes

The representation of biotypes proposed by Pende (1955) is a pyramid (fig. 12.1). The square base is the essentially hereditary foundation of the individual. It can vary in the functioning of conditional factors, such as the penetrance of genes, or of environmental or alimentary factors. On that base, four facets arise in the human being, united by their edges:

- the *morphological facet,* called morphotype or *habitus corporis*
- the *physiological facet,* rather close to temperament in the old doctrine of medicine of the humors
- the *thymopsychic facet,* corresponding to the affective and emotional instinctive sphere

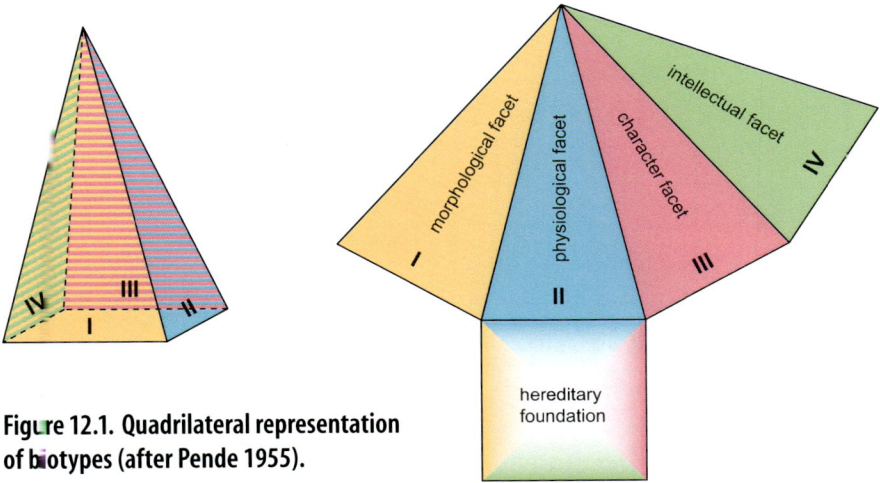

Figure 12.1. Quadrilateral representation of biotypes (after Pende 1955).

- the *noopsychic facet,* comprising the imaginative sphere of the intellect and make-believe

It is very rare that the four facets are equal, symmetrical, or even harmonious.

The first two reflect the somatic aspects of the individual, which are intimately linked to one another:

- the shape of the body
- its manner of functioning

The determination of this morphophysiology is mainly neuroendocrine.

The two other facets represent the psychic constitution, structural aspects of the personality:

- the *thymopsychic facet* corresponds to character. It is the emotive personality, the basis of our psychological structure. It concerns affective, emotional, and sentimental behaviors strongly tied to the soma and temperament, as in observations of psychoanalytical, psychosomatic, or even of somatoemotional liberation techniques.
- the *noopsychic facet* involves activity of the upper psychic field as well as human, spiritual, and moral functions: ideas, abstractions, intellectual creations, self-criticism, and free will.

For Pende and Marcel Martiny (1955), this is relatively independent of somatic biotype. For other authors, the functional and spiritual dynamism of the human being constitutes a unitary whole.

Equivalents

Most often, biotypology considers the human being according to a quaternary principle, already in use in the constitutional doctrines of Hippocrates and Galen. There are also more specific approaches that use endocrinology and neurophysiology to complete the classifications. Different schools describe the same reality with slightly different concepts or points of view. The different schools are summarized in figure 12.2.

	Pende	Hippocrates	Sigaud	Martiny	Sheldon	Vague
Sthenic Types	lanky sthenic	bilious	muscular	cordoblastic	–	thin android
	stocky sthenic	sanguine	respiratory	mesoblastic	mesomorph	obese android
Asthenic Types	lanky hyposthenic	nervous or melancholic	cerebral (habitus phthicicus	ectoblastic	ectomorph	thin gynoid
	stocky hyposthenic	Lymphatique ou pituiteux	digestive	entoblastic	endomorph	obese gynoid

Figure 12.2. Equivalents in biotypology.

Clinical Concerns

The biotypological approach is in the preclinical field. Human constitution is not an illness, and we don't confuse a premorbid constitution with a morbid state. Biotypology indicates the weak points as well as the strong points of the somatopsychic structure. It concerns the connections of the body and the soul and establishes a bridge between people's spiritual values and their organic structures, along with the functions of animal life. According to the aspects considered, we can achieve different points of view on the individual.

The Somatic Entity

Anatomical Aspects

Figure and Size

At its simplest, the size of an individual allows us to distinguish two categories: large and small. The arrangement of different parts of the body allows for a first approximation. Based on what determines the figure as slender or stocky, we can determine two somatic qualities: a lanky or a stocky tendency.

■ The *lanky* person is characterized by development of the body influenced by:

- height rather than breadth
- in the transverse plane rather than in the sagittal plane
- The trunk is relatively short in relation to the lower limbs.
- The thorax is long in relation to the abdomen; the sides are in an expiratory position, with the infrasternal angle closed.
- The neck is long and thin.
- The musculature is slim and elongated.
- The figure is slender, relatively flat in profile, and narrow and thin in varying extremes.

■ The *stocky* person, by contrast, is characterized by a development of the body influenced by:
- breadth rather than height
- In the sagittal plane, the trunk has a globular form.
- The trunk is relatively long in relation to the lower limbs.
- The neck is short and thick.
- The silhouette is stocky, relatively bulging when seen in profile, and fat and dilated to varying degrees.

Bipolar Deformation

For Viola (cited by Pende 1955) and the Italian constitutionalist school, human structure is governed by two systems:

■ the autonomic nervous system, connected to the viscera and which controls "vegetative life"
■ the central nervous system, which, in synergy with the nerves and voluntary muscles, controls "relational life"

In their own way, the proportions of two systems teach us about the connections that maintain the two polarities of the individual (fig. 12.3). The two biotypes are fashioned from these two systems, according to the law of bipolar deformation:

■ The first system is represented by the trunk. The more developed the volume of the trunk is, the more developed the organs of vegetative life are.

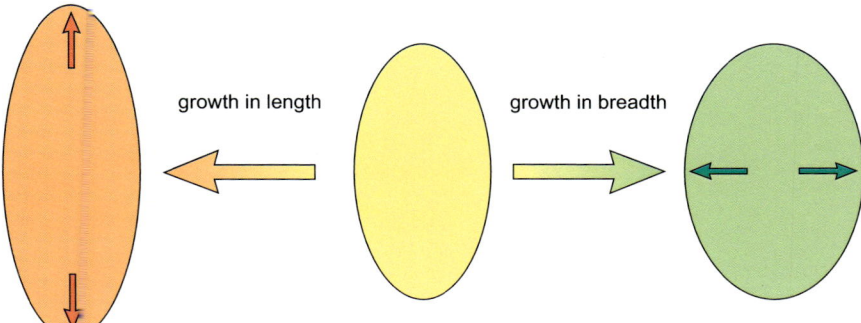

Figure 12.3. Bipolar deformation.

■ The second system is represented by the limbs. Development in the length of the limbs shows development of the organs of relational life.

In the ideally proportioned human body, the two systems are harmoniously balanced. Development influencing the vegetative life system translates a weak capacity for action in the surroundings. The person is rather destined to assimilation and is the anabolic type, of infantile morphology, and often vagotonic. Development influencing the relational life system is translated as the great evolution of human adaptation to the surroundings. The individual is destined to action and is the catabolic type, active and often sympathicotonic—displaying abnormal irritation of the sympathetic nervous system.

Biometry

A biometric indicator, simple and weak, allows us to determine whether an individual is of the lanky or stocky type. It involves the skelic index, developed by Manouvrier, who evaluated the proportions of the trunk and the lower limbs, which reflect the development of the systems of vegetative life and relational life:

$$\text{skelic index} = ((\text{standing height} - \text{seated height}) \times 100) \div \text{seated height}$$

A result greater than ninety represents a lanky morphotype. Less than eighty-five indicates a stocky morphotype. Between eighty-five and ninety is a medial type.

231

Stature

The total mass of the individual can be taken into account. It can be normal, exaggerated, or deficient, described as mediosomia, hypersomia, and hyposomia, respectively. We find macrosomic lanky or stocky types as large as those with gigantism; there are also microsomic types as small as those with dwarfism (fig. 12.4).

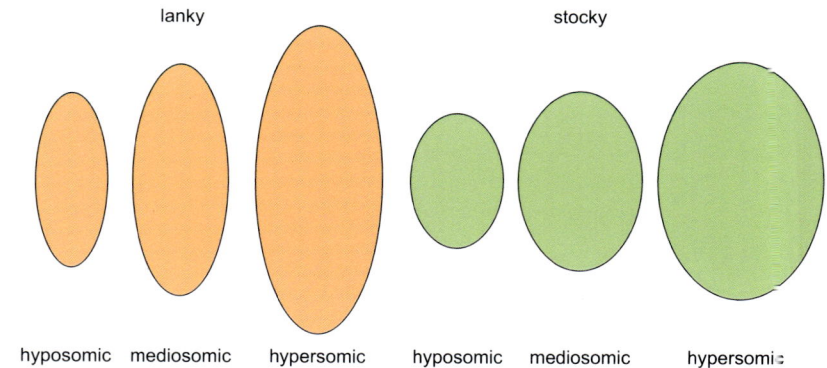

Figure 12.4. Somatic mass.

Functional Aspects

Sthenotype

Purely external morphological knowledge should be accompanied by functional knowledge. Pende (1955) introduces the notions of solidity and sthenia, with the opposites softness and asthenia. They permit us to characterize a morphotype independently of its form and mass. Sthenotype appraises the quality of all functions of the constitutional type (fig. 12.5). It is a consideration of vital potential and informs us about neuropsychic reactions, neurovegetative factors, functioning of the endocrine glands, and the metabolic activities linked to them. Sthenia translates as the capacity to react to the metabolic plan. Sthenic individuals possess capacities of adaptation that are not seen in asthenic individuals. Whatever the general morphology, a subject can have a sufficient or deficient energetic quality, a sthenic or asthenic character. Evaluation of sthenia is made based on elements of clinical and functional semiology. In effect, certain organs, systems, and tissues are more directly indicative of potential vital energy:

- the skin
- the muscular and osteoligamentous systems
- the respiratory and cardioarterial systems
- the blood
- the reticuloendothelial system
- the gonads
- certain endocrine glands: pituitary and adrenals

	Signs of Sthenia	Signs of Asthenia
Osseous and muscular systems	well developed	deficient
Tissues in general	firm, good quality	flabby
Skin	with color	cold
Hair	developed	thin, scant
Chin	firm	soft
Face	well proportioned	eyes with little expression
Sensitivity to temperature	slightly sensitive	sensitive

Figure 12.5. Semiology of sthenotype.

Growth

According to Pende, the growth of individuals is dependent on the homeostatic action of two neurohormonal constellations:

- One favors anabolism, increase of mass, and development of systems of endomesodermic origin dedicated to nutrition.
- The other, antagonistic to the first but collaborating with it, favors

233

catabolism and the development of systems derived from the ecto-derm appropriate for "relational life."

Endocrine connections rule the being and the energy. Metabolism is then oriented toward catabolism or anabolism. This bipolar principle is found again at the level of the autonomic nervous system. The opposite action and the collaboration of the two systems guarantee an indispens-able balance in maintaining normal functioning. The orthosympathetic and parasympathetic synergy is expressed in the balanced neurovegeta-tive system, asymptomatic and capable of adapting the vital functions to internal and external conditions.

The Four Basic Morphotypes

In combining the different anatomical and functional aspects, we can determine four morphodynamic types:

- the stocky hyposthenic
- the stocky sthenic
- the lanky sthenic
- the lanky hyposthenic

In each category there is a mediosomic form, a hypersomic form, a hyposomic form, and neuroendocrine subcategories. These are inter-esting to discuss because they may allow us to understand certain somatopsychic and psychosomatic correlations. In practice there are numerous mixed types, which makes a rigorous clinical assessment dif-ficult. Nonetheless, some main diagnostic principles can be determined. Faced with morbid aggression, the behavior of the basic biotypes is especially interesting.

Stocky Hyposthenic Adult Biotype

Morphology

- The general aspect of the body is round and atonic. The chest is short, while the stomach is voluminous, high, and protuberant, as in a child.

234

- Height is often short.
- Weight is especially exaggerated, with a certain tendency toward adiposity. The fat has often accumulated on the cheeks, neck, breast areas, stomach, flanks, and limbs. It is a flaccid watery fat, falling in big folds.
- The skin is pale. The thick and soft dermis indicates myxedema.
- The limbs are short and endowed with poorly developed muscles, masked by watery fat. Cellulite is common.
- Hands are large and short and have short, pudgy fingers, as if infiltrated with water.
- The face is moon-shaped. The eyes are small with straight palpebral slits and drooping eyelids. The round brow is noticeably receding and low. The cranial perimeter is of a medium size.
- The inferior level of the face is large. The rising rami of the mandible are wide. The chin is round, large, and often receding. The teeth are malformed and irregular, subject to caries, with the incisors short and the canines slightly pronounced.
- The neck is big and short, with the nape sticking out (due to cellulite, scleredema, or a large increase of adipose tissue), giving the head a general impression of bovine morphology to the body.
- The hair, eyebrows, and beard are scant and fine (fig. 12.6).

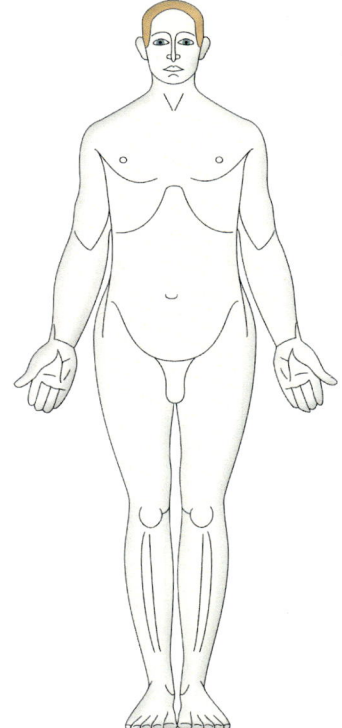

Figure 12.6. Stocky hyposthenic adult.

Functions

- The lymphatic tissue and the lymph are very well-developed. This biotype corresponds to a phlegmatic, lymphatic, and pituitary temperament in older people.
- The parasympathetic mainly dominates the neurovegetative system.
- In the cardiovascular system, this group of individuals presents a hypoplasia of the cardioarterial system. One notes an atony of the venous system, with a tendency to varicosities, as in atony of dermal capillaries. The right heart is prevalent over the left heart; arterial pressure is especially low, whereas venous pressure is elevated. This creates a tendency to acrocyanosis and chilblains. The skin is mottled, and edemas of the distal parts of the body are common.
- Renal function has slowed down.
- In the digestive system, the stomach has a large capacity, associated with an excessive appetite. The pancreatic, exocrine, and endocrine insulin functions are exaggerated, favoring alimentary assimilation. The physiological tendency is toward atonic obesity of the gynoidal type. The liver is in a state of "functional torpor."
- In the endocrine system, the hypofunctioning of the anterior pituitary gland notably affects growth hormone. Posterior pituitary vasopressin is probably in excess. Likewise, the hypofunctioning thyroid and a deficiency of adrenalin and steroid secretion by the adrenals and the gonads translate in both sexes as signs of immaturity of the primary and secondary sexual characters. Despite this, fertility is high, especially in women.
- Muscular strength is weak, and movements are slow.
- In the circulatory system, there is anemia and an increase of lymphocytes.
- This biotype corresponds to an infantile temperament. There is a predominance of anabolism, with materials augmenting the construction of living material, in effect the digestive tract and the lymphatic system.

Metabolism

- The basal metabolic rate is normal or a bit depressed, and the metabolism associated with exertion is lowered.
- Despite strong digestive capacity, cardiomuscular nitrogen metabolism is reduced, such that fatty anabolism is enhanced. Glycemia usually stays low, however.
- Common hypercholesterolemia involves few atheromatous lesions. The cholesterol moves toward other areas, such as the biliary ducts.
- Oxalic and uratic precipitations are common in the urine.

Diagnostic Concerns

Stocky hyposthenic individuals are parasympatheticotonic. They present a hormonal tendency to pituitary and thyroid hypofunctioning. They are generally slow, inactive, and easily depressed. The organic reactions of this biotype are readily and quickly generalized due to their weak tonicity, tied to their lack of maturity and wide plasticity. They are maladapted to morbid aggressions.

They have a rather marked tendency to form stones, much more in the biliary system than in the urinary system. They are predisposed to articular afflictions. Older women are predisposed to rheumatoid arthritis and polyarthritis. Acute articular rheumatoid arthritis and its cardiac consequences affect the young, which practitioners should watch for. This biotype possesses good recuperative abilities in the case of an acute affliction or shock. The infant and child of this biotype quickly become dejected but rapidly rebound.

Very sensitive emotionally, any aggression can destabilize their visceral system, which is a suitable approach for verification. Their complaints are especially chronic, and if structural manipulations are indicated, they are best accomplished in several minutes, at the end of a session, after having worked on the visceral, circulatory, and reflex aspects.

Stocky Sthenic Adult Biotype

Morphotype

- Height is often below average, with excessive weight. There are some individuals of tall stature.
- The volume of the trunk, especially the thorax, is exaggerated. It is very large and extremely short, with the sternocostal angle quite open.
- In women, there is exaggerated development of the mammary glands.
- The skin is dewy and very vascularized.
- The limbs are relatively short, robust, and muscular, and at times athletic. The shoulders are strong.
- The head is well developed, connected to the trunk by a short and large neck with a powerful nape, like the neck of a bull.
- The face is large and tends to be hexagonal and a bit angular due to the developed mid-respiratory stage. The eyes are rather small and the nose prominent, often convex and voluminous. The chin is strong and often protrudes.
- The teeth are large, with strong pointed canines.
- In adults, there is abundant hair on the thorax and limbs, linked to hyperadrenalism, and an exaggerated redness, seen as congestion of the facial skin (fig. 12.7).

Functions

- This biotype clearly differs from the hyposthenic stocky type:

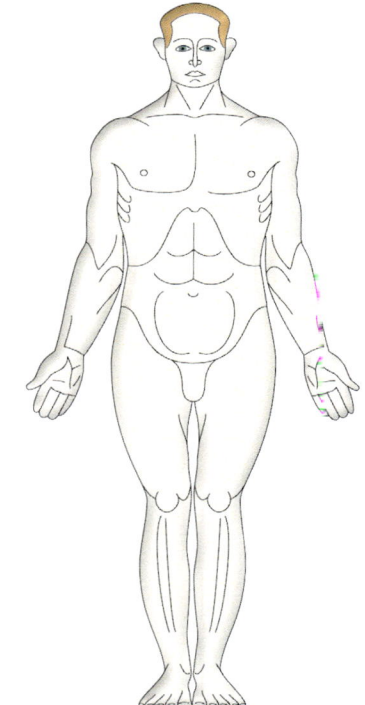

Figure 12.7. Stocky sthenic adult.

- The osteomuscular systems and the cardioarterial system are particularly dominant, with the left heart prevailing over the right heart.
- Systolic arterial pressure is commonly above normal.
- Hematopoiesis is excellent, with polyglobulia.

- This biotype corresponds to the impulsive type or apoplectic habitus of the ancients.
- The reticuloendothelial system, the source of strength and youth, functions in excess. It is responsible for allergic reactions or exaggerated defense to acute infections or poisoning.
- Good muscular development and impulsion allow a good general level of strength and activity.
- Movements are slightly differentiated by the relative shortness of the limbs.
- In the endocrine system, this biotype is dominated by hyperfunctioning adrenocortical and genital steroid hormones, with relative deficiency of the thyroid.
- The internal genitalia are very fertile and overly developed. The genital organs and the secondary sexual characters are well developed.
- Often and precociously, at the age of perimenopause, women have a tendency for menorrhagia and virilism of the adrenal type.
- According to Pende, individuals of tall stature suggest panhyperpituitarism.
- The autonomic nervous system has slight sympathicotonic predominance.
- This biotype corresponds to the temperament of an adolescent or young adult. Aerobic catabolism predominates, with the respiratory and circulatory systems predominant.

Metabolism

- The excess of cholesterol, uric acid, and bilirubin in the blood translates as a tendency to atheromatous arterial lesions as well as renal or subcutaneous precipitation of uric acid.

- The excess of corticosteroids and/or mineralocorticoids generates a certain degree of sodium retention with a loss of potassium.
- Likewise, there is an increased risk of hyperglycemia, no doubt due to pancreatic dysfunction and probably an excess of action by growth hormone, ACTH, and glucocorticoids.

Diagnostic Concerns

The stocky sthenic type is sympathicotonic. They present a hormonal tendency to hypothyroidism and hyperfunctioning of the adrenals, gonads, and pancreas. Because of the strong reactivity of their connective tissue, they are predisposed to ailments of collagen, hypertrophic scars, and visceral fibrosis. Their other pathological predispositions are mainly allergic accidents, arterial hypertension, and gout.

Their strong reactivity makes them ideal candidates for all acute manifestations. Their reactions will be directly generalized, the tissular plasticity being at its maximum. Lumbago and vertebral restrictions of all sorts are common in this biotype, and the etiology is rarely purely mechanical. Mechanical visceral etiologies are often real causes of somatic dysfunction in stocky sthenic individuals.

Watch for nourishment as a source of many therapeutic failures or recurrence. Meat, simple sugars, and acidic condiments such as vinegar maintain inflammation in this hearty eater.

Lanky Sthenic Adult Biotype

Morphotype

- The general aspect is robust, toned, and harmonious, as in an ideally proportioned adult.
- Height is generally taller than average, with the weight a bit low.
- Skeletal and muscular development are excellent. The shoulders are large and wide, the flanks sometimes narrow.
- The limbs have well-designed muscles that are both globular and long.
- The neck and the limbs are slender, and the hands and feet are long but robust, with gnarled fingers and toes.

- The lower limbs are large in relation to the trunk and to the upper limbs.
- The lower half of the body, especially in women, is richer in fat than the upper half, especially with hyperthyroidism.
- The cranium, well endowed with hair, is well developed in all its dimensions. Most often it is of the mesocephalic or dolichocephalic form.
- The three levels of the face are about equal.
- Overall, this biotype has a strong musculature and scant fat reserves (fig. 12.8).

Functions

- The large development of long limbs and of the musculature gives the impression of both strength and precision.
- The skeleton is rich in calcium.
- Hematopoiesis is excellent, and the development of arterial circulation is significant.
- From the neurovegetative point of view, sympathicotonia dominates.
- In the endocrine system, the thyroid and anterior pituitary, especially growth hormone and gonadotrophins, dominate the hormonal balance. Likewise, there is good adrenocortical, medulloadrenal, and genital gland functioning. According to Martiny (1955), even the pineal gland is hyperfunctioning.
- The liver in this biotype is hyperexcitable. Its work is stimulated around-the-clock by thyroid, medulloadrenal, and growth hormones. A strong load of

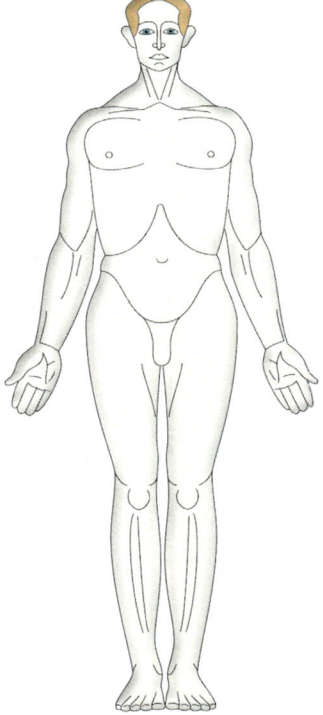

Figure 12.8. Lanky sthenic adult.

241

bilirubin is added to this high degree of activity due to the destruction of red blood cells and muscular activity, and bile secretion is abundant. This is the choleric type described by the ancients.

- This group requires high doses of vitamins B, C, and K.
- This biotype corresponds to the temperament of a mature adult. Anaerobic catabolism is predominant, with a preponderance of systems in which this reaction is made by local tissular oxygen in the muscles.

Metabolism

- The basal metabolic rate is elevated without exaggerated heat wastage. This biotype has a catabolic tendency after considerable physical activity, and a relatively weak digestive capacity.
- Muscular performance is elevated.
- There is relative insulin deficiency with difficulty in accumulating fat and some tendency for hyperglycemia.

Diagnostic Concerns

Lanky sthenic individuals are sympathicotonic and remarkable for their balance of health. They are characterized by a hormonal tendency for pituitary and thyroid hyperfunctioning. Their principle fault is to be mentally unstable. They have a predisposition to the late onset of diverse spasms, Raynaud's phenomenon, and arthrosclerosis. Due to their very high metabolic rate, they are also prone to ailments of the detoxification organs, the liver and gallbladder.

This biotype responds very well to osteoarticular manipulations. It is necessary to systematically check the lower limbs, which can have a cluster of somatic dysfunctions. Carefully investigate the painful area, and in the case of a local dysfunction, do not hesitate to manipulate it. People of this biotype readily retract at the tissular level. Psychologically, they do not tolerate our disinterest in their symptoms or painful regions.

Craniosacral manipulations, when they are indicated, are generally poorly received psychologically. These individuals find them too static, and they doubt their efficacy. It is thus necessary to perform them, if possible, at the end of a session and to spend little time on them.

Lanky Hyposthenic Adult Biotype

Morphotype

- The morphology of the whole body is reminiscent of a prepubescent adolescent.
- Height is often quite tall, sometimes medium, but the general delicacy and fragility of the figure is striking.
- Thinness is typical and is difficult to correct. The subject has a tendency to lose weight with the slightest external affliction.
- The proportions of the stomach in relation to the thorax and the upper limbs differ according to the endocrine formula of the individual.
  - If gonadal deficiency is predominant: the lower limbs are too long in relation to the chest, which is short and narrow.
  - If hyperthyroidism is predominant: the upper limbs and the thorax are long in relation to the lower limbs and to the height of the stomach.
  - If adrenal deficiency is predominant: the thorax is flat and collapsed, the shoulders are narrow and sloping, the stomach is ptosed and concave, and the sternocostal angle is acute.
- The limbs are delicate and thin.
- The hands are long and lightly muscled. The palms have many lines, are poorly designed, and are slightly deep and delicate. The fingers are long and thin.
- The muscles and the skeleton are hypoplastic and soft, and the articular ligaments are hyperlax.
- The cranium is most often large and dolichocephalic.
- The face is somewhat developed and angular.
- The chin is narrow and short. The whole face is triangular, with exaggerated development of the cerebral level and deficiencies of the nasal and buccal levels.

- Most subjects have a long, thin, and convex nose.
- A pointed palatoglossal arch and mandibular retrognathism are very common.
- The teeth are most often pointed: the molars are of small diameter, the incisors trapezoidal, and the canines blunt.
- Hair is often abundant and fine. A low hairline on the brow is a sign of hypogenitalism.
- The neck is long and thin, especially at the nape, and sometimes cylindrical like a swan's neck. The Adam's apple is sometimes jutting and infantile, and in other cases excessively prominent (fig. 12.9).

Functions

- The length of their limbs makes these individuals incapable of using their muscles for significant and prolonged exertion.
- The left heart and the arteries are poorly developed. Blood pressure is low, but emotional jolts can cause momentary systolic hypertension.
- In the digestive system, the stomach is generally atonic and elongated, with hypersecretion and exaggerated peristalsis. The pylorus, duodenum, gallbladder, and even the colon can be ptosed.
- Assimilation is poor:
  - Blood analysis shows low levels of cholesterol and fats.
  - Lack of vitamin B1 produces diverse pain, anoxemia, and constipation accompanied by abdominal distention.

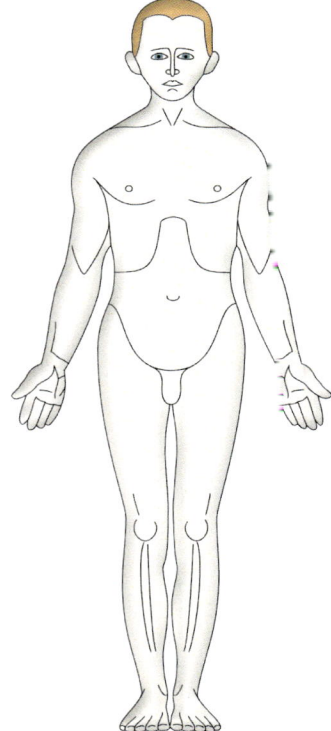

Figure 12.9. Lanky hyposthenic adult.

- Deficiency of vitamin B2 causes cracked lips and mucous membranes as well as a tendency for eczema.
- Deficiency of vitamin B6 causes asthenia and fatigue when walking as well as frequent insomnia.
- Deficiency of vitamin B3 causes some cutaneous problems and a tendency for nervous depression.
- Spasmophilia is common, with hypocalcemia and an increase of vagal tonus.

- In the endocrine system, the thyroid is often hyperfunctioning but unstable. The parathyroids, adrenals, insulin, and genital hormones are always deficient. The pressures of the thyroid and adrenal hormones alternate with an increase in vagal tonus or a lowering of sympathetic tonus.

- Hematopoietic function is mediocre; relative lymphocytosis is common.

- This biotype corresponds to the temperament of an aged person. Cellular excretion is important, and the subject may struggle with an excretory obstruction. It is necessary for the vital organs to rely on excretion. Fighting sclerosis is imperfectly directed by the nervous system.

Metabolism

- People of this biotype are characterized by their weak digestive capacity and strong catabolic tendency, which has two types:
  - Where anabolism is weak, there is increased catabolism and an excess of thyroid hormones. Basal metabolic rate and metabolism with exertion are both elevated, which causes heat loss, hypocalcemia, and hyperreflexia.
  - Where anabolism is weak and catabolism is reduced, there is a pituitary gland deficiency with an adrenal deficiency in androgens and deoxycorticosteroids. The secretion of thyroid hormones is normal; muscular tissue and blood composition are deficient, with only the lymphatic tissue hyperplastic and persistent.

- Glycemia is low and increases with difficulty. There is a tendency to hypoglycemia and exaggerated sensitivity to insulin.
- Hypocholesterolemia is common.

Diagnostic Concerns

Lanky hyposthenic people are generally parasympathicotonic. They present decreased secretions in one or several endocrine glands, usually the adrenals and gonads, generally called *hypocrinism*. They often try to compensate for this tendency with an increase in thyroid activity, which is not always lasting. It is a fragile biotype, and lanky hyposthenic people are rarely sick but always "out of sorts." They are sensitive and rather easily depressed. These individuals correspond to the *habitus phthisicus* of the ancients.

There is a certain degree of pleuropulmonary fragility in this biotype. Their tendency for respiratory ailments is expressed primarily by a predisposition to pneumothorax at a young age, and by a susceptibility to *Mycobacterium tuberculosis* in those with low immune system activity. Based on the laxity in their visceral attachments, they have a marked propensity for ptoses. With age, their myofascial tissues tend to retract notably. They are also predisposed to neurovegetative problems, more or less aggravated by their endocrine dysfunctions. Thyroid instability thus creates a foundation of anxiety, adding to their emotivity and favoring the appearance of cenesthopathic[1] problems. Their complaints generally concern chronic afflictions.

Even if they tolerate structural manipulations well, we must avoid treating the whole body this way. It is preferable to precede structural manipulations with tissular, reflexive, or fluidic techniques to warm and relax them. This biotype needs to have a faultless craniosacral mechanism to assure their neurovegetative equilibrium.

---

1. Cenesthopathy: trouble with the internal sense of bodily existence, consisting of an abnormal bodily sensation, more annoying than painful. It is not accompanied by depression or delirium, and resists therapeutic and psychiatric medications. It is considered to be a sensitivity hallucination.

The embryological biotypes are described in box 12.1.

Box 12.1. Embryological Biotypology

Pende's four basic biotypological categories tally with the embryological biotypes described by William H. Sheldon (1954) and Martiny (1955). Martiny's studies provide a profound explanation of individual morphogenesis and of the sthenic or asthenic components.

According to Martiny, the stocky distortion is attributable to hereditary or congenital predominance of the *endodermic layer* and of the elements derived from it: digestive epithelia from the pharynx to the rectum, the tonsils, the thymus, the parathyroids, the liver, the pancreas, and the islets of Langerhans. The endodermic or stocky biotype is infantile and hypoevolved, with more mass in the trunk and abdominal viscera than on the limbs and head. The organs of vegetative life clearly dominate over those of relational life (Viola, cited by Pende 1955), and anabolism is stronger than catabolism (Pende 1955).

The *mesoderm* is the embryonic layer that forms the structures of strength, combat, and defense: striated muscles, the skeleton, ligaments, aponeuroses, the heart, blood vessels, red blood cells, the spleen, lymph nodes, and the adrenal cortex. Normally there is a natural synergic endomesodermic association. In this case, the synergy of the two systems produces a sthenic biotype. If the mesoderm does not sufficiently balance the dominant endoderm, the result in an adult is the stocky hyposthenic biotype.

If the activity of the *ectoderm* predominates in relation to those of the endoderm and the mesoderm, there will be a predominance of tissues of ectodermic origin: the central nervous system and the peripheral neurovegetative complex, epithelia of the sense organs, epithelia of the mouth, teeth, epidermis, mammary glands, posterior and even anterior lobe of the pituitary gland (the latter is partly of endomesodermic origin), the pineal gland, and the adrenal medulla. This results in an ectodermic biotype, with hypoentodermism and hypomesodermism corresponding to the lanky hyposthenic type, which is characterized by deficient development and activity of the nutritive organs, the musculoskeletal framework, the blood, cardioarterial structures, genital structures, and the reticuloendothelial system.

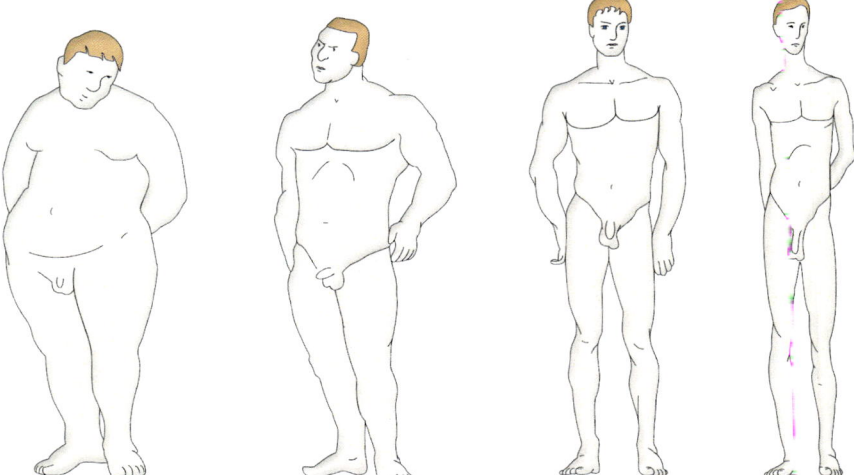

Figure 12.10. Embryological biotypes.

When the ectoderm is dominant but accompanied by sufficient development of entomesodermic organs, it results in the lanky sthenic biotype. Martiny calls this type *chordoblastic*. He theorizes that the notochord, part of the mesodermic layer, has an inductive role, balancing and coordinating harmonious functioning of the three layers. Even in this case, however, the relationship of body length to size persists, and the relational system prevails over the vegetative system (fig. 12.10).

The Psychic Entity

Definitions

Personality

Personality is defined as the dynamic organization of the intellectual, affective, volitional, physiological, and morphological aspects of the individual. This organization arises from innate and acquired factors. It is formed partly from temperament and partly from subjective experiences, expressing itself as character and behavior. Personality governs adaptation and the individual's response to variations in the environment.

Personality Structure

The structure of the personality represents the individual's profound, stable, and definitive psychic organization. It involves four notions:

- individuality
- autonomy
- stability or consistency
- specificity of motivations

Personality Orientation

Two modalities of personality orientation exist: toward the outside and the external environment (extroversion), and toward the inside and intimacy with the self (introversion). It is not necessary to consider this parameter as a static state that is fixed in the personality, but as a dynamic orientation, a process in motion.

Extroversion

The extroverted personality is entirely defined by relations with the outside world. These individuals need presence and contact. They easily lose their stability when alone. Perfectly integrated in society, extroverts are attached to concrete ideas and actual objects, beings, and events. They rarely believe in the existence of invisible forces. They follow the customs and rules of their age and culture. They easily externalize their feelings, which, like their thoughts, accord with those of the community. They follow their instincts and indulge in sensuality and food. They are candidly straightforward and readily show themselves as generous. Cordial and amiable, they are often brilliant conversationalists with easy, witty replies.

Introversion

Introverts live within themselves and are detached from the outside world. Internal events and the internal reverberations of external events are what matter to them. They barely trust the data from their senses. What they feel within the intimacy of their being appears much more real. They believe in invisible and secret forces hidden in the soul. They live on the sidelines of the world. They are unsociable and often resist the status quo. They need solitude. Readily misanthropic, they have very personal feelings and opinions that differ from those of the majority. They fear human contact and avoid it. They find it difficult to externalize their feelings and thoughts. They do not readily follow their own instincts, and sometimes fight them. They can be seduced by the idea of an ascetic life: sexual abstinence, frugality, sobriety, etc. Introverts barely open their hearts, seeming cold and reserved. They are always modest about their feelings and do not easily divulge their thoughts. They are not always capable of expressing themselves: either they don't have the words or they lack witty comments to share.

Character

Character is the entirety of observable traits in an individual that defines a manner of behavior. It emanates from the base structure of the personality, the affective and behavioral exteriorization of relational life. Character is the permanent basis that people always resort to in similar situations. It is partly determined by the socioaffective environment. Character relies on four components:

- emotivity

- activity
- reverberation
- field of conscience

Emotivity

Emotion is an agitation produced by the individual from the shock of a perception or a thought. It liberates varying amounts of energy. Emotivity, also called *psychic sensibility* or *psychoesthesia*, corresponds to the ability for emotions to be released in the organism by environmental influences. Depending on the situation, we use the terms *psychohyperesthesia, psychohypoesthesia,* or *psychodysesthesia.*

Activity

Activity, also called *volitivity,* is the capacity to exert an influence on the environment. Active individuals live to act, and difficulties encourage them to act. In the same circumstances, inactive individuals become discouraged. Will, a determining element of activity, gets its energy from emotivity. The value of activity is shown through the power of an exerted action, which is itself determined by two elements: *strength* and *continuity.* Depending on the degree of volitivity, we use the terms *hyperbulia* or *hypobulia,* which is very different from *abulia,* when all will is absent.

Reverberation

The "response time" of the individual is the time period between a stimulus and the response. It defines the notions of *primarity* and *secondarity.*

Primary Reverberation (Primarity)

The action has a short pathway, and the response is almost immediate. Primary reverberation individuals react at once and rapidly to any stimulus. They have much spontaneity and naturalness, but they are impulsive. Their intelligence is lively but not very deep. Their reactions last for some time, and their goals are short-range. They love change, have a tendency to live day to day, and often seem capricious.

251

Secondary Reverberation (Secondarity)

Secondary reverberation or *secondarity* is the inverse tendency. In this case, the action has a long pathway. Excitation is delayed in the organism, with the response slowed by a braking influence. Secondarity never lets itself succumb to its first response. These individuals lack natural spontaneity. They calculate everything and know how to keep "cool." Reason dominates their hearts. Their intelligence is more deep than vivid. Reactions are prolonged. Their goals are long-range. They love durability and have the spirit to follow and persevere. They easily remember what makes them loyal, but they can also have spiteful tendencies.

Character Modulation

The three components described above have different manifestations depending on the field of conscience and the egocentric or allocentric nature of the individual. The fullness of the field of conscience has a narrow or wide scope:

- Egocentric individuals are incapable of leaving their own center of vision.
- Allocentric individuals, by contrast, understand the situation of others by being able to put themselves in their shoes.

Note: it is important not to confuse these terms with *egoism* and *altruism.* An egocentric person may be an altruist, and an egoistic person may be allocentric. The first are capable of loving those near them like themselves, but without understanding it. The second, able to guess all of the psychological behavior of others, can use that quality to exploit them.

Intelligence

All the elements of character influence intelligence. We can artificially separate intelligence from character. Intelligence can be considered the *synthesis of all abilities that give us the means to know the world.* The creative, fundamental element truly is thought.

Somatopsychic Bonds

The physical and psychic aspects of human beings are not independent things; numerous observations attest to this. It is not easy to determine the causality and the structure of these extremely complex bonds, as witnessed clinically. Somatopsychic systematizations differ according to the schools of biotypology. Beyond differences of points of view and vocabulary, however, they blend, allowing development of an image of psychic functioning for each type of individuals.

Mind-Illness Correlations

Research in psychosomatic medicine tries to analyze the links between illness and psychology. Generally, psychosomatic expression of an illness is due to the emotional repercussions of a shock or tension. By contrast, modification of metabolic activity can induce specific psychological behavior. Medical semiology describes numerous psychic phenomena provoked by certain physiological alterations. Studies have allowed us to establish causal relationships between corporal functions and psychology. For example:

- Modified physical activity has a euphoric effect. Exaggerated effort can overwhelm us and slow us down.
- Respiratory exercises, like those used in certain psychotherapy techniques or in the practice of yoga, provoke sensations of liberation and psychic expansion; conversely, respiration that is voluntarily maintained beyond ideal values of rhythm and amplitude can generate anxiety and a troubled conscience.
- Any excessive change in metabolic equilibrium (glucose, urea, etc.) leads to psychic problems with nervousness and fatigability, then delirious states, and finally an alteration of consciousness that can result in coma.
- Psychic emotions and tension have enormous consequences for the body. In return, physical tensions bring up psychic tensions. We all know that a deep tissue massage, correctly done, is emotionally relaxing: it surely relaxes the body, but it also calms the spirit.

253

Links between soma and psyche are established by the paths of the autonomic nervous system and metabolism in general. The links are complex, and their direction is not unambiguous. Thus depression, anxiety, and stress accompany physical symptoms of which interpretation can vary.

In Western cultures, fatigue, weight variation, and irregularities in the cardiac rhythm are considered physical manifestations of a mental problem. In Asian cultures, sadness, loss of self-esteem, feelings of guilt, and the absence of pleasure are the mental repercussions of a physical problem.

Other Correlations

Certain physical data are linked to specific character traits. There is a parallel between the psychic expression of character and the significance of specific corporal structures. In this way, biotype also seems to be a good indicator of personality.

Typological research has established groupings of stable or regular psychophysical relationships. Endocrinology has furnished certain points to support these studies. For example, it is possible to establish some links between certain particularities of the skin, subcutaneous tissues, and osseous structure with alterations concerning emotivity and activity. Causality is not established in this correlation. It only concerns correspondences frequently observed statistically.

Another somatopsychic relationship is figurative. The functions and organs of the body have symbolic significance. Respiration symbolizes contact with the world, the heart relates to the emotions and love, the head represents spiritual existence, and so on. Various systematizations have been proposed to try to connect pathologies or the organs with corresponding symbols. At this level, somatopsychic relationships go beyond the framework of causality to become a mode of expressing a "sign."

The Principle of Expansion and Retraction

Biological Principle

For certain French morphopsychologists like Louis Corman (1988) or Claude Sigaud (1890), the shape of a living being expresses adaptation of the organism to the environment in which it is placed. Analysis of this shape allows us to discern the reaction mood of the individual (fig. 12.11). The *self-preservation instinct* is characteristic of life. It is especially developed in those whose vitality is declining and for those whose lives are placed in danger, meaning when the individual must conserve strength to survive. The true instinct of life is the *expansion instinct*. It pushes toward conquest of the external world and action within the environment. In the surroundings of life, some contradictory influences come together. Individuals possess two adaptation possibilities—expansion and retraction:

- In a favorable environment, the human shape expands with the instinct of expansion.

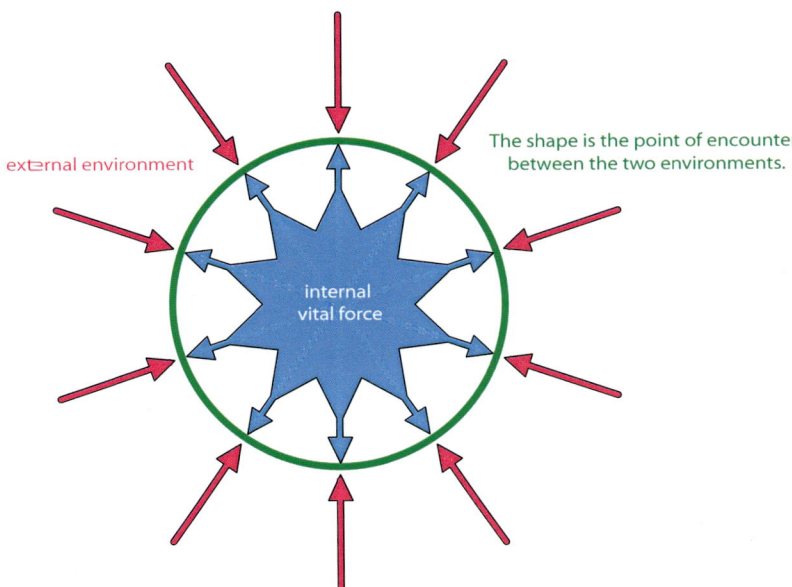

external environment

The shape is the point of encounter between the two environments.

internal vital force

Figure 12.11. Shape as the result of interaction.

255

- In a hostile environment, individuals curl up on themselves and retract due to the instinct of self-preservation.

In identical conditions, some subjects expand while others retract. The external appearance of the organism, especially visible in the face, reveals the predominant reaction tendency and allows us to define two groups. The *dilated type* corresponds to expansion in a favorable environment. The dilated face is large and shaped like a circle, an oval, or a rectangle with rounded corners (fig. 12.12). The pattern is round, the lines curved, and plumpness is common. The complexion is clear, colored by the flow of blood to the skin. The sensory receptors are somewhat open to the external world. The mouth is rather large, the lips fleshy, and the nostrils enlarged. The eyes are large, prominent, and wide apart.

The *retracted type* corresponds to taking shelter, as in an unfavorable environment. The retracted face is generally long, narrow, and shaped like an inverted triangle or a narrow rectangle (fig. 12.13). The face shows straight and angular lines. The structure is a bit fleshy and bony. The complexion is pale. The sensory receptors are slightly open, at times hooded, and in truth closed. The lips are pinched and the nostrils half-closed. The eyes, sunken and close together, appear small.

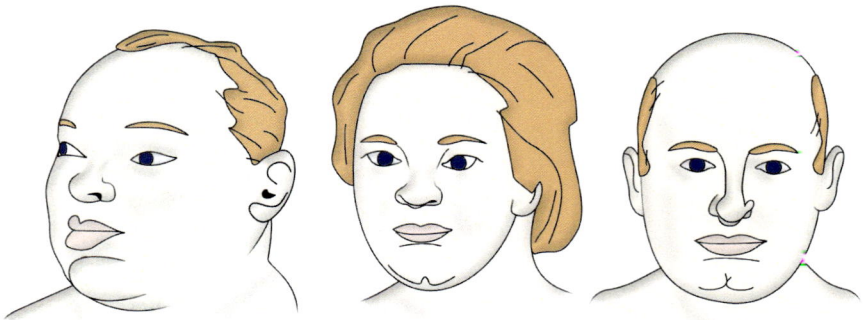

Figure 12.12. Dilated faces (after Corman 1988).

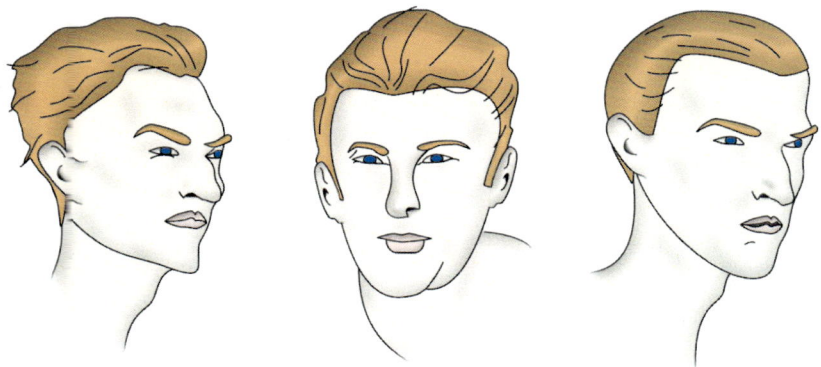

Figure 12.13. Retracted faces (after Corman 1988).

Psychic Expression of Expansion and Retraction

In all the areas of relational life, Corman studied the expression of the predominance of the expansion instinct or the self-preservation instinct.

Dilated Type

Individuals of the dilated type are endowed with a personality oriented toward extroversion. They externalize without holding back their instincts. They are fond of food and drink, sensual, combative, and quick-tempered. In terms of character, their activities are supported by the vitality of expansion and by primary reverberation. When they feel resentment toward someone, they quickly explode into a heated anger, which dissipates rapidly. Their affective life is abundant. Dilated people are sociable and amiable with everyone. Usually in a good mood, they cannot do without company.

Retracted Type

The personality of retracted individuals is oriented toward introversion. Their activities hinge on the vitality of self-preservation and secondary reverberation. Retracted individuals have restrained instincts that are resistant to being induced externally and manifest only with an internal impulse. Their affective life is limited to the narrow field of immediate family. They are slightly good-natured but don't really like society.

257

They are reserved, taciturn, and secretive. When someone physically bumps into them, instead of reacting with sudden anger, they fold up and reflect on their injuries.

SUMMARY

These two types are complementary. They see that the other has worth, precisely because of what they themselves lack.

- Dilated people are worthy for the fullness of their external lives and for their excellent integration in social groups. However, they lack individuality, independence of character, internal principles, and the will to pursue their actions.
- Retracted people are worthy, by contrast, for their individuality, independence, refusal to be swayed, the personal character of their ideas, and their capacity for making decisions. On the other hand, they lack adaptation to the present, flexibility, common sense, and speed in their actions.

Equilibrium is necessarily a blending of the dilated and retracted types.

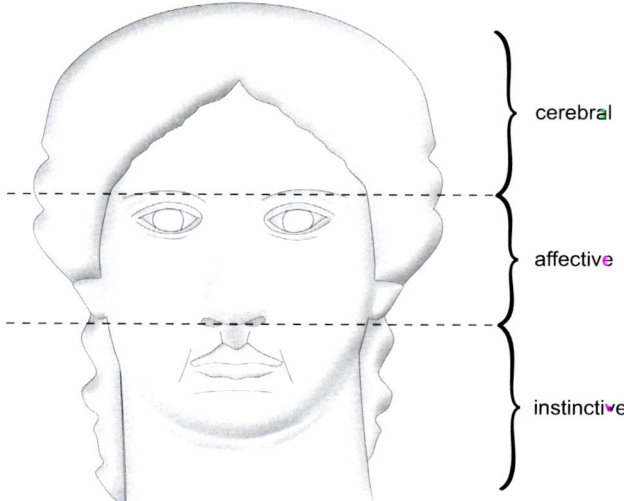

Figure 12.14. The three levels of the face.

258

The Levels of the Face

This principle of expansion and retraction can be extrapolated to the analysis of certain proportions of the body. The proportions of the different levels of the face are rich in information on somatopsychic correlations (fig. 12.14). The height and volume of each zone must be examined. When one level of the face is predominant, we generally find a preponderance of the corresponding psychic tendency. Conversely, weak development generally accompanies a deficiency of that psychic frame of mind.

Superior Zone: Cerebral

The superior zone stretches from the hairline to the top of the nose. It contains the encephalon, the organ of thought and the seat of all intellectual life. It corresponds to thought, conscious life, intelligence, rationality, and spirituality.

Median Zone: Affective

The median zone is from the eyebrows to the upper lip. It contains the eyes, the nose, and the ears. It represents reception of the external world and receives sensations. It is the frame of mind for affectivity, sensibility, emotivity, and contact with others. This zone maintains privileged connections with the thorax: the respiratory rhythm that enlivens it. Likewise, the emotions and the soul are linked, and they are displayed in the eyes.

Inferior Zone: Instinctive

The inferior zone is situated between the nostrils and the chin. It is the vegetative level, where physical sensations, organic needs, and instincts arise. It responds to action, sexuality, and will. This zone maintains close connections with the abdomen. The mouth is a link with both alimentary and reproductive needs.

The German School

Ernst Kretschmer, a German psychiatrist, analyzed the links that could exist between psychiatric pathologies, temperaments, and morphotypes.

Kretschmer's Morphotypes

Kretschmer (1925) considers four basic morphotypes, which he designates *leptosomatic, pyknic, athletic,* and *dysplasic.* Their physical characters can be summarized:

- Leptosomatic or asthenic: growth is normal in height, reduced in breadth. Leptosomatics are rather lanky. The shapes are dry and angular, the visceral cavities reduced, the trunk long, and the limbs thin and slender.
- Pyknic: They present a relative predominance of horizontal dimensions over the vertical ones. *Pyknic* come from the Greek *pyknos,* which means "stocky"; it is the stocky biotype. The shapes are round and opulent, the visceral cavities voluminous, the trunk padded with fat, and the limbs short.
- Athletic: They possess a powerful skeleton and strong, well-defined musculature. The shapes are robust as though hewn with a hatchet. The trunk is cylindrical, the breadth powerful, and the limbs strongly muscled with paw-like hands.
- Dysplasic: Nature has not been kind to these individuals. They are a varied and heterogenous group comprising all the deformities and hereditary endocrine aliments.

Kretschmer's Temperaments

Kretschmer defines two opposing temperaments, cyclothymic and schizothymic, between which there are many intermediate states.

- *Cyclothymic:* individuals are extroverted, their spirit turned toward the outside, in good contact with reality.

- *Schizothymic:* individuals are introverted, their spirit turned inside, folding on themselves; typically dreamers and logicians.

Kretschmer's Typology

Combinations of physical and psychic factors allowed Kretschmer to define four types (fig. 12.15). According to his classification, leptosomatic individuals are *schizothymic,* while pyknic individuals are *cyclothymic.* Besides these two forms, Kretschmer also outlined the *epileptoid* constitution.

Type	Physique	Personality	In the Movies
Pyknic	small and round	expansive, joyful, spontaneous, realistic	Danny DeVito
Leptosomatic	tall and thin	reserved, cool, a dreamer	Clint Eastwood
Athletic	broad and muscled	impulsive, quick-tempered	Harvey Keitel
Dysplasic	poorly developed, scrawny, anomalous	asthenic, feels inferior	Mr. Bean Woody Allen

Figure 12.15. Kretschmer's four morphotypes.

Cyclothymic Pyknic Constitution

Their natural tendency is to oscillate between *joy* (soaring) and *sadness* (depression), and between mobility and clumsiness. Endowed with a degree of intuition, their posture is open, natural, and soft, usually adjusted to the circumstances. These individuals are the rotund, good-natured type, with an expansive sense of humor and somewhat pathological sociability; they alternate between joyous excitation and melancholic depression. When they are balanced, we call them *syntonic,* meaning realistic, practical, and well-harmonized (fig. 12.16).

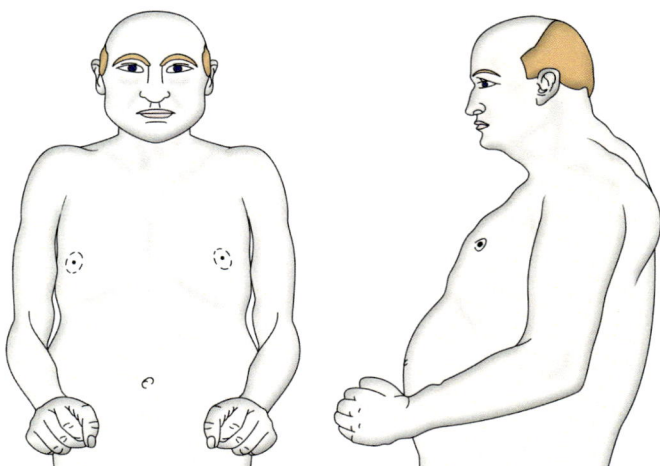

Figure 12.16. Kretschmer's pyknic type.

Schizothymic Leptosomatic Constitution

The psychic tone of these individuals comprises oscillations between *sensitivity* (hyperesthesia) and *coldness* (anesthesia). According to Kretschmer, their temperament is seen alternately in two modes of expression: *capricious hastiness* and the *rebellious stubbornness*. They are reserved people who use reflection to calculate their adaptation to the environment. Their posture often appears inadequate for the circumstances: reserved, lazy, slothful, and rigid. They have an arched back, keep their humor locked away, are silent, solitary, and laboriously sociable, oscillating between sulky irritability and scornful indifference. When they are balanced, we call them *intermediary,* meaning energetic, tenacious, systematically logical, and calm (fig. 12.17).

Epileptoid Constitution

The epileptoid constitution corresponds to athletic and dysplasic types. Their tendency varies between *viscosity* (calm and dull) and *explosivity.* Body language is moderated, the imagination restrained, and language laconic. Athletic individuals are not nervous, giving the impression of considerable affective stability. Under the influence of accumulated

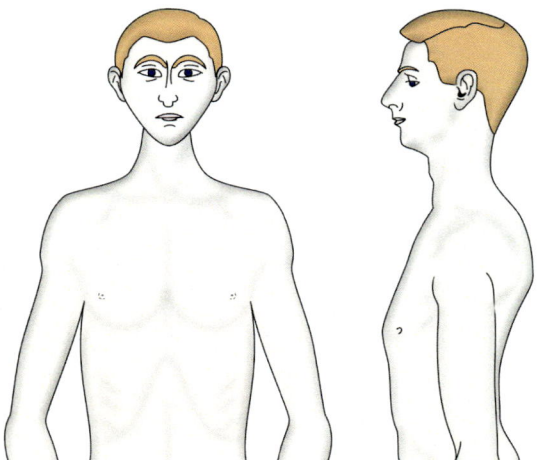

Figure 12.17. Kretschmer's leptosomatic type.

excitations, however, emotions discharge in an explosive way. These individuals are predisposed to convulsive manifestations. They are the "sentimental brute" type, with vigorous, impulsive, and opinionated passions, ranging from exacting tenderness and jealousy to furious and violent hatred (fig. 12.18).

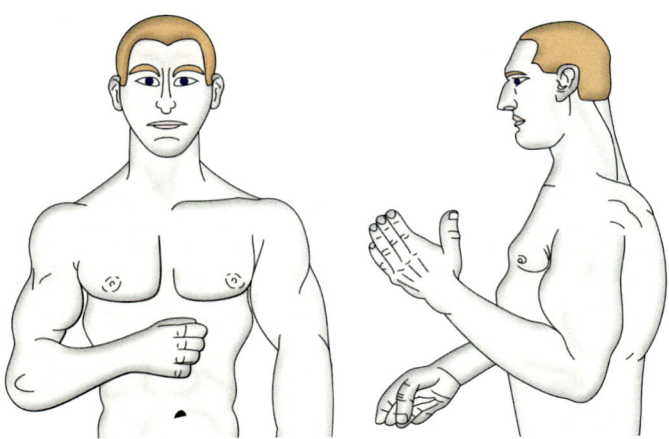

Figure 12.18. Kretschmer's athletic type.

Precision

German psychiatry's anthropometric classification has raised some important points of discussion, but its strengths are in its findings. Kretschmer's originality is in the classification of psychic types that he proposes. It rests on the distinction between cyclical psychosis (a cycle of alternating states of depression and excitation) and precocious dementia. Remember that Kretschmer was a psychiatrist. He was studying mentally ill people when he was inspired by the correlations between mental afflictions and physical constitution.

He affirms that the two major forms of morbid behavior, schizophrenia and bipolar disorder, are only alterations of normal behavior. Related to schizophrenics are the schizoid characters (capricious, eccentric, opinionated, strange, defiant, etc.). The schizoid character can precede the appearance of psychosis or be found in its origins.

The cycloid character is common in families with an incidence of bipolar disorder. Hypomanic characters (excited, unsettled, joyful, boisterous) and subdepressive characters (inhibited, heavy, discouraging) are found in this group, as are some cycloid depressives with heightened agitation and depressive inhibitions.

This theory supports the idea that, from normal personality to psychosis, there are only quantitative transitions in sequence:

normal	→	pathological	→	psychotic
schizothymic	→	schizoid	→	schizophrenic
cyclothymic	→	cycloid	→	bipolar disorder

The Embryological School

The embryological typology of William H. Sheldon (1954) provides the notion of type and introduces the morphological "component" or "dimension." The germ layers of the embryo determine the morphological tendencies of the adult. Sheldon distinguishes three types:

- endomorphic
- mesomorphic
- ectomorphic

They correspond in large part to Kretschmer's pyknic, athletic, and leptoscmatic types. The psychological correspondences are respectively:

- viscerotonia
- somatotonia
- cerebrotonia

Viscerotonia

Viscerotonia characterizes beings in which the visceral functions predominate. Individuals are carried away by pleasures that provide tranquility and digestion. A certain degree of slowness arises from this behavior. They have a slack personality, endowed with a large capacity for compensation, adaptation, and relaxation. Their tendencies are toward extroversion and primary reverberation.

Somatotonia

Somatotonia is found in people whose locomotory functions surpass the other functions. They need to move and expend energy to maintain psychic balance. They are persevering and tenacious, with behavior that is much firmer than that of viscerotonic individuals. Their reaction time is moderate, and they are endowed with a great psychic robustness. Their reactions are generally explosive despite seeming emotionally stable on the surface.

Cerebrotonia

Cerebrotonia characterizes individuals whose intellect is always on the move. They find balance in the imaginary and satisfaction with their large need for reflection. Their psychic reactions happen at maximized speed, but their behavior is unpredictable. They have a tense and contracted personality that they control at all times. Frequently inhibited and timid, their spirit is always awake. Easily fatigued, they need good-quality sleep to recharge themselves. Their personality is clearly introverted and has tendencies of secondary reverberation.

The composition of these character structures is outlined in figure 12.19.

265

Viscerotonia	Somatotonia	Cerebrotoria
1. flaccid behavior	1. tense, firm behavior	1. timid, inhibited, contracted behavior
2. easy bearing	2. adventurously sporty	2. pronounced physiological excitability
3. slow reactions	3. very rapid reactions	3. very rapid reactions
4. gluttonous	4. needs physical exercise	4. enjoys solitude
5. enjoys guests	5. wants to dominate	5. awakened spirit, precise observations, application
6. enjoys tranquility	6. enjoys taking risks	6. emotively reserved
7. enjoys conventions	7. easygoing	7. mimicry and controlled gestures
8. social	8. combative	8. antisocial
9. congenial to everyone	9. enjoys competition	9. inhibited social behavior
10. wants sympathy and appreciation	10. psychically robust	10. difficulty acquiring customs or routines
11. oriented to the environment	11. claustrophobic	11. agoraphobic
12. equality of emotional experience	12. lacks scruples	12. unpredictable behavior
13. tolerant	13. arrogant in speech	13. humble in speech
14. vain	14. dislikes physical pain	14. sensitive to pain
15. sleeps deeply	15. enjoys noise	15. sleeps poorly, fatigable
16. lacks zest	16. seems more mature than his or her age	16. juvenile behavior
17. immediate affective contact	17. horizontal psychic split, extroverted	17. vertical psychic split, introverted
18. relaxed and social when drinking	18. argumentative and aggressive when drinking	18. stable when drinking
19. wants company in grief	19. seeks activity in grief	19. seeks solitude in grief
20. imaginatively orientated to infancy and family relations	20. oriented to goals and activities of childhood	20. oriented to advanced age

Figure 12.19. Somatopsychic correspondences of Sheldon (1954) and Kretschmer (1925).

266

Personalities of the Four Basic Morphotypes

Pende (1955), citing the psychiatrist Maxime Laignel-Lavastine, evaluates psychic aspects by:

- the *characterogram*, which represents the whole of instinctive, affective, and volatile tendencies
- the *psychoideogram*, the whole of the characters of the ideative sphere
- the *ergotypogram*, the behavior of individuals in their life work
- the *sociotypogram*, the behavior of individuals in their social connections

Each of the four basic biotypes thus possesses socio-, psycho-, and ergocharacterological characteristics. Some mixed transitory states of these diverse psychic constitutions exist.

Stocky Hyposthenic Adult Biotype

- They are extroverts with predominant viscerotonia.
- Individuals of this biotype have sluggish, atonic, and asthenic functioning, called *bradypraxism*.
- With a passive and tranquil nature, they are rarely combative, and their reactivity is weak. Calmness, apathy, and sedentary lifestyle aid the relaxation of their psychic tension. Hypoesthesia is the rule.
- Psychomotor reactions are slow.
- The natural tendency is toward pleasures of sleep, food, and drink, with a weak libido. Women of this biotype take the initiative sexually.
- Social qualities are cool, patient, and regulated.
- Intelligence is dormant and analytical.
- People of this biotype lack the strength to concentrate but possess good imaginative capacity. They often prefer to live in a dream world.
- This biotype displays these characters: obedient, patient, methodical, diligent, meticulous, timid, and endowed with great kindness based in abandon and passivity. They can adapt to monotonous work (fig. 12.20).

267

Stocky Sthenic Adult Biotype

- The dominant character trait is extroversion. Somatotonia is the rule.
- Individuals of this biotype are not very sensitive and are rough-hewn, energetic, and nomadic. They are combative, hot-tempered, impulsive, and readily sensual.
- They love the outdoors (hunting, exploring, etc.), meat dishes, and strong drink. They also have excellent esthetic sensibility.
- This biotype does not have great resistance to physical exertion. They systematically seek out activity.
- Due to their cycloid tendency, they are subject to depression despite their elevated tonus.
- Psychomotor reactions are not very rapid but are strong and long-lasting.
- Social qualities are courage, passion for life, and love of a battle. They adapt easily to varied and irregular kinds of work.
- Slightly profound, their intelligence is essentially analytical, objective, and concrete (fig. 12.21).

Lanky Sthenic Adult Biotype

- They are introverted and somewhat obscured by their numerous possibilities.
- In terms of temperament, they are sthenic in all functions, but with a tendency toward exhaustion.
- They have quick reaction time and are more muscular and nervous than psychic.
- The character is balanced and positive. They are readily dominant over others and themselves.
- Sexuality is powerful but controlled, with a slight predisposition for men to be gay. Women are often hyperestrogenic and rich in somatic and psychic heterosexual signs.
- They are straightforward, frank, and lack respect for others. They have little sense of humor.
- They have paranoid or epileptoid tendencies.

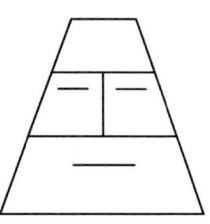 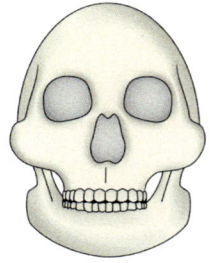 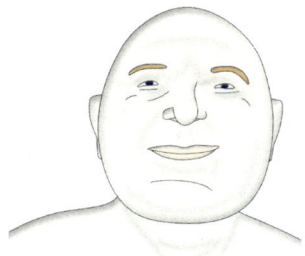

Figure 12.20. Face structure of a stocky hyposthenic adult.

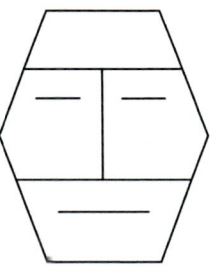 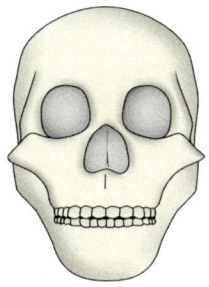 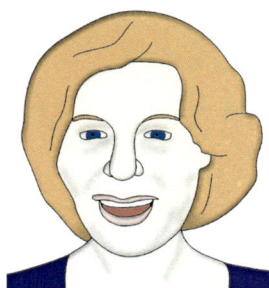

Figure 12.21. Face structure of a stocky sthenic adult.

- They have violent and tenacious emotivity and a passionate nature, which is relatively well controlled in individuals with very active thyroid and adrenal functions.
- In those with a predominant pituitary gland, this emotivity hides behind false coldness.
- For these reasons, this biotype seems more inclined than others to crimes of passion and violent murder.
- Their intelligence is often remarkable, lively, intuitive, artistic, and synthetic.
- In their social lives, they are predominantly masterful, quick to make decisions and adapt.
- As Kretschmer observed, this biotype is the most predisposed to schizophrenia (fig. 12.22).

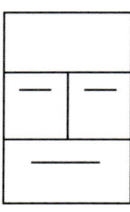 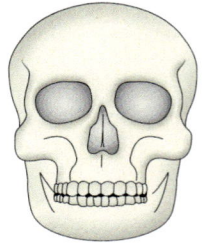 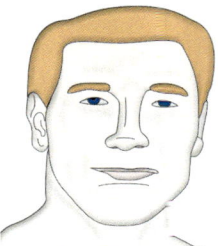

Figure 12.22. Face structure of a lanky sthenic adult.

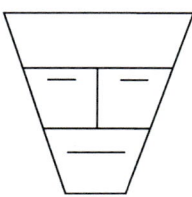 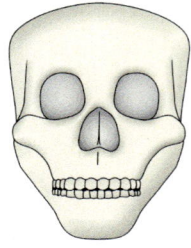 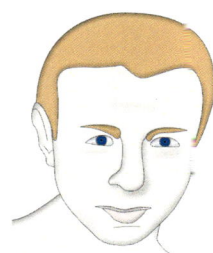

Figure 12.23. Face structure of a lanky hyposthenic adult.

Lanky Hyposthenic Adult Biotype

- Characterologically, lanky hyposthenic individuals are hypersensitive introverts. Their vitality is measured. Their emotivity is marked and modulated by fatigability.
- Psychically, they are cerebrotonic. They have great mental activity and lively intelligence augmented by a good imagination. Individuals in this biotype have a good sense of the abstract and a certain degree of goodwill. However, they are readily depressed, introverted, and schizothymic.
- Mystic and metaphysical tendencies are common. Haunting ideas as well as mental and affective dissociation are often observed.
- Psychomotor reactions are excessive and rapid but unstable because exhaustion is rapid. There is more speed than motor ability.
- Overall, they are pessimistic, lively, imaginative, sentimental, and romantic.
- They make intellectually schizoid workers (fig. 12.23).

270

Evaluation of Personality

The impact of patients' personalities on their therapeutic support is often very significant. In practice, evaluating personality is done throughout the consultation with all the information that patients communicate. Certain semiological elements allow us to discern individual profiles. Individuals may present various traits of different personalities without a pathological personality.

Evaluation of personality requires caution. Not only are hasty judgments often erroneous, but it is sometimes necessary to have several consultations for patients to reveal their true colors. Likewise, I have seen that in a period of crisis, characteristic traits may be exaggerated or truly distorted.

Criteria and Limits of Normality

The notion of normality, which depends on the largest percentage of behaviors, implies a *collective ideal.* All deviations from a statistical mean are considered pathological. In psychology, normality cannot be prescribed based on largest percentages. That would risk confusion between psychological balance and social conformity. The notion of normality, which is articulated around a functional criterion, is defined as the optimal functioning of an individual, taking into account his or her specific psychological characters. In this case, normality adheres to the fact that personality traits are numerous, less intense, and flexible through different events and stages of life. Decompensation toward pathology corresponds to a break in the equilibrium among the different reactional and adaptive modalities of the individual without changing the basic structure.

Pathological Personalities

Pathological personalities are permanent states characterized by quantitative deviations in relation to a personality called "normal." According to the psychiatrist Kurt Schneider (1959), *the quantitative anomalies of the personality only become pathological when they involve suffering, whether of the individual or of society.* In principle, psychic symptoms do not exist as they do in neurotic or psychotic states. The pathological personality is stuck in a predominant mode of functioning that is the origin of psychic suffering or significant social maladaptation. Character traits are less numerous and very marked.

There is great diversity in the nomenclature for pathological personalities. These theoretical classifications have an especially didactic goal because, in practice, an individual can present character traits belonging to several pathological personality types.

Clinical Examples of Pathological Personalities

It is desirable to know the psychological details of certain pathological personalities in order to best evaluate somatic symptoms and to avoid some pitfalls.

Hysterical or Histrionic Personality

Hysterical individuals are not always aware of what they are doing—their possibilities for introspection are reduced. This type of personality, more common in women, is characterized by:

- *Histrionic behavior* dominates the picture and is often the first thing we see. Hysterical individuals seek to please, to seduce, and to corner the attention of spectators. Their vocabulary is readily emphatic and lacks naturalness. Eminently an actor, always performing, they can change roles when their audience changes.
- *Mythomania:* sensitive to external influences, they live through others by substitution and through successive identifications. They are very disposed to dreaming, and mythomania is characterized by denial of reality and refuge in the imaginary. At times, there is a mix of reality and lies, of invention and suggestibility, with mystifications, all supported by strong conviction.
- *Seductive behavior:* it is possible to confuse hysteria with hypersexuality. They attempt seduction with manipulation and provocative posture, whether in an erotic mode concerned with physical attraction or in an infantile and nonerotic mode.

272

- *Emotional liability* and *intolerance to frustrations:* their affectivity is versatile and unstable but not simulated. Their feelings, even if exaggerated, are experienced with intensity. They are often irritable, capricious, and impulsive as well as incapable of distancing themselves from the annoying events of daily life. Thus emotional discharges are spectacular scenes of crisis with tears or anger. Frustrations can also cause depression and anxiety. The general tendency is dissatisfaction.
- *Egocentrism:* hysteria has the tendency to bring everything back to itself. Hysterical individuals indulge only in the self without respect for others. Others only exist for the satisfaction of their needs as narcissistic support.
- *Affective dependence:* hysterical individuals avoid authentic affective relations; however, they constantly need others:
  - to be worthy through altruistic tasks—their personal sacrifice is a measure of their dependence on others.
  - to put themselves in charge in order to get the protection, reassurance, and approval of the group. In this case, they are particularly immature and infantile with a generally timid, unobtrusive, and inhibited posture. Social integration is poor, conflicts are denied, and sexuality is almost nonexistent.
- *Problems with sexuality* are displayed in the hysterical personality:
  - Women can display hyperfemininity. Their seductive coquetry masks their sexual inhibitions. They seek out a multiplicity of sexual adventures, often deceptively. Failure is a repetitive behavior, and they avoid long-lasting commitments.
  - They may also avoid all forms of sexual relations, or not take pleasure in them. Hypoactive sexual desire can then express deep rejection of their gender. They prefer platonic friendships and reject those who try to become sexual. To try to mask their questionable way of life, they invent romantic and secret love stories, often an imaginary or real veiled theme in childhood.

The psychopathological decompensations presented by patients are of two sorts:

- *Somatization:* all hysterical personalities have a tendency to somatize. Somatization can be moderate or transitory, with character and sexuality problems appearing first in the clinical picture. In ill adults, somatization is more marked because it is the only solution for conflicts: fatigue, pain, neuropathological crisis, or manifestations of hysterical conversion are then rediscovered.
- *Depression:* asthenic and anxious, depression happens in reaction to frustration and surrender. Often short-lived, in the context of affective blackmail (suicide attempts) by young women with hysteria, depressive decompensations tend to become more severe and more rambling with age. An aged hysteric may appear as a chronic and invalid hypochondriac.

In men, the hysterical character is rarer and poorly tolerated socially. Being histrionic translates as boastfulness, bragging, or embellishment of favorable adventures, or hysteria seeks to mask weakness. Their desire to please and perpetual virility quest easily induce philandering along with multiple and unsatisfying relationships. Frequently they present sexual difficulties such as impotence and premature ejaculation. At times they sever heterosexual relationships, preferring male friendships or alternately displaying homophobia. In men, the hysterical character is often associated with psychopathological unbalanced traits: instability, impulsivity, minor delinquency, alcoholism, drug addiction, etc.

The Therapist's Position

The tendency toward somatization of hysteria makes any therapist a potential savior. This relationship, however, does not proceed without difficulty. You will successfully play the savior, and then be helpless and truly incapable. You may face, by turns, the tinted docility of admiration and clearly expressed somatic complaints that nothing can alleviate. When this happens, do not let yourself be too soft or deprecate yourself, and do not let yourself be seduced. It is important not to give in to either antipathy or charm. Don't let yourself be drawn into the multiple levels of the consultation. It is necessary to practice an attentive and patient listening with kindly neutrality that will not be mistaken for indifference.

Hysteria is not simulated; it is simply an accessory of the patient's problems that are rooted in unconscious conflicts. The hysterical personality rises from the pathological resolution of conflicted sexuality, or repression of aggressive and sexual urges.

Paranoid Personality

The paranoid personality is characterized by *self-overestimation,* which is manifested most of the time by arrogance and pride. Personally infallible, paranoiac individuals judge others severely and often scornfully, and they readily attempt to redress perceived wrongs. They never question their own opinions. Never wrong themselves, they feel misunderstood and stubbornly push their own way of seeing things on everything and everyone. At times, fake modesty and a conceited front mask the paranoia.

The paranoid personality is also marked by *absence of an internal critic* and *duplicity of judgment,* which are truly consequences of this ego hypertrophy. Their thought process is rigid and systematized. Permeated by unalterable principles, these individuals are seen as overbearing and intolerant toward others.

Finally, *distrust* and *irritability* mark their relations to others. Their distrust is manifested by a disposition to doubt others and their affirmations or intentions. Unjustified doubts about the fidelity of friends, spouses, or collaborators are frequent. Their irritability is omnipresent, to the point that even innocuous information can have personal and intentional significance. They feel surrounded by a malevolent and envious universe, which makes them hypervigilant.

Social maladaptation is the rule. Paranoiac individuals have a difficult life because they are combative. Their reactions to perceived situations, such as persecution, are variable:

- They can make aggressive demands with complaints, procedures, threats, and revolts: these paranoid personalities are called *combative* or *aggressive*.
- On the contrary, they can react by elaborating on the goodness of the world according to a theoretical system: these paranoid personalities are called *wishful* and display passionate idealism.

If possible, the company of these shady, egocentric, aggressive, jealous, and readily tyrannical individuals and their entourages are to be avoided.

Their posture is heightened and rigid, and they display demanding and vindictive behavior. Their intellectual level is generally very high. Because of their isolation, they are often self-taught, and their level of social success can be surprising.

Most paranoid personalities never decompensate and conserve the integrity of their intellectual capacities. They can even acquire enviable social positions in professional, political, or religious fields. People close to them—spouses, children, and subordinates—suffer along with them because of their character.

From the psychopathological point of view, paranoid individuals can:

- present *hypochondriac complaints.* You risk exposing yourself to accusations of negligence or incompetence, and sometimes procedural claims.
- have *thrilling reactions* related to frustration: morbid jealously, inheritance battles, humiliations, etc.
- more rarely evolve toward delirium.

The Therapist's Position

Several degrees of paranoia exist. Faced with paranoiacs, it is important not to become paranoid ourselves. Not all paranoid individuals are worthy of the fear elicited by their pathology. A bit of tact and prudence can help avoid disagreements with these individuals, who can be rather likable in other ways.

Paranoid individuals manage themselves with restraint with much finesse They are shrewd and will be watching you at every turn. Scrupulously follow formalities, because any lapse in etiquette may be perceived as a sign of distrust or mockery. Observe regimented politeness, but do not be obsequious, because they will sense your lack of sincerity and suspect that you are bored by their distrust.

At diagnosis, they may react extremely harshly. Discretion is indispensable for any therapeutic decision. Always express as clearly as possible what you propose for their therapeutic plan. If you must draw attention to an inconsistency, emphasize the parts that do not appear to be part of their behavior, but avoid confronting them about personality or self-image. Any perceived criticism is insupportable and will expose you to disproportionate reprisal.

Psychasthenic Personality

The psychasthenic personality is characterized by a distressing feeling of *incompleteness,* with a marked tendency to reservation and doubt. Hesitation and doubt in consciousness lead to mental rumination. Individuals are subject to lucid and guilty introspection, inhibition, a sense of being powerless to act (abulia), and hyposexuality. Fatigue is constant and particularly marked in the morning, with a sudden onset. It tends to continue throughout the day. All decisions and concrete activity require painful effort. Psychasthenic individuals try to reassure themselves with minutia, precision, and perfectionism on the basis of rigid moralism. They equate intellectualism with action: the all-powerful thought. They love to ask themselves their own questions. This tendency for contemplative daydreaming allows them to escape from everyday reality.

To fight their abulia, psychasthenics sometimes uses stimulants (tobacco, coffee, alcohol, amphetamines), without succumbing to major drug addiction. Their anxious introspection is often concurrent with hypochondriac preoccupations and nosophobic fears. Obsessional neurosis can develop against this uneasy and painstaking backdrop. Their hypersensitivity to physical and psychological stresses is a frequent source of depressive decompensation with renewed outbreaks of asthenia in the form of illness or shock. Psychasthenic individuals suffer from passivity, which is a means of defense against intense aggressive tendencies.

The Therapist's Position

Psychasthenic individuals are neither simulators nor manipulators. It is not necessary to deny their fatigue, which is very real, nor minimize it. Recognize it as real fatigue. Little by little, make them aware that their state of mind does not have a physical source (if that is the case), and that their tremendous weariness is only psychological, since they are *nervously* and *psychically* tired.

These patients are worth listening to, even if their sluggishness is irritating. Be patient, and you can urge them to reconsider their problem. They can be counseled to arrange some periods of rest or take some exercise like walking to become oxygenated, and they can be encouraged to do the work of psychotherapy.

Kretschmer's Sensitive Personality

The sensitive personality combines paranoid and psychasthenic personalities with depressive traits. Psychic suffering is intense but silent. These individuals keep the tension of their feelings within. They are hyperemotive, painstaking, tormented, complicated, timid, and perpetually unsatisfied with themselves. Pride and distrust are present. Asthenia readily replaces hypersthenia of the paranoid type. Hypersensitive and touchy, these individuals are very vulnerable. They present hyperesthesia in their relationships with others and extreme sensitivity to the reactions of others, and they struggle in the face of life's difficulties and affective shocks. They are incapable of exteriorizing their deep feelings. They have a tendency to interiorize them by folding in on themselves and analyzing them at great length. They present numerous traits of the paranoid personality: affective coldness, idealism, distrust of others, and sometimes aggression. Their internal critic emerges with feelings of guilt, responsibility for their failures, and an overestimation of their noxiousness. They are indecisive, taking initiative only with difficulty, and have poor confidence in themselves. Their humor is depressive, with sadness, asthenia, and pessimism. Suicide risk is high with this type of personality. They also display some hypochondriac complaints.

Delirious decompensation is rather rare, but it can happen after a succession of existential ordeals. This could be the case after rejection, intolerance in a circle of friends, isolation, or professional stagnation, which multiply frustration and humiliation and exacerbate the feeling of failure. These individuals therefore have the impression they are being bullied. They attribute pejorative and malevolent behavior to those close to them, such as work colleagues or superiors. Any of these feelings can decompensate in major depressive episodes of anxiety, suicide attempts, or severe hypochondria.

The Therapist's Position

Kretschmer's sensitive personality is a mix of two other personalities, so your positioning depends on the relative proportion of paranoid and psychoasthenic elements. You need to adapt to the major tendency at the time of the consultation. It is important to win their confidence while keeping a relational distance so as not to create impassioned contact.

Obsessive Personality

People with obsessive personality get their bearings from a well-structured character with:

- Constant worry about *order* and *cleanliness* accompany considerable meticulousness, harsh punctuality, and unyielding perfectionism. In the moral domain, they faithfully attend to their obligations with a sense of duty and painstaking respect for their responsibilities.
- *Frugality* can advance to stinginess and even greed. Difficulty with sharing and giving and the resulting desire for possessions often drive them to hoard provisions or collections.
- *Stubbornness* creates tenacity and perseverance in these individuals, who are not impressionable and are readily authoritarian.

Cold, dry and unconcerned, these individuals have a tendency to intellectualize and not to allow affective associations to arise that might make them suffer. They express themselves concisely, which can sometimes be pedantic as they search for the exact word. Their psyches are well partitioned and seem to be a juxtaposition of memories, feelings, and actual displays without links among them. These individuals can be remarkably adapted, however, and function without anguish or psychological crisis.

The development of an obsessive neurosis in this basic personality is relatively rare. On the other hand, it is common to observe especially in women in the latter part of life, the sudden onset of bouts of depression. In addition, this type of personality is found in people with colon pathologies and in those with myocardial infarctions or coronary disease.

Individuals with obsessive personality drive themselves in reaction to unconscious mechanisms that resolve anal eroticism and sadistic aggression in the anal sadism stage. Psychological habits are built contrary to repressed desires. Thus excessive cleanliness is a reaction to an interest in filth. Submission and exaggerated politeness take the place of an intensely aggressive subconscious. Certain other urges may also have been displaced and refined: interest in money and manipulating objects (tidying up, collecting things), which can replace the interest that obsessive children have in playing with their feces.

The Therapist's Position

Obsessive people have a fundamental need to anticipate and organize things, which we need to respect. They generally come to consultations with stacks of well-organized medical records. Often they have drawn up a list of past and present symptoms. This list, which they offer to you, of course, and which you put in your records, is a kind of unspoken contract. They will watch to see how rigorous you are in your art and that the contract is fulfilled.

Even if these patients have clearly summarized their medical history, that does not exempt you from the interview. Show some interest in their work and tell them that their organization and thoroughness are much appreciated, but that you need to ask a few things to be precise on certain points. In the case of multiple questions or chronic and older pathologies, explain up front the relative chances of success. Do not promise anything that you cannot guarantee. Try to set out the number of sessions you think they will need to resolve the problem. Determine the onset dates to estimate the evolution of the ailment or symptoms. They like to be able to get a fix on things, and they are reassured when they feel there is a certain degree of planning. When their problem is resolved, tell them that you hope to see them in a specific number of months to verify their condition or to prevent a recurrence. They will appreciate that you are making plans for them and that you are allowing them to look ahead.

Obsessive people live in perpetual tension. They hope to control everything, verify everything, and make sure that everything is perfect. Specifically, it is important not to talk ironically about a serious problem that they have or make light of their manias. Obsessive individuals believe they are acting in the best interests of perfection in the world around them. Sometimes humor can help them to progress to a condition of well-being in the framework of an already established relationship of trust.

It is necessary to help them discover the pleasure of relaxation. You can certainly reach it technically, but you can also achieve it if your positioning is reliable, rigorous, and predictable. At least then they will feel that they can relax in your presence.

Phobic Personality

The phobic personality is characterized by *inhibition* and its consequences, such as *timidity, reserved demeanor,* and *lack of dynamism.* As a general rule, phobic individuals try to proceed unnoticed, refuse to be involved, and avoid certain situations. They escape their anguish by projecting it outside themselves, fearing external dangers. They suffer from hypermotivity and are in a constant state of alert with regard to their affective life and instinctual subconscious.

Avoidance behavior can become a flight from danger: rejecting means of transport, trips, hospitals, and so on. Inhibition can also be translated as paradoxical *contraphobic behavior:* defiant attitudes, confronting dreaded situations, overcrowding, and so on. Anticipatory avoidance is tied to some overcompensation and shifting mechanisms. For example, fear of sexuality could be dealt with by brash behavior in a variety of areas, more obviously when devoid of any direct sexual implications.

The Therapist's Position

Phobic individuals have a hypersensitive personality and really fear being criticized. They fear ridicule and thus avoid entering relationships with others if they are not assured of unconditional benevolence. It is necessary to gain their confidence and be fully understanding and empathetic. Do not speak ironically about their conditions. Due to their hypersensitivity and feelings of inferiority, even a little humor can cause a serious wound.

If you have the opportunity, ask them for advice in an area where they could provide information, for example in their profession. People with phobic personalities believe that their advice is of no great value. The fact that you ask them for it will aid in establishing a relationship of trust.

Reassure them and urge them to get additional help. Individual or group psychotherapy and certain medications can sometimes help these patients in a spectacular way.

Schizoid Personality

The schizoid personality is expressed by withdrawal into the self, inability to express feelings directly or form close relationships with others, and by the absence of affective warmth. Behind the coldness, which is only indifference on the surface, is hidden an intense imaginary life with some degree of ambivalent hypersensitivity.

Schizoid individuals are solitary, distant, dreamy, and introverted. They often appear impassive, detached, and difficult to understand. Due to their disinterest in the outside world, they do not easily connect with others and have no close friends. They do not spontaneously seek the company of others and usually choose solitary activities. They are equally indifferent to praise and criticism. Their incapacity to get pleasure creates an absence of sexual desire. Even though most schizoids never decompensate, their existence is often marginal and presents some behavioral peculiarities.

The Therapist's Position

Note that even though we see the root *schizo*, which means "split," *schizoid personality* does not mean *schizophrenic*. Schizophrenia is a mental illness involving delusions and disturbances of the intellectual faculties. Schizoid individuals are simply cut off from the world.

Schizoid individuals have a great need for solitude. They do not speak much, but they possess numerous tacit qualities. If you want them to share elements of their internal world, don't bore them with conversation or questions. Don't wait for them to express intense emotions. Encourage them to speak and show them that you are attentive and patient. Respect their silences. If you know how to put them at ease, they will certainly disclose some of their vast internal richness.

Cycloid Personalities

These are pathological variants of the normal cyclothymic temperament. Cycloid individuals are warm and extroverted. They can have the aspect of being permanently hyperthymic; in that case it is called hypomanic personality. These personalities can also be manifested by the oscillations between hypomania and depression. Even though they may be depressed, cycloid individuals nonetheless remain syntonic.

The Therapist's Position

Cycloid personalities poses relatively little problem for therapists, especially during the hyperthymic phases. Of good humor, they gladly mask the somber components of their existence. Even when sick, they generally know how to make their caregivers appreciate them in spite of their problems.

During the depressive phases, they are more authentic but persist in minimizing their distress and continue to conceal their fears and anxieties. These individuals rarely expose themselves during the first consultation; don't to be fooled by the jovial image they present.

Anxiety and Anxious Personality

People with anxious personality are in a painful state of constant anxious tension with emotional instability as its foundation. Their sleep is light, agitated, barely restful, and interspersed with nightmares. They are highly sensitive to even minor frustrations, often accompanied by muscular hypertonia, exaggerated osteotendinous reflexes, tachycardia, and dyspnea after minor effort. They have a pessimistic view of the world. They are sad, readily complaining about failure and misfortune. Fundamentally, feelings of incapacity, inferiority, and insecurity explain their common tendency for depression.

Anxiety is a normal emotion. Everyone is anxious to some degree when a situation presents risk. Because anxiety is not very pleasant, we seek ways to avoid it:

- Certain people try to avoid losing control of the situation: preparing carefully for examinations, lectures, and classes, or arriving early at the airport or train station.
- Other people, in contrast, avoid putting themselves in situations they judge too stressful: refusing to show up for an examination, to begin speaking, or to take a trip. So people with anxious personality avoid, or are anxiophobic, causing inhibition, isolation, timidity, blockages, and refusal to take responsibility. They continually stand aside and adopt avoidance behaviors when faced with agonizing situations. This can lead them to considerably reduce their activities and relationships, and it causes difficulties in their social and professional lives.
- Sometimes they display hyperactivity with defiant behavior. These individuals have forced themselves to face what they want to escape. They adapt their behavior by overcompensating: taking on challenges, high-risk sports, etc.

The Therapist's Position

For the anxious personality, the world is a machine where any part can fail at any moment and cause a breakdown. If you show them that you are reliable, they will respond with less worry. This will put your relationship on a good footing from the outset. It is often the details that help these anxious individuals calm down. They want to talk with you before deciding to make an appointment. Even if that takes up your time, agree to the request, decipher their fears, and reassure them about your support. Sometimes after treatment they will phone you to get some information on an actual reaction that disturbed them. Be patient and understanding, tell them if you think the reaction is normal, and give them a bit of simple advice; you will have gained several degrees of reliability.

You can also help them put certain fears into perspective. Sometimes this can be done with humor, but again, not with teasing or irony. People with anxious personality are always deliberate, even if that can be exasperating for the people around them or for their therapists. You don't have to become their slave. They may attempt to draw you into their incessant prevention routines, calling you with minor concerns about themselves or family members. After even a minimal injury, they will be afraid of possible consequences. Don't let yourself get caught up in their point of view. Make your diagnosis and present your opinion on the matter.

Generally, individuals with anxious personality react strongly to surprises, both good and bad. Do not surprise them. If you think that you must use certain osteoarticular manipulations, it is better to forewarn them; be reassuring, try to relax them with kindness, but specifically do not use surprise with this type of patient.

Do not share your own concerns or worries with them. For some practitioners, the temptation can be great to use their own annoyances as a point of reference to put those of our patients in perspective. In general, this approach is quite strong and not therapeutic—except perhaps for the therapist—and it is the worst of approaches for anxious individuals. They already have enough of their own worries; sharing yours will be upsetting, and they will regard you as something new to worry about. Likewise, avoid topics of conversation that could be painful. For them, life and suffering already evoke danger. For further support, you may even recommend that they not watch television news. Broadcasts of daily catastrophes may reinforce the feeling that the worst is not only possible but probable.

Sociopathic Personality

This personality anomaly involves difficulties adapting or permanent maladaptation to the norms and laws of society. The terms *psychopathic imbalance, sociopathy,* and *antisocial personality* currently designate this form of social deviance, seen especially in males and in disorganized sociofamilial surroundings. This personality is characterized by a way of living marked by *instability, impulsivity,* and *maladaptation.* Patients are often seductive and well-spoken, and they are happy to give an incomplete or edited version of their history. These omissions can be the consequence of memory loss, voluntary deceit, or mythomania.

Almost always, their childhood has been disturbed with irregular schooling, indiscipline, violent anger, nervous breakdowns, petty theft, episodes of truancy, and sometimes running away. In adolescence, they have had repeated conflicts with authority figures (parents and teachers), successive scholastic failures, and have mixed with marginal and delinquent people. It is often when they have their first sexual experience, run away, attempt suicide, drink to excess, and experience drug addiction and homosexual and heterosexual prostitution. The constraints of military service are generally poorly tolerated and can bring on excitomotor nerve crises, insubordination, and desertion. In adulthood, instability persists and is expressed by difficulties in job functioning (frequent changes of profession or employer, temporary or marginal jobs), recurrence of delinquency, or parasitism on a partner or family members. Egocentrism and affective instability are common (separation, divorce, abandoning family, transitory affairs, etc.). These individuals have few ties, flee from conflicts and responsibilities, and may leave on an adventure "to see the world."

Intolerant of frustration, they react in an immediate way, uncontrolled and disproportionate to the conflict or restrictive situation. Acting out is their normal method of impulsive discharge. Incapable of foreseeing the consequences of their actions for themselves and others, they express neither shame nor remorse. On the contrary, they blame bad luck and readily establish themselves as victims of society or the people around them who have thrown up obstacles to the immediate realization of their desires. Incapable of drawing from past lessons to avoid repeating their mistakes, they often commit many more offenses.

Behind this apparent insensitivity, there is profound internal uneasiness. Enemies are everywhere. They try to overcome it by perpetually changing their environment and occupation. They lose themselves in alcohol, drugs, or the search for stimulating excitement, such as risk-taking in dangerous situations, sports, or illegal activities.

Mythomania sometimes infiltrates their behavior. When reality is opposed to their desires, they flee from it. They are fed by illusions and fool themselves as much as they deceive others. Confusing fantasies with reality, they exploit to their advantage valorizing roles that satisfy their egos: usurping titles or identity theft to facilitate loans, swindles, and parasitism.

They are often more amoral than wicked, and the practice of paraphilia is generally episodic. However, the pernicious dimension can express itself in certain individuals who derive pleasure from scandal, provoking or making all sorts of malicious denunciations.

The Therapist's Position

This is a dangerous personality, and these individuals are extremely difficult to heal. They respect nothing and systematically seek to find you at fault. They are not among your loyal patients, although some therapists may think they are. They readily make one or more appointments and don't keep them, without informing you and without apology. How you are treated is up to you, but they are usually skilled at playing you from the outset, in particular in terms of contracts. For example, it is best to say, "I'll give you another appointment, but it's the last time. If you don't come, we're done; I won't be able to see you again."

They are irresponsible individuals, incapable of honoring their promises. They can be violent and know no remorse. If, in very rare cases, you manage to win their confidence, it is nearly impossible to obtain their respect. It is very difficult for this personality to advance.

Narcissistic Personality

This personality is characterized by overestimation of the self. Individuals with narcissistic personality have no limits to their self-confidence. They consider themselves unique and think everything is owed to them. They are at ease, thoughtless, and without scruples. They need to be excessively admired and have a constant need for attention. They demand to be recognized as exceptional and by high-ranking people. They make the distinction between sycophants, whom they scorn, and the powerful, from whom they seek favors. They need to put themselves first. They love dominating and being in command. They are intolerant of criticism, and their demeanor is haughty. They lack empathy and despise the feelings of others.

Narcissistic personality is rare and mainly involves men. They can present sexual problems in terms of abstinence. If they fail at a heterosexual relationship, they may have a tendency to try a homosexual relationship.

Their ambitions know no bounds. Wanting to succeed at any cost, they can take advantage of others. They can proceed from excessive idealization of other people to devaluing them. At the same time, they can alternate between overestimating the self and self-devaluation.

The Therapist's Position

Narcissistic individuals readily consult well-known therapists to calm their hypochondriac anxieties. They are touchy and demanding patients. In dealing with them, scrupulously respect customs and formalities. Narcissists consider themselves more important than you, and they expect some respect. Don't show up late or greet them impersonally, but don't be too familiar either. What might be an insignificant detail for you may be seen by them as a lack of respect. Do not hesitate to compliment them whenever you can do so sincerely, but don't use flattery. You appear to them as someone intelligent who can recognize their worth. They will be less tempted to try to impress you, and you will carry more authority if you make a complimentary remark. If you must make a critical remark, be precise, and don't say it unless it's essential. This can be a chance for them to modify certain behaviors, but don't expect them to modify their vision of themselves and the world. Even if they are irritating or truly unbearable, don't systematically contradict them, and don't be hostile or wound their self-love.

Be wary of their attempts to manipulate you. Narcissists are charming beings who can easily mesmerize others. Their charm, confidence, and the unimportance that they assign to others make them dangerous manipulators. They will always try to persuade others to their points of view.

It is necessary that narcissists know precisely what you are willing to tolerate and what you will not. They will then have fewer tendencies to try your patience. For example, suppose that your appointment book is full, and your new appointments have a certain waiting period. If you grant these individuals the favor of seeing them ahead of other patients, you can guess what they'll try to do next time. Only do it if you can repeat the favor every time. Even so, don't expect any recognition for it. Narcissistic people never feel indebted, even if you have done them a favor.

Chapter 13

Orientation for Manual Diagnosis

If you don't hear the whispers of your body, you will hear its screams.

— CHINESE PROVERB

This chapter is intended to provide nothing more than a working canvas. It is not meant to dictate a way of working.

Generalities

Manual diagnosis requires precise organization. For the beginner, the problem is often in knowing where to start. The orientation for diagnosis provides a panorama of the patient's mechanics. It requires that you divide the patient into a grid, using a series of tests that will determine the most problematic regions.

We must never turn our focus in a specific direction without having good reason to do so. Clinicians must adapt to the patient and to what we discover in the examination without any preconceived judgments. Diagnostic orientation is like a sieve that retains only the fundamental diagnostic possibilities.

The orientation for diagnosis constitutes the first part of the clinical mechanical diagnosis. It is a manual examination of the patient, quick and thorough, with the following goals:

- to realize the physical condition of the patient's joints and mechanics
- to draw up an inventory of locations of dysfunctions and imbalances for the entire physical structure
- to determine the zones of the body that are the most destabilizing and the most disturbing to the individual as a whole
- to prepare for the specific diagnosis that will be made on the elements in question

This examination must investigate all the components of the mechanics of the body:

- the musculoskeletal system
- the visceral system
- the craniosacral system

This quick examination is presented according to the logic of physical movement, system by system, element by element.

At the end of this chapter, in order to perform the tests more easily, I have created a summary of the logic of positioning, according to the basic positions—standing, seated, and supine—in order to put the tests into practice more easily.

Anyone can freely adapt these tests, replacing some with others, without a problem. The most important aspects to grasp are the principles and methods of examination. Anyone can build their own sequential routine to arrive at the essential findings. One real imperative emerges: to carry out an examination of detection; consequently, the tests must be sensitive but not necessarily specific. The goal of this first stage of examination is to not overlook a dysfunction. The tests used are almost of a binary nature: according to their findings, they implicate or exclude as problematic the mechanical structure being examined.

Sensitivity and Specificity

Sensitivity and specificity are indicators, expressed as percentages, that indicate the predictive value of a test. *Sensitivity* is the probability that a test is positive if the subject has a dysfunction. It represents the capacity of a test to identify the mechanical elements that are disturbed. *Specificity* is the probability that a test is negative if the subject does not have a dysfunction. It represents the capacity of a test to identify healthy subjects. An increase in one of the indicators is most often to the detriment of the other: if sensitivity increases, specificity diminishes, and vice versa. Depending on the goal of the test, we have to favor one or the other:

- Screening tests favor sensitivity. They allow maximum detection of abnormalities and miss only a small number of sick or dysfunctional elements. Of course, screening must be followed by more specific tests to confirm the problem since screening does not have the goal of providing a more precise diagnosis.
- Diagnostic tests favor specificity. They allow us to affirm and name a dysfunction or pathology.

Listening

Diagnostic Orientation

The various listenings are tests for the general orientation of the diagnosis. They require manual sensitivity and skill. Well utilized and well understood, they constitute very good diagnostic tools. They also permit us to verify the efficacy of a treatment. Indeed, their modification is almost instantaneous when we correct the element responsible for the dysfunctional chain.

General and regional listenings are tests during which our attention is oriented toward the patient as a whole. They are not concerned with a segmental assessment of mechanics but a general evaluation using several parameters. Our *mental focus* must be as broad as possible. We are only seeking to evaluate how the patient's body, as a unit, is in balance or out of balance.

The principal interest of these tests is to determine *probable diagnostic orientations.* This period of orientation allows you to locate the mechanical problems that are most significant for the organism. It constitutes the first stage, before the routines that list the dysfunctions more precisely.

Specific diagnosis comes next, to clarify and name the dysfunction. These listenings do not determine how we continue with the diagnosis, but they bring a particular light to the diagnosis. The result of the listening allows us to make subtle distinctions about the significance of each dysfunction. It is a fundamental piece of information during the differential diagnosis.

The questions that these general tests raise, in substance, are:

- How does the patient achieve balance?
- On which side is the most destabilizing dysfunction for the organism located?
- How and where are the imbalances expressed? Which parts of the individual seem to be the seat of the greatest imbalance?
- Are the tensions for the individual expressed more posteriorly or more anteriorly?

These initial listenings are based on the spontaneous reactions of the patient. We perform them before testing the mechanics in any given position. Mechanical tests are more challenging and momentarily disturb the equilibrium of the deeper tissues. It is preferable to perform them secondarily, in each of the basic positions, after the listening tests.

NOTE

Certain therapists, after many years of practice, succeed in obtaining very subtle information from general and regional listenings. I cannot advise you strongly enough to use the greatest caution and respect for progression in the use of these tests. For the beginner, these tests must clearly answer the simplest questions. When you are able to rely on the information obtained, your questions can become more complex and subtler.

The listening points out the imbalances of the body. The body shows its weak points without error. The touch and especially the interpretation of the therapist is another story.

Wanting to go through these steps too quickly in this type of test generally has serious consequences for elaborating the diagnosis that follows.

General Listening

This first evaluation, based on the general listening of the body, takes into account the tissue reactions of the patient. Sick tissue and mechanical dysfunction disorganizes the tissue equilibrium of the whole body, creating new axes of mobility and motility for the different mechanical structures. The organism is always attracted to the side of the dysfunction or fixation. Our hands remain passive and must gather information without interpreting it too quickly. As therapists, we must be stable so as not to transmit our own tissue imbalances to the patient.

The body cannot be imbalanced on several fixed points at the same time. The predominant dysfunction constitutes a relatively fixed point, around which the body must adapt mechanically. It is this point that is determined by the listenings. Because of the perpetual adaptations and mechanical compensations that the human body makes, this predominant dysfunction evolves through time and is therefore not unchanging. The osteopathic consultation must attempt to ascertain how individuals present to us here and now, and how they must be treated on the basis of this data.

Standing

The patient is standing, and you stand behind him. Place one hand on the vertex and the other at the lumbosacral junction (fig. 13.1). Ask him to close his eyes to eliminate all visual references. The patient's body is now ready to express its internal tensions. The tissues will move toward the most disturbed region on the mechanical plane. Your hand detects this imbalance. It is generally in the first seconds after the eyes are closed that the tissue imbalance shows itself. This is a tissue attraction; the hand must feel it to interpret it. It must not be confused with a postural reaction, which is generally of much larger amplitude.

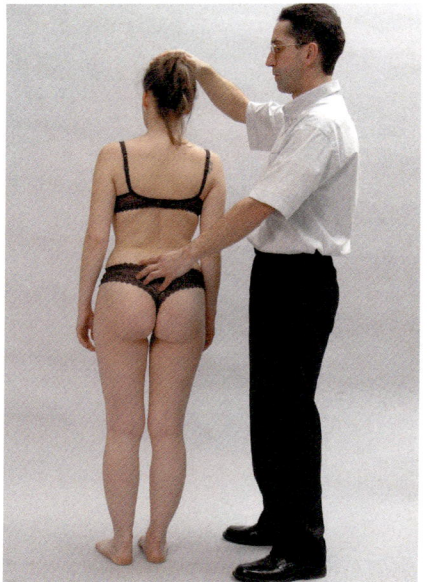

Figure 13.1. General listening while standing.

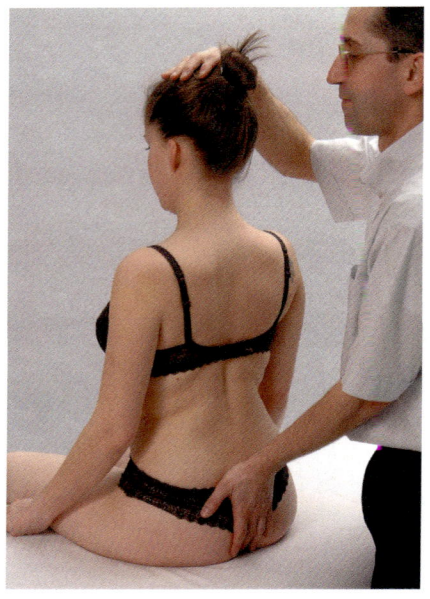

Figure 13.2. General listening while seated.

Seated

The patient is seated. Stand behind her, one hand placed on the vertex and the other on the posterior surface of the sacrum (fig. 13.2). The procedure is exactly the same as above; the patient closes her eyes to allow you to note the listening. The difference between seated listening and standing listening is in the exclusion of the lower limbs and their potential imbalances.

PRACTICAL ADVICE

In order to make this listening highly effective, it is good to adopt a standard position in relation to the patient. By always positioning yourself on the same side, your hands will be placed the same way on each patient, and your visualization will always take place from the same point of view. Your hands must be passive; they are going to reveal the movement by amplifying it. You are not inducing but listening.

Your mind and your intellect must be silent throughout the entire process of perceiving. It is not a matter of interpreting but of noting all attractions in the tissues through your hands. Decoding is only done in the second stage.

Results of Global Listening

Global listening allows us to evaluate the mechanics of the body according to the main axes. They allow us to draw a rough sketch, possibly ever to locate the mechanical dysfunctions that have the greatest impact at the time of the examination. They allow us to decide whether it is on the right side or the left side, the front or the back, and sometimes whether it is the visceral contents or the craniosacral mechanism. This stage of the diagnosis only involves paths that must be more thoroughly investigated.

In the case of a *lateral dysfunction,* tissues are pulled and constrain the body in a pattern of lateral flexion on the side of the mechanical problem. The greater the tendency for lateral flexion, the farther from the midline the location of the dysfunction is.

During the seated listening, a significant lateroflexion, similar to rolling on the ischium, reveals either a significant somatic dysfunction or the orthopedic aftereffects of surgery in the lower limb, on the same side of the ischium that is affected.

When the tissues engage in a *flexion pattern,* the problem is more anterior, frequently related to the visceral system. The greater the tendency for flexion, the lower the location of the dysfunction is.

If the pattern involves extension, the problem is more posterior, often located along the axis of the somatic system:

- When it concerns a vertebral somatic dysfunction, it translates as rather pure posterior-anterior movement of the head and the top of the trunk.
- Coccygeal dysfunctions create significant movement, a real tendency to pull slightly toward the thigh, as if the back of the head sought to touch the sacrum.

- Beware of drawing conclusions too quickly. In the case of metabolic disorders of the liver or kidneys, we can also notice a paradoxical response in extension.

An impression of *sinking to the level of the cephalic hand* directs us more toward restrictions of the longitudinal structures of the body. Most often, a dysfunction of the craniosacral system is encountered. A fixation of the dura mater of the spinal column, the nerve roots, or the peripheral nerves also creates this sensation, often coupled with a feeling of slight unilateral compression of the vertebral column.

It could also be a fixation in the deep myofascial chains of the trunk, also called the *central tendon.*

Regional Listening

Cervicothoracic Balance

Test

This test is done standing, with the practitioner standing behind the patient (fig. 13.3). Place one hand on the vertex, with soft and light support, in contact with the fascia. Without increasing your pressure, move the head and the cervical spine into a right lateral side-bend, then repeat to the left. Compare the amplitudes and the resistances found to determine whether there is a deficiency in lateral side-bend to one side or the other. If this is the case, analyze whether the limitation in the cervicothoracic

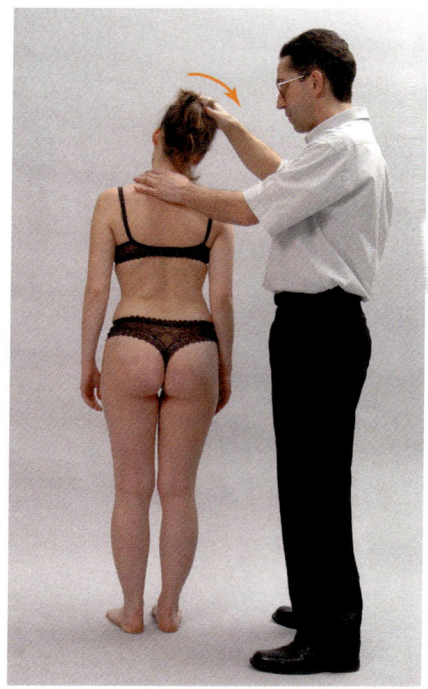

Figure 13.3. Cervicothoracic balance.

side-bend is caused by an excess of contralateral tension (traction difficulty) or by too great an ipsilateral resistance (difficulty compressing).

Results

The side on which a lateral side-bend is limited is not necessarily the side of dysfunction. When the primary dysfunction is located on the opposite side, there are tensions that limit the side-bend. When the primary dysfunction is located on the same side, there is difficulty in compressing the spine on the side with the limited side-bend. This test of general orientation thus allows us to differentiate between a predominant dysfunction within the musculoskeletal system or within the visceral system. For example, suppose that you have found a limited right lateral side-bend:

- If the limitation is due to tension that is too strong on the left side, this directs your diagnosis to tension placed on a deep myofascial chain, generally of visceral origin. You are dealing with a dysfunction of an organ or viscera, thoracic or abdominal, located to the left of the midline.
- If the limitation in the side-bend is linked to difficulty compressing the tissues on the right side, this directs you more along the osteoarticular slope. It concerns a somatic dysfunction, costal or vertebral, on the right side.

Listening to the Trapezius and Scapular Regions

Technique

Place your hands wide open on the cervicoscapular junction on the right and left, in a way that encompasses the trapezius, clavicle, and scapula as well as the thoracic outlet (fig. 13.4). Observe the movements that happen spontaneously during thoracic respiration and compare their amplitude and symmetry. Then, exert light pressure toward the lower part of the body, on both sides simultaneously or one side after the next. Observe tissue resistance to your movement. Then let it come back upward, observing the speed and the quality of the return.

Results

This listening shows the dysfunctions that can have repercussions on the neck, the cervicodorsal transitional area, and the upper limbs. With simple contact, a feeling of rigidity or significant density under one of your hands often suggests an ipsilateral parietal problem. On this side, the thorax seems a bit more voluminous, even to the point of being extremely rigid. This finding generally confirms the previous test of cervicothoracic balance. You see this when there is a costal or vertebral somatic dysfunction on the same side, or when there are significant fixations of visceroligamentous elements of the diaphragmatic pleura.

Unilateral resistance to your compression reveals neuromeningeal tensions on the same side, either of the cervical plexus, the brachial plexus, or of the ipsilateral dura mater of the spinal column. Sometimes this tension results from a dysfunction of the cranial base. The muscular tone is greater on one side, and frequent spasms of the trapezius prevent your hands from moving downward.

Listening to the Lower Limbs

Anterior Fascial Structures

The patient is lying down, and you are standing at the foot of the table (fig. 13.5). Place your hands on the dorsal surface and on the instep of the feet, with light fascial contact. Gradually apply tension to the fascial chain in the caudal

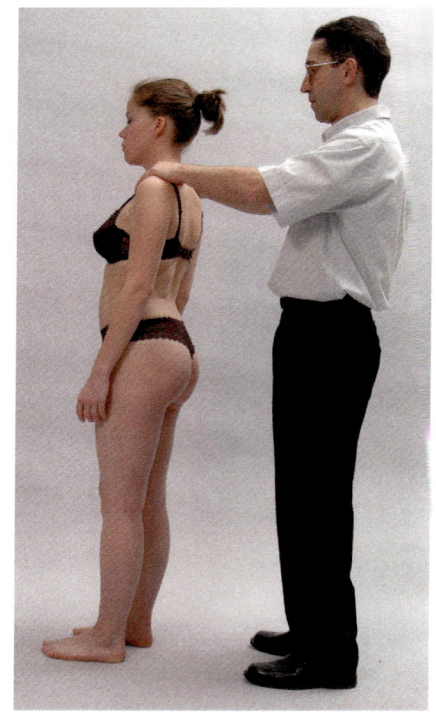

Figure 13.4. Listening to the trapezius and scapular regions.

direction until you obtain joint mobilization of the foot and ankle in the direction of plantar flexion. Analyze the ease or difficulty of this tension. At the maximum level of fascial tension, suddenly let go. Analyze the speed at which the foot returns toward dorsal flexion; the foot that displays the quickest return indicates the side where the dysfunction is predominant. It is possible to analyze the fascial chain's gradual application of tension to locate the level of the dysfunction. The sooner the tension occurs, the closer to the foot the dysfunction is.

Posterior Fascial Structures

In the same position, place your hands on the posterior surface of the heels and the Achilles tendons, still in contact with the fascia (fig. 13.6). Gradually apply tension to the posterior fascial chain in the caudal direction until you obtain a reaction in the lumbosacral joint. The side

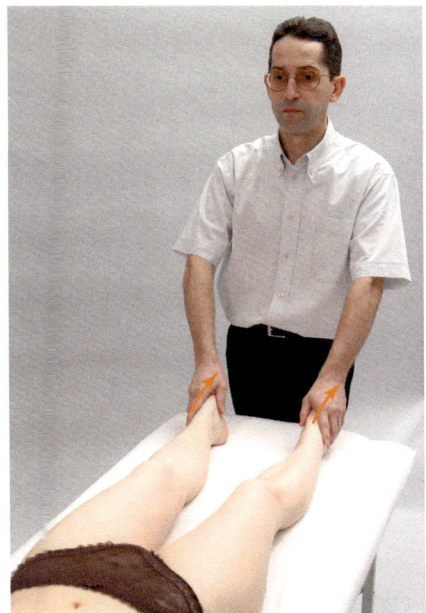

Figure 13.5. Listening through the anterior fascial structures of the lower leg.

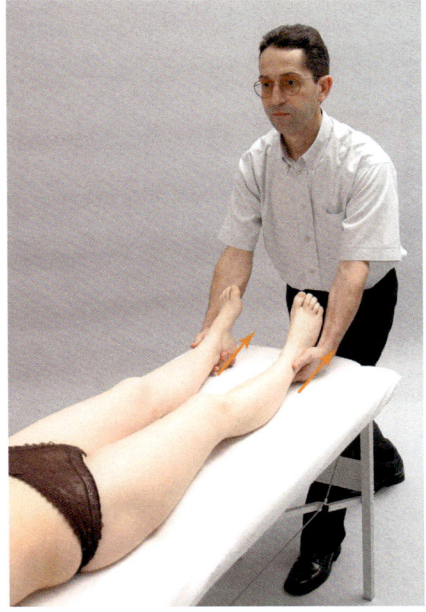

Figure 13.6. Listening through the posterior fascial structures of the lower leg.

that shows the least elasticity is the one with the dysfunction. As with the previous listening, it is possible to precisely identify the level of the disturbance by analyzing the moment when the tension first appears in the fascial chain.

Results

The test of reactions and tensions in the anterior fascial chain tells you the *side* and eventually the *level of the dominant mechanical dysfunctions*. Most often, it concerns:

- dysfunctions of the mechanical visceral abdominopelvic region, quite easily perceived up to the diaphragm
- myofascial-joint imbalances of the lower limb

The test of the posterior fascial chain also indicates the side and the level of the strongest mechanical disturbances. It most often indicates:

- somatic dysfunctions affecting the lower limbs, the pelvic bowl and even the axis of the spinal column
- lateralized mechanical dysfunctions of the dura mater or of the lumbosacral plexus

REMARKS

Listenings from the lower limbs can help verify the effectiveness of a treatment. It allows us to measure the impact of a visceral or neural manipulation on the freeing of the restrained myofascial chain.

Listening to the Upper Limbs

There are two modalities for this test, both of which generally give the same information: the seated position or the supine position. According to the capability of the patient, it is informative to do both.

Seated Position

The patient is seated facing you, with the upper limbs bent perpendicular, elbows at the side of the body (fig. 13.7). With your hands supinated, place your palms underneath the bent elbows and gently lift upward along the axis of the humerus. The weight of the arms is removed at the level of the scapulohumeral joint. Maintaining this contact effort, create traction in the anterior direction and analyze the ease of movement. Any restriction on one side signifies a predominant dysfunction on that side.

Supine Position

The patient is supine, upper limbs to the side (fig. 13.8). Stand at the head, grasp the wrists by the dorsal surface, and lift the upper limbs overhead. In contact with the fascia, apply tension to the posterolateral chains of the upper limbs, keeping the arms below their maximal overhead position. Analyze every restriction of mobility and every loss in elasticity while in this position of tension. Noticing a significant resistance on one side is a sign of fascial restriction.

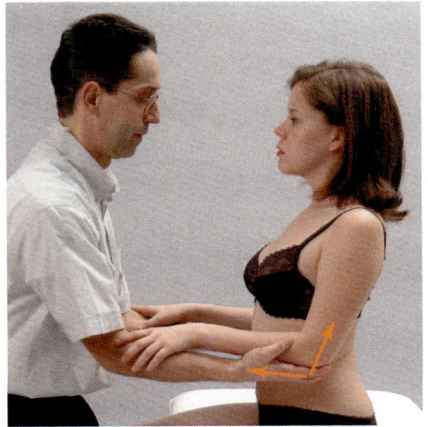

Figure 13.7. Listening to the upper limbs in seated position.

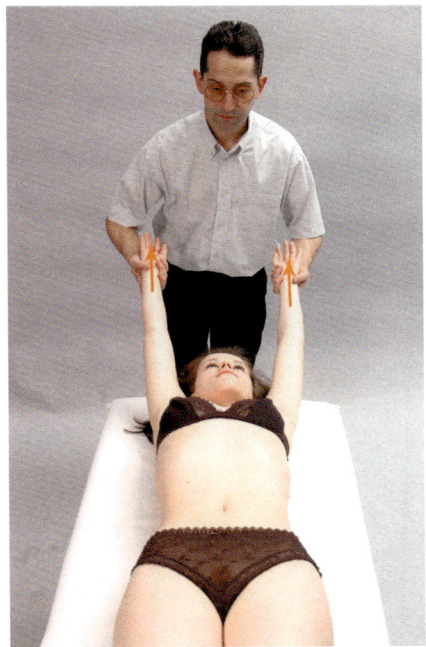

Figure 13.8. Listening to the upper limbs in supine position.

Results

- Every perceived restriction during the two listenings must make you suspect a significant mechanical dysfunction, generally on the same side. It could involve the upper limb itself, the shoulder complex, the ipsilateral hemithorax, the cervical spine, the brachial or cervical plexuses, the pleura, the lung, the heart, the pericardium, or even the visceral sheath of the neck.
- In the supine position, hepatic dysfunctions, which have an impact on the muscular chains of the shoulder and of the upper limb, are easily perceived in the process of listening.
- In the seated position, the weight of the visceral elements below the diaphragm plays a dominant role. This listening also provides information about the mechanics of the viscera and of the supramesocolic organs suspended from the diaphragm.

By increasing the tensions, the inherent gravity of the seated position allows us to perceive the most subtle fixations that are sometimes not found in the supine position.

Routines

This is the when we detect dysfunctions. Routines search for their locations without concern about their exact nature. Routines must be supplemented by specific tests, performed on the most problematic zones, which will then be treated. There is no point in performing specific tests on structures that will not be treated; it is a waste of time. What point is there in knowing that a given vertebra has a right ERS dysfunction if this vertebra is not related to the pathogenic pattern we are currently concerned with? On the other hand, drawing up a list of dysfunctions that the patient presents allows us to measure their quantitative and qualitative significance.

Routines prepare for prioritization of the dysfunctions to establish the most probable pathogenesis. This panorama of dysfunctions constitutes a major diagnostic orientation.

PRACTICAL ADVICE

Day after day, osteopaths forge their own routines. Those that I present are easy to use but can be adjusted. Nevertheless, routines must respect certain key principles:

- The patient's "grid" must cover the totality of the mechanical systems of the body.
- The whole set of tests must flush out the most significant dysfunctions with a minimum of time and effort.
- The routine must have a maximum efficacy and must establish a system applicable from one patient to another, allowing for standardization.
- The organization of the different tests must avoid disunity and being scattered during the clinical examination.

Musculoskeletal Routines

General Rule

The tests that constitute the routine are simple and quick: they tell us if the joint is moving freely or not. If it is free, you will have nothing further to do. If it is not free, you know only that there is a dysfunction, but not its exact nature nor its impact on the body.

The Spine

The spinal routine must explore all the vertebral levels from the atlanto-occipital junction, to the sacrococcygeal joint, passing through the twelve pairs of costovertebral joints. Perform it preferably in weight-bearing seated position.

C0–C1: Flexion-Extension Test

Place your index finger or third finger in the parotid region, between the ramus of the mandible and the anterior side of the transverse process of the atlas (figs. 13.9 and 13.10). Be gentle because this zone is naturally sensitive; the parotid gland and the facial nerve come between your finger and the surfaces of the bone. Place your other hand on the top of the cranium at the level of the sagittal suture in front of the obelion. Apply slight craniocaudal compression, and make small flexion and extension movements of the head on the atlas. When in extension, your palpating finger should feel an opening or space. With the rolling and gliding of the occipital condyles on the atlas, the ramus of the mandible seems to slip forward. When in flexion, the feeling is the opposite. The space closes, and your palpating finger seems to be pushed away from the contact zone. If there is a fixation of the atlanto-occipital joint, you can feel neither opening nor closing with your finger.

C1–C2: Rotation Test

Place the pad of your index finger on the mastoid, the pad of your middle finger on the transverse process of C1, and the pad of your ring

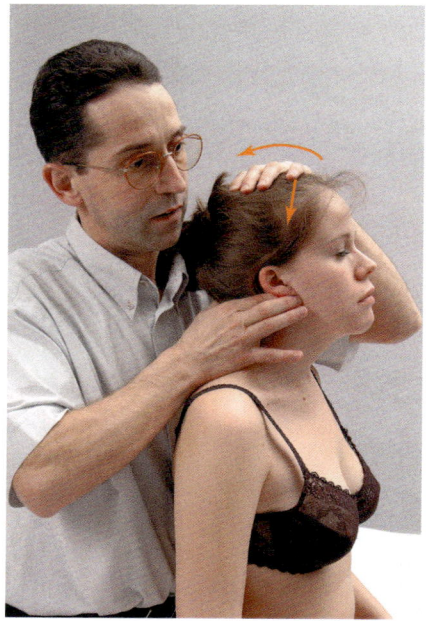

Figure 13.9. C0–C1 flexion-extension routine.

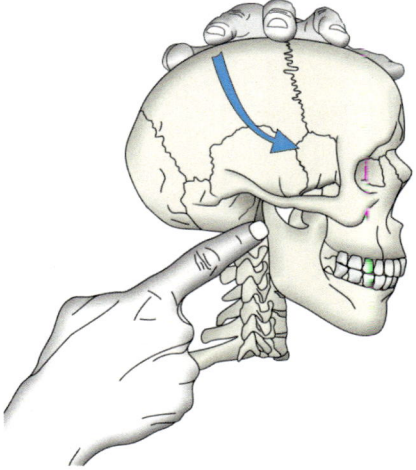

Figure 13.10. Finger contact for C0–C1.

finger on the articular pillars of C2 (figs. 13.11 and 13.12). Place your other hand on the top of the cranium. Apply slight compression and flexion of the head on the cervical spine. Then, take the head into right rotation, then left rotation. When you make the head turn to the side opposite your palpating fingers, you can feel your finger pads moving away from each other, creating space between your fingers. When you have the head turned to the same side as your palpating fingers, you can feel your finger pads and fingers getting closer to each other. In the case of C1–C2 fixation, your index finger and your middle finger seem to be bound together. They turn at the same time but do not get closer or farther away from each other.

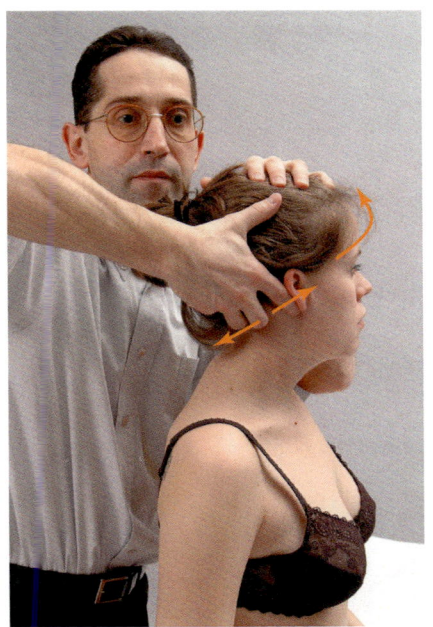

Figure 13.11. C1–C2 rotation routine.

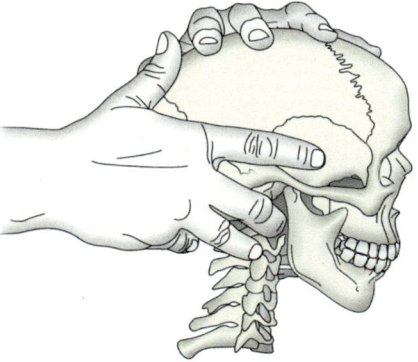

Figure 13.12. Finger contact for C1–C2.

C2–C7 Lower Cervicals: Lateral Side-bend Test

The test is performed in slight flexion of the cervical spine to disengage the posterior articular pillars and facilitate identification of different vertebral levels (figs. 13.13 and 13.14). Place the index finger and middle finger of one hand behind the posterior articular pillars of C2–C3. Placed on top of the cranium, your other hand mobilizes the neck in a right lateral side-bend, then left. On the concave side of the neck formed by the lateral side-bend, your finger pad perceives the retreat of the articular process. If your fingers are close to the midline, you can also feel the spinous process move away toward the side opposite the side-bend. When there is a fixation at one articulation, the whole joint seems locked in place. The articular process does not retreat, and the spinous process does not follow.

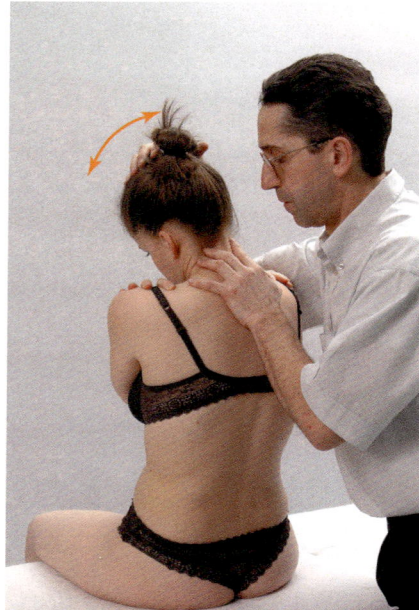

Figure 13.13. C2–C7 lateral bending routine.

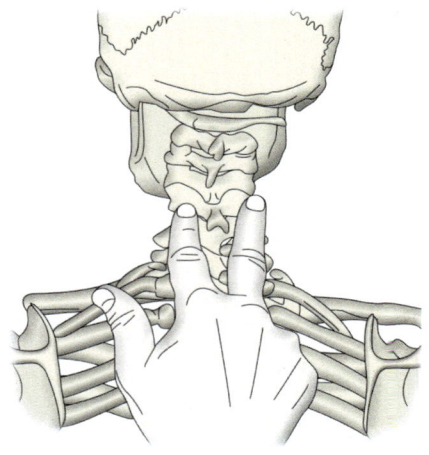

Figure 13.14. Finger contact for C2–C7.

Thoracic Vertebrae: Lateral Side-bend Test

The subject is seated on the table, arms crossed over the chest and hands on shoulders, legs slightly apart, and the trunk slightly flexed. Stand behind the patient and to one side, the finger pad of the medial side of your thumb against the lateral surface of the T1 spinous process. The general principle of the test is to verify the movement of the spinous process while you impart lateral flexion movement at the segment of the spinal column being tested. In a position of slight flexion of the trunk and in the absence of a dysfunction, lateral side-bend of the spine normally generates vertebral rotation in the same direction. The palpating thumb should notice a contralateral movement away of the spinous process. Conversely, when a dysfunction exists, the vertebra does not allow rotation, and the spinous process remains fixed. This lack of movement, an integral part of somatic dysfunction, is called *vertebral fixation*. It translates under your fingers as a feeling of resistance, hardness, or density that is a contrast to the suppleness and fluidity of the levels that are mechanically free. For the movement of the spinous process to be most effectively perceived by your thumb, you must reach maximum amplitude at the level tested. Your push toward the lateral side-bend must always be oriented along a straight line that passes through the level tested (fig. 13.15). When you test with your thumb, you must do the test twice, one side after the other.

Some therapists prefer to test with the index finger and the middle finger on either side of the spinous process. They can thus verify mobility by comparison at the same level, in right side-bending and then in left side-bending. Be careful, however, with this hand position, as it is a little more difficult to obtain perfectly symmetrical movement.

For levels T1 to T4–T5, place your hand on the top of the patient's head and your elbow on the shoulder. With the lever thus created, it is easy to obtain a good lateral side-bend of the superior thoracic spine (fig. 13.16). For levels T5 to L1, place your forearm across the patient's shoulders. Create a lateral side-bend by leaning on your elbow toward the level you are examining (fig. 13.17).

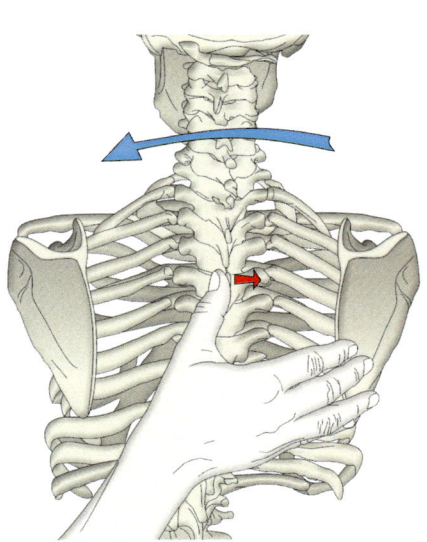

Figure 13.15. Contact with the thoracic spine.

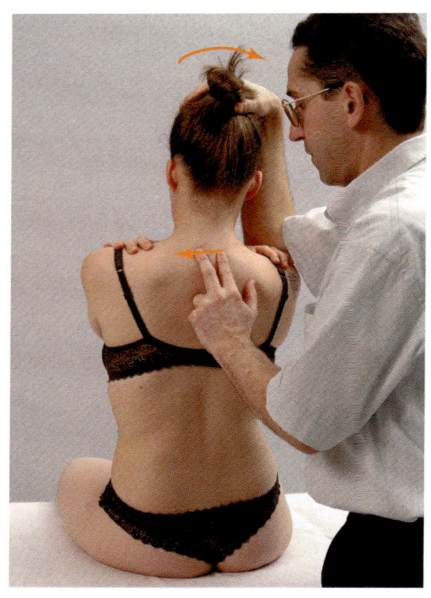

Figure 13.16. T1–T4 routine.

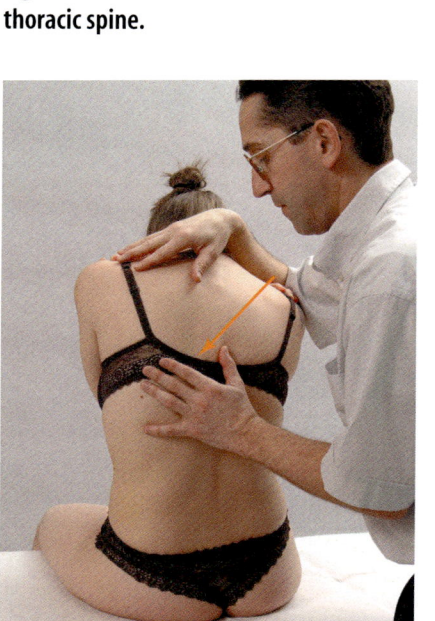

Figure 13.17. T5–L1 routine.

L1–L5 Lumbar Vertebrae

The positioning is the same as for the lower thoracic spine. The push of your elbow is directed in the same way but a bit lower. Without hesitation, you must aim at the opposite coxofemoral joint to mobilize the lower part of the lumbar spine (figs. 13.18 and 13.19).

The Sacrum

By virtue of the numerous axes and the large variety of sacroiliac movements, beginning osteopaths are often disappointed when they

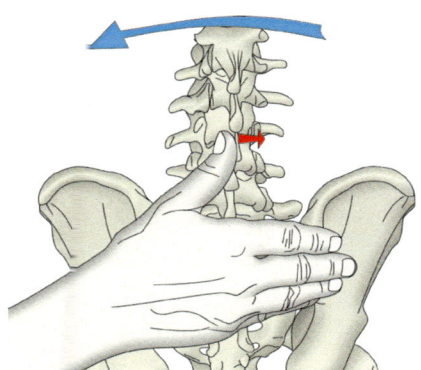

Figure 13.18. Contact with the lumbar spine.

Figure 13.19. L1–L5 routine.

simply want to know if the sacrum is free or not. Indeed, too often the sacrum and the sacroiliac joints are tested immediately in detail before they have been tested globally.

The sacrum is a special kind of vertebra. It is the only part of the body where the axial skeleton is directly opposite the appendicular skeleton. It is found within a complex system of levers that can make it move in different ways. Osteopathic biomechanics and their clinical applications allow us to define a large diversity of axes and movements. Even so, all movements happen in the same joint: the *sacroiliac joint*.

Before learning *how* this joint is dysfunctional, one of the first questions that arises is *if* this joint is dysfunctional or not. To answer this question, we can use a quick test without predicting the nature of the dysfunction (ilium-sacrum, sacrum-ilium, physiological, or nonphysiological). With slight differences, the sacrum has largely the same possibilities for movement as the other vertebrae. Rotation and side-bending movements are thus an excellent means for quick diagnosis. Keep the positioning of the patient that you used for the lumbar spine and let your forearm rest across and on top of the shoulders. Lay your posterior hand flat, longitudinally on the posterior surface of the sacrum. The heel of your hand rests on the base of the sacrum, while the pads of your index and ring fingers are placed at the inferolateral angles of the sacrum. Make the patient move into a lateral side-bend of the trunk to the right. The right inferolateral angle, on the side of lumbar concavity, rises in the cephalic direction, while the left inferolateral angle, on the side of lumbar convexity, moves downward in the caudal direction (fig. 13.20). Then, make the patient move in a lateral side-bend toward the left. Now the left inferolateral angle rises while the right inferolateral angle moves downward. If you feel these movements, the sacrum is free at the level of the inferior part of the joint. It can glide on the long arms of the L-shaped sacroiliac joint. If it is fixed on one of the two longer arms of the joint, movement upward or downward is hampered on that side.

Next, take the patient into rotation of the trunk toward the right and analyze what happens. You should feel the right base of the sacrum retreat backward, pushing the heel of your hand backward, while the left side of the base of the sacrum moves forward (fig. 13.21). Repeat the maneuver, making a left rotation. The base of the sacrum now retreats backward to the left and moves forward on the right. If these movements happen easily, the sacrum is free at the level of the superior part of the joint. It can glide on the short arms of the L-shaped sacroiliac joint. If it is fixed on one of the two short arms of the joint, anterior or posterior rotation is hampered on that side.

The Sacrococcygeal Joint

The sacrococcygeal joint is often forgotten in vertebral tests. Dysfunction of the sacrococcygeal joint, however, is highly pathogenic for the whole body mechanism.

Position the patient in anterior flexion of the trunk until he or she rolls on the ischia and the buttocks lift from the table (figs. 13.22 and

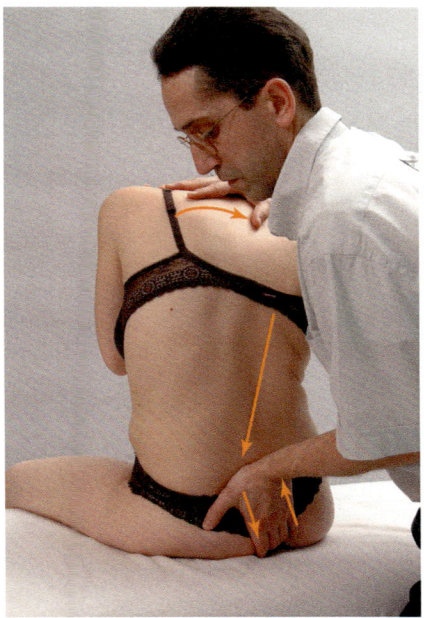

Figure 13.20. Lateral flexion routine for the sacrum.

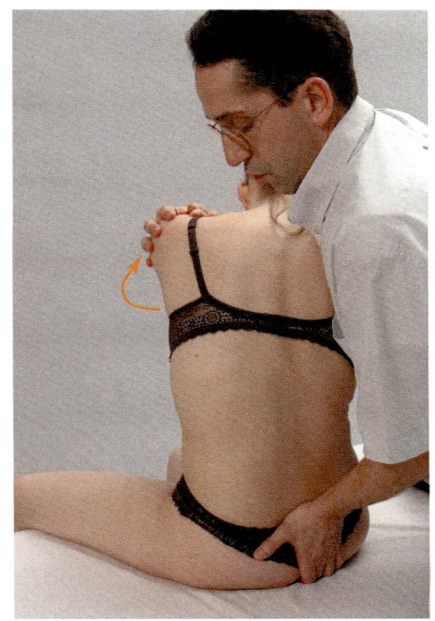

Figure 13.21. Rotation routine for the sacrum.

13.23). Over the underwear, slide a finger or two toward the apex of the coccyx, following the dorsal surface of the coccyx in the crease of the buttocks. The only difficulty is in going far enough; it is necessary to identify the small tuberosity of the apex of the coccyx and place the finger pad on it. Bring the patient into a bi-ischial support, and from the coccyx apply slight compression along the main axis. While maintaining this compression, mobilize the apex of the coccyx toward the front, toward the back, toward the right, and toward the left. Note that these are not big movements but rather more like initiating movement. Do not look for a large range of motion but rather easy quality of movement.

All restrictions are suspicious. In this case, the coccyx must be the object of a more in-depth examination as part of a specific diagnosis for the pelvic diaphragm. This detailed examination leads to establishing a

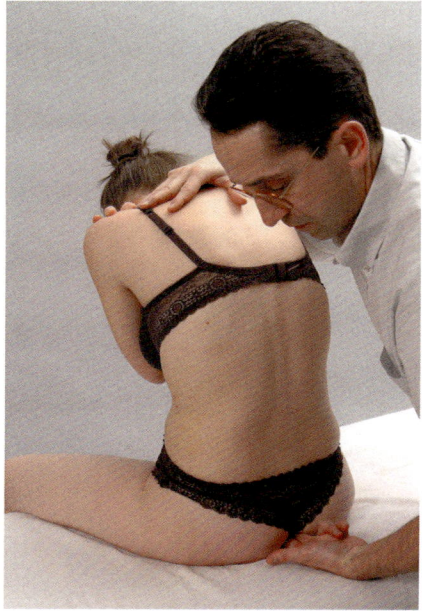

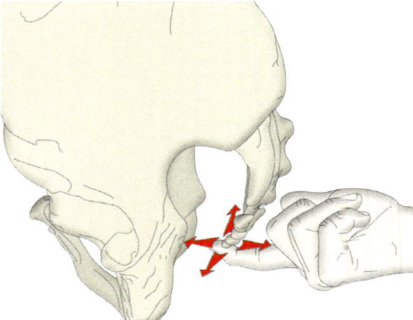

Figure 13.22. Sacrococcygeal routine.   **Figure 13.23. Sacrococcygeal routine.**

tally that allows us to determine the appropriateness of proceeding with tests via the rectum.

Costovertebral Joints

The patient is seated on the table, arms crossed over the chest and hands on the shoulders, legs slightly apart, and the trunk slightly bent. Stand behind the patient slightly to one side. On the opposite hemithorax, place the pad of your index finger on the posterior surface of the transverse process of the first thoracic vertebra, and place the pad of your middle finger on the posterior arc of the first rib (figs. 13.24 and 13.25). With the other hand around the front of the patient's trunk, grasp the tip of the scapula of the opposite shoulder. Gently pull the shoulder toward the front until you feel that the movement connects to the costovertebral joint complex that you are examining. Normally, if play in the joint is free, you should feel that during the rotation; the rib

314

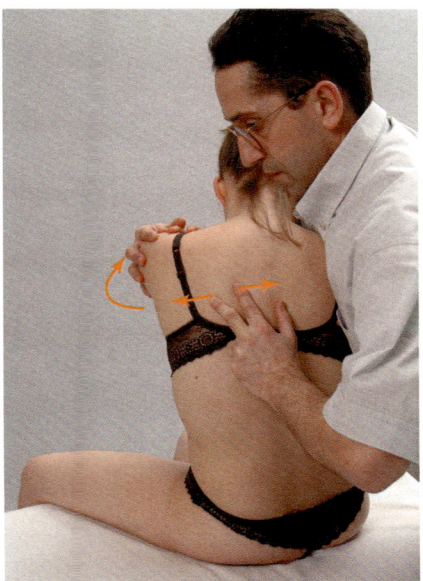

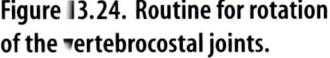

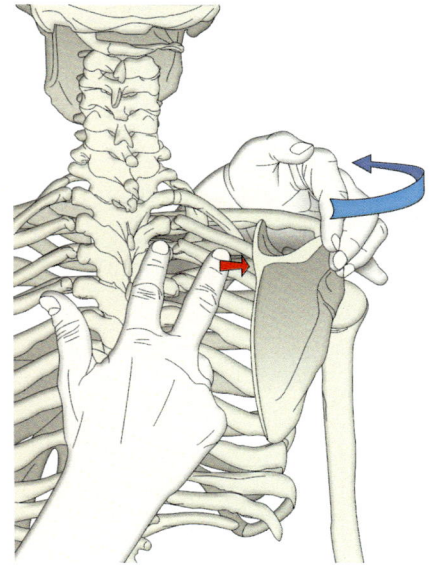

Figure 13.24. Routine for rotation of the vertebrocostal joints.

Figure 13.25. Finger contact for the vertebrocostal joints.

seems to move farther and more quickly than the transverse process. This translates into a feeling that your palpating fingers are moving apart. When there is a costovertebral or costosomatic joint fixation, this feeling disappears; the rib and the vertebra seem as one. The fingers do not move apart but appear to rotate simultaneously.

Proceed from the top to the bottom. Progressively, press with your index finger from one transverse process to the next, and press with your middle finger from one rib to the next. Do not be misled by the level of the spinous process compared to the rib. By relying on the bony prominence of the ribs and the transverse processes, your fingers will always be on structures belonging to the same joint.

Practical Advice

- During vertebral or rib routines, it's important to know at which level your fingers are and which level you are testing.

■ When you find a fixation, mentally note at precisely which level it is. This information is very important in establishing links between cause and effect when looking for the pathogenesis.

Inferior Pole

The Foot: Play in the Arch

In architectural terminology, the foot is often seen as a set of vaults or arches. From the mechanical point of view, the best model suggested for the foot is, without doubt, the foot truss, proposed by P. W. Lapidus (1963) and expanded on by Émile De Doncker (1977). The foot behaves like a truss, deformable when not bearing weight and self-locking when bearing weight (fig. 13.26). A quick way to test the mechanical integrity of the foot is to observe how this truss, classically called the *arch of the foot,* behaves. The play in the foot truss necessitates the functional integrity of all the joints in the foot. If it is capable of widening and flattening smoothly, we can say that all the joints are free.

The patient is in the supine position, and you are at the feet. You can do the test on both feet simultaneously to judge symmetry, or you can test one foot after the other.

■ *Rounding the arch:* place your thumb transversely underneath the sole of the foot, at the place where the foot is hollowest. Place your fingers flat on the dorsal surface of the metatarsals. Take the metatarsal heads in the direction of plantar flexion while you stabilize the metatarsal region with counterpressure from your thumb in the cranial direction (fig. 13.27).
■ *Flattening the arch:* place your thumb transversely, under the plantar surface of the heads of the metatarsals. Place your fingers on the dorsal surface of the metatarsals. Mobilize the metatarsal heads toward dorsal flexion while holding the metatarsals with counterpressure from your fingers in the caudal direction (fig. 13.28).

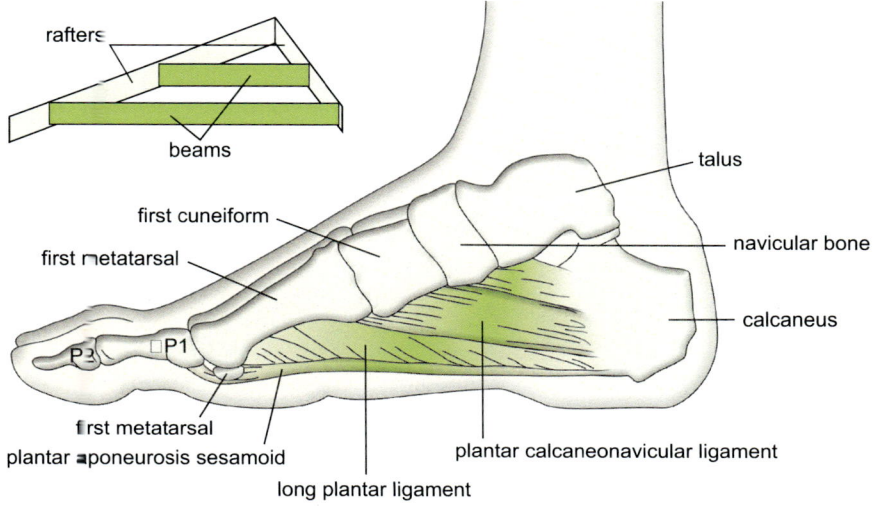

rafters

beams

first cuneiform

first metatarsal

P3 □P1

first metatarsal
plantar aponeurosis sesamoid

long plantar ligament

talus

navicular bone

calcaneus

plantar calcaneonavicular ligament

Figure 13.26. The foot truss.

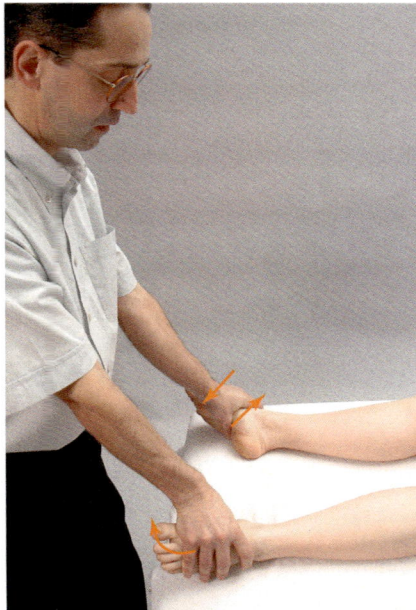

Figure 13.27. Routine for rounding the arch.

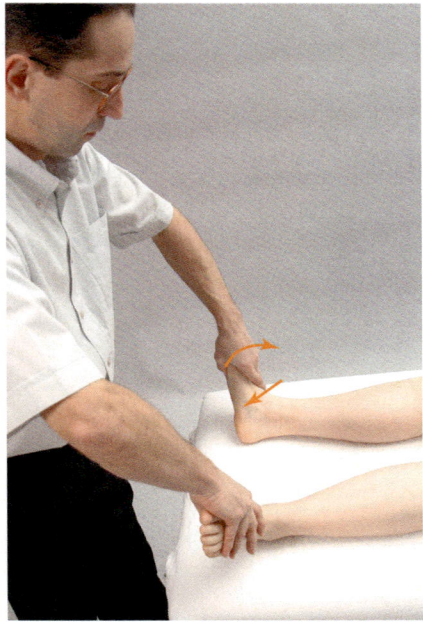

Figure 13.28. Routine for flattening the arch.

Results

Any difficulty noted either during flattening or rounding of the longitudinal arch of the foot is synonymous with dysfunction. It can be located at the level of the subtalar joint or the metatarsal, intertarsal, or tarsometatarsal articulations. These articulations must then be examined in depth to determine the site and the nature of the somatic dysfunction.

The Ankle

The patient is in the supine position, and you are at the feet. You can proceed in a symmetrical and comparative way (fig. 13.29). Place the heel of your hands on the anterior surface of the distal end of the lower legs. Exert gentle and gradual compression toward the table. This encourages gliding anteroposterior movement successively at the tibiotarsal joint and then at the subtalar joint (fig. 13.30). When you reach

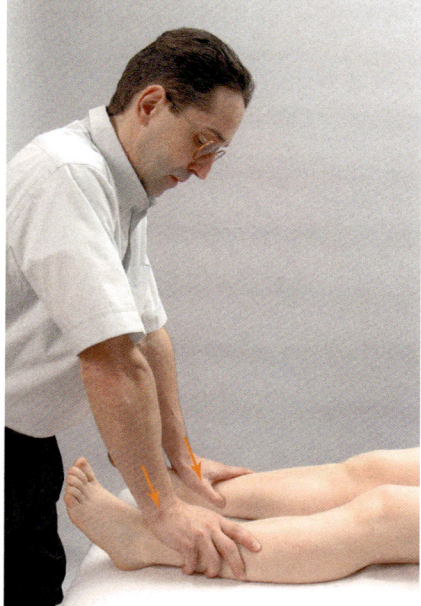

Figure 13.29. Routine for the tibia-talus-calcaneus junction.

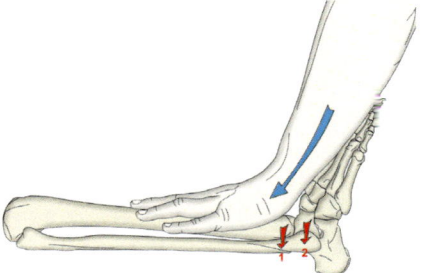

Figure 13.30. Gliding movements at the back of the foot.

the maximum possible movement, gently let go and analyze the speed and quality of the return movement. Normally, if both levels of the joint are free, the gliding is symmetrical and easy, and the return happens evenly and at the same speed on both sides. In the case of a fixation at the ankle or at the back of the foot, you will feel a significant resistance at the moment the movement starts, and sometimes even a "brick wall" feeling with no possibility of movement. You may also feel a speedy return, more significant on the side of the mechanical dysfunction. This indicates that some myofascial tensions are involved in the dysfunction.

The Knee

The routine tests of the knee call for a dual assessment: one for density and the other for global microdeformability. The subject is in the supine position with the legs straight. Standing at the level of the feet, test both knees at the same time to compare the palpatory information. Look for small movements of anteroposterior glide at the level of the femorotibial joint.

- Tibia-femur glide: place the palm of your hands on the anterior tibial tuberosity. Exert gentle and gradual pressure on the tibia toward the table. Comparatively assess the elasticity and deformability of the knees when placed under this constraint. Note the ease or resistance found on each side during this maneuver (fig. 13.31).
- Femur-tibia glide: move your hands next to the lower end of the femur. Again, exert gentle and gradual pressure toward the table. Note the ease or difficulty that you find during the test. Compare the two sides.

Any discomfort, blockage, restriction, or sensation of density that increases beneath one of your hands during compression should be considered abnormal. Suspect a somatic dysfunction of the knee on the same side; examine it precisely using more specific tests.

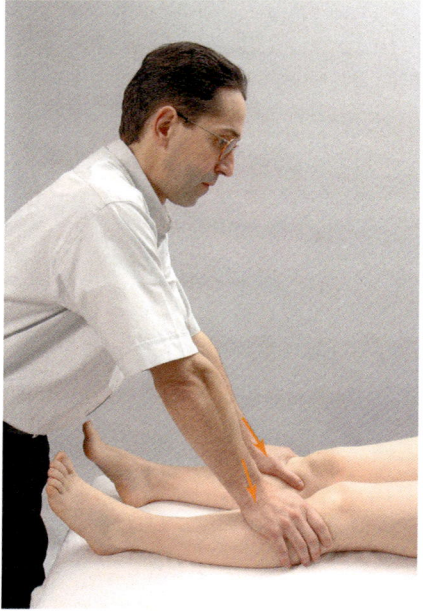

Figure 13.31. Tibia-femur glide routine.

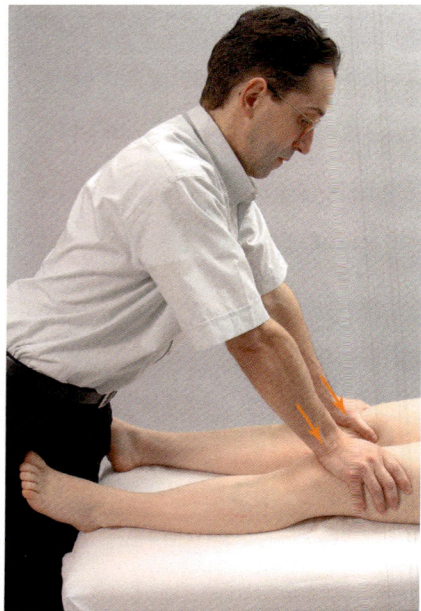

Figure 13.32. Femur-tibia glide routine.

The Hip: Rotators Test

First Test

The patient is in the supine position, and you are at the feet. Place the palms of your hands around the outer surfaces of the ankles, supporting them at the level of the Achilles tendon. Slightly lift the heels off the table, keeping the patient's lower limbs in extension. First, transmit a movement of internal rotation to the entire lower leg until both of your hands feel the same resistance. Then compare the amplitude obtained on the right and the left. If there is a difference in amplitude, the restricted side shows stronger tone in the external rotator muscles (fig. 13.33).

Second Test

Switch the placement of your hands at the feet. Cross your lower arms and take hold of the internal surfaces of the heels. Mobilize the lower leg toward external rotation. Compare amplitudes. Limitation in external rotation of one side shows stronger tone in the internal rotator muscles of this side. External rotation deficiency is often contralateral to internal rotation deficiency (fig. 13.34).

The hip rotation test is sensitive, but it is not specific to dysfunctions of the coxofemoral joint. The hip has a large number of external rotator muscles and only a few internal rotator muscles. When there is an imbalance, it is often the external rotators that cause it, and the amplitude of internal rotation is restricted. Any restriction in mobility observed during this test must lead you to investigate not only the hip but also all the elements that can be the cause of this mechanical destabilization: the base of the lumbar spine, the pubic symphysis, the back of the foot, the dorsolumbar transitional region, and neighboring

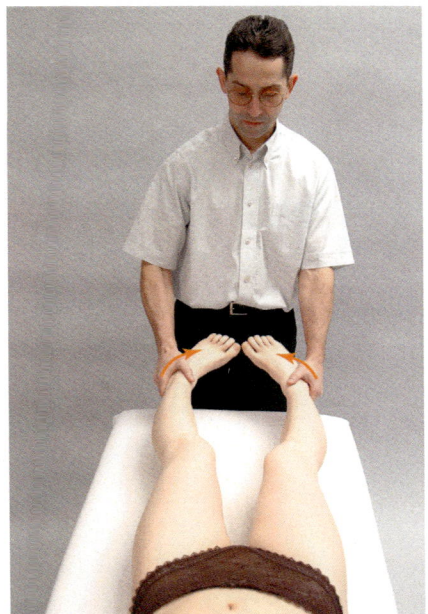 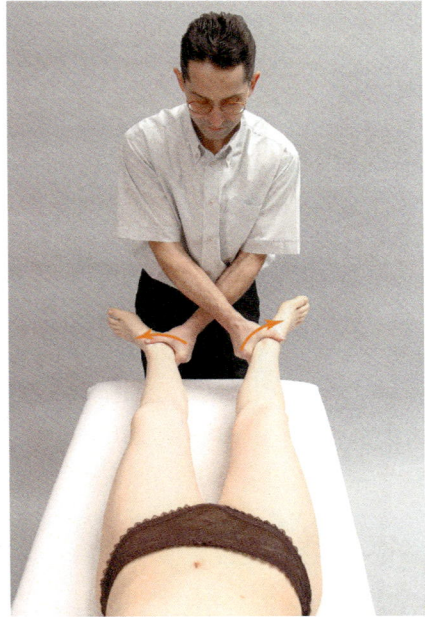

Figure 13.33. Coxofemoral internal rotation routine.

Figure 13.34. Coxofemoral external rotation routine.

myofascial and visceral elements (the obturator region, vesicles, the prostate, etc.).

The Ilia: Alternating Rotation

The patient is in the supine position. Stand at the side of the table, at the height of the knees, facing the patient. Place the palm of your hands on the anterior superior iliac spine (ASIS), centering your pectoral girdle above the patient's pelvis (fig. 13.35). Mobilize the iliac bones gently but firmly. Push the ASIS backward largely along the sagittal plane. Alternately examine the mobility of each side. In slowly releasing your pressure, also monitor the return of the ASIS toward the front. Note the ease of mobilization of each ilium in each direction. Any restriction or resistance to movement indicates sacroiliac dysfunction. But be cautious: it is not necessarily a primary somatic dysfunction; this test is also indicative of secondary dysfunctions and fixed adaptations.

The Pelvis: Lifted-knee Test

Also called the standing stork test, the lifted-knee test is very useful for detecting any somatic dysfunction of the sacroiliac joint. The patient stands facing a wall or a piece of furniture, placing the hands or leaning on them so that the upper limbs form a ninety-degree angle with the thorax. Stand behind and place the pads of your thumbs on the posterior superior iliac spines (PSIS). Then ask the patient to alternately lift one bent knee, then the other, above ninety degrees of hip flexion (fig. 13.36). Physiologically, the ilium makes a posterior rotation on the side of the elevated knee and an anterior rotation on the side of the supporting leg. From the point of view of palpation, this translates to a descending movement of your thumb on the side of the elevated knee and an ascending movement of your thumb on the other side. You can repeat this test, shifting your thumb placement to the base of the sacrum and, finally, under the inferolateral angles of the sacrum. Physiologically, the sacrum makes a lateral side-bend on the side of the supporting leg.

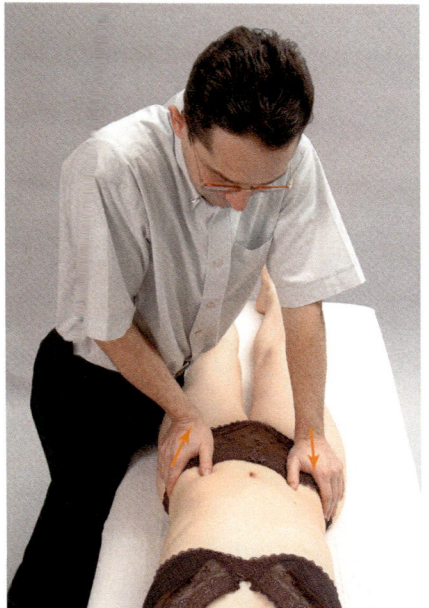

Figure 13.35. Alternating iliac rotation routine.

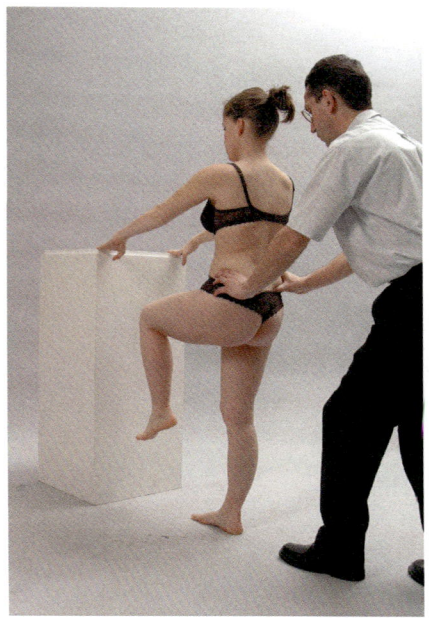

Figure 13.36. Lifted-knee routine.

With regard to spinal curvature, this test is particularly useful when there is acute lumbago. Even in a case of very painful blockage, the patient generally retains the ability to lift the knee.

Superior Pole

The Temporomandibular Joint

Standing behind the seated patient, place your middle fingers at the level of the external auditory meatus. With your index fingers, locate the mandibular condyles just in front of the auditory canal (figs. 13.37 and 13.38). Then ask the patient to open the mouth wide while you follow the movement of each condyle with your index finger. Next, ask the patient to close the mouth, and check to see if the return movement is harmonious or not. Normally, the play in the two temporomandibular joints should be perfectly synchronous and symmetrical. Note every

323

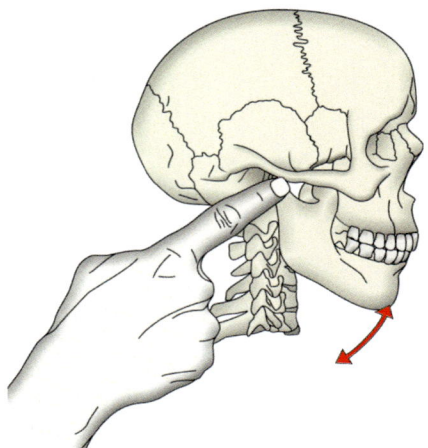

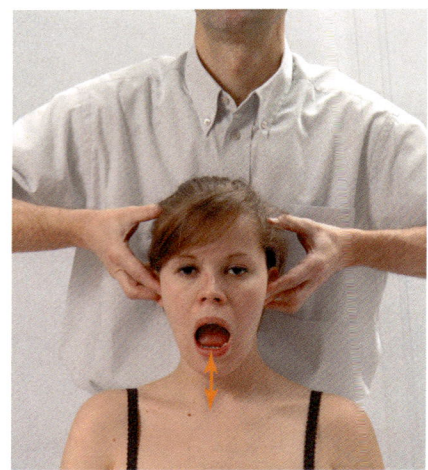

Figure 13.37. Finger contact for the temporomandibular joint routine.

Figure 13.38. Temporomandibular joint routine.

shift, delay, and lack of movement during these opening and closing movements. Clicking, cracking, or even pain during movement are also good signs of somatic dysfunction of the temporomandibular joint

The Sternoclavicular Joint

Standing behind the seated patient, place your middle fingers on the anterior surfaces of the proximal ends of the clavicles and your index fingers immediately above on the superior border. Ask the patient to shrug the shoulders, then to let them down (fig. 13.39). In the absence of a fixation in the sternocostoclavicular joint or the scapulothoracic joint, during the elevation of the distal tip of the shoulder you will feel that the proximal ends of the clavicles glide downward. They rise back up with the return movement.

Next, ask the patient to roll the shoulders forward (fig. 13.40). On the rolling movement, the proximal ends move slightly backward; they move back to their original position during the return movement.

These clavicular movements are disrupted or completely absent when there is a fixation of the scapula, restriction of the deep fascia

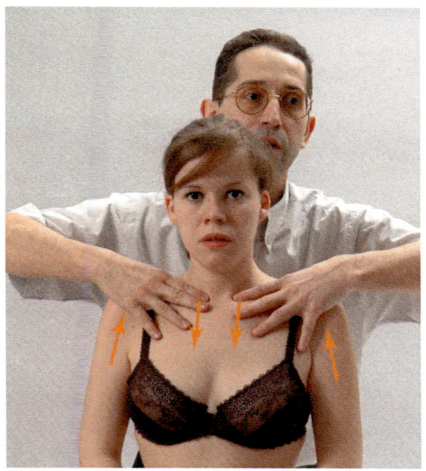

Figure 13.39. Elevating the tip of the scapula routine.

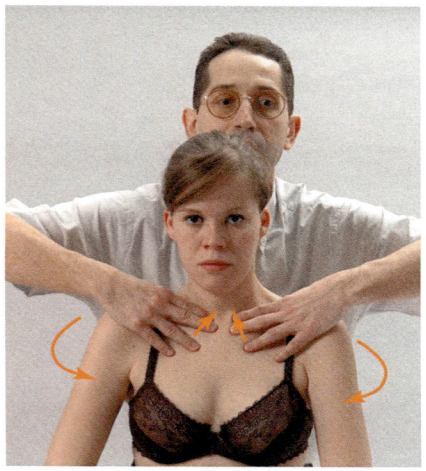

Figure 13.40. Rolling the tip of the scapula routine.

of the shoulder, or when there is a somatic dysfunction of the sternoclavicular joint.

The Acromioclavicular Joint

Now place the palms of your hands on the external surfaces of the shoulders. Between your thumb and index finger, take hold of the distal end of the clavicle. Stabilize the head of the humerus between the heel of your hand and the pads of your little fingers. Gently mobilize the distal end of the clavicle toward the back and then toward the front (fig. 13.41). Any restriction in anteroposterior movement suggests a somatic acromioclavicular dysfunction, or a fixation of the coracoclavicular ligaments or the subclavius muscle.

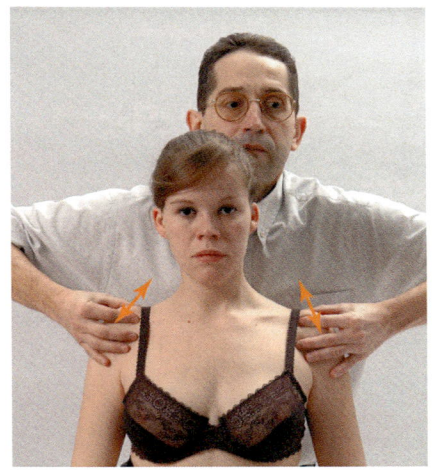

Figure 13.41. Acromioclavicular glide routine.

325

The Scapulohumeral Joint

The patient is seated with forearms relaxed and hands on the thighs. Standing behind, wrap your hands around the outer surfaces of the heads of the humeri and hold them between your finger pads and the heel of your hand. Mobilize both humeral heads simultaneously toward the front, then toward the back (fig. 13.42). Normally, the amplitude,

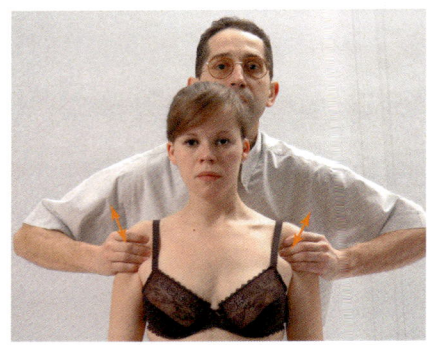

Figure 13.42. Anteroposterior glide routine for the glenohumeral joint.

resistance, and ease of movement are symmetrical. Any resistance to mobilization on one side compared to the other suggests a somatic scapulohumeral dysfunction or myofascial tension involving this joint.

The Elbow

The patient is seated, elbows bent, forearms supinated and resting on the anterior surface of the thighs. Place your hands just above the bend in the elbow, on the anterior surface of the proximal part of the forearm. Exert soft pressure on the forearm toward the table. Continue your pressure until the humerus glides downward at the level of the scapulohumeral joint. Slowly let the tissues come back, and compare the two sides (fig. 13.43). Normally, the movement

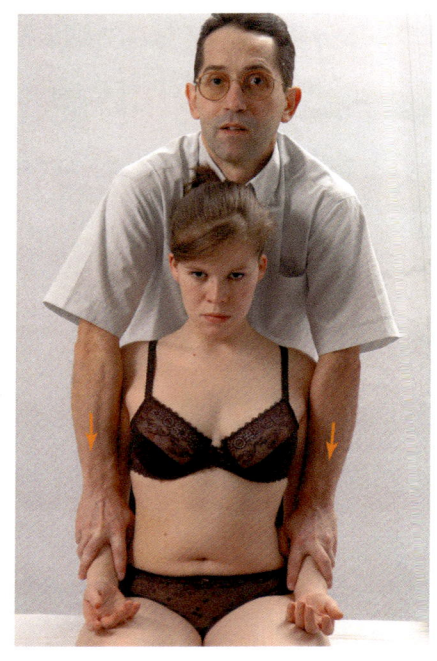

Figure 13.43. Elbow decompression routine.

is fairly ample and symmetrical; there is no sudden stop. Analyze resistances that you find carefully. At first, information comes from the elbow. The feeling of freedom or blockage is produced by the capacity for separation of the humeroulnar and humeroradial joints. At the end of the movement, you should sense the freedom of the shoulder joint in the vertical direction.

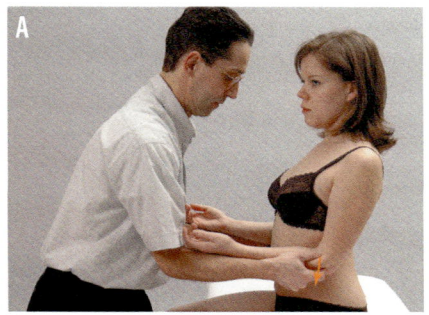

The Radial Head

The patient is seated, elbows bent, hands placed on your forearms. You are facing the patient with your forearms supinated and your hands supporting the elbow

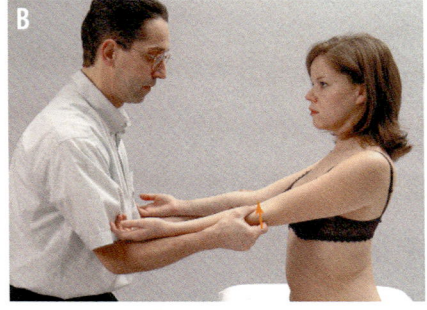

Figure 13.44. Radial head routine.

region. With your thumb and index finger grasping it, monitor the radial head (fig. 13.44). Bring the elbows into extension and monitor the movement of the radial head, which should glide slightly forward. Then move the elbows into flexion and verify that the radial head now glides toward the back. The test is comparative. Note any restriction to mobility and any asymmetry at the level of the radial head.

The Forearm

The patient is in the supine position, forearms straight and pronated. Stabilize the patient's hand between your finger pads and your palm. Then place your thumb on the dorsal surface of the distal end of the radius and push it in the direction of the table. You thus provoke radio-ulnar and radiocarpal gliding in the palmar direction (fig. 13.45). Next, shift your thumb onto the ulnar styloid and do the same thing. Compare each glide with the opposite side (fig. 13.46). Any restriction in

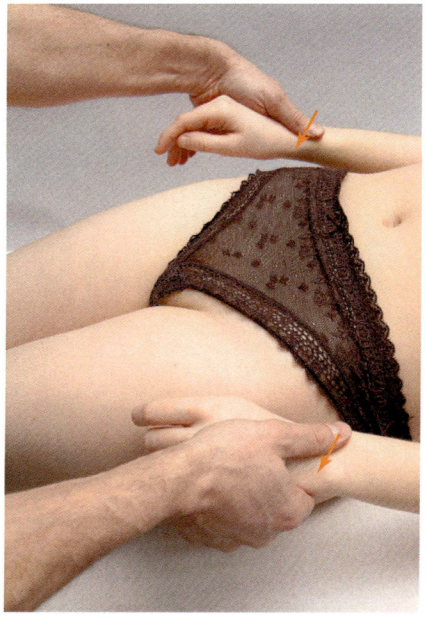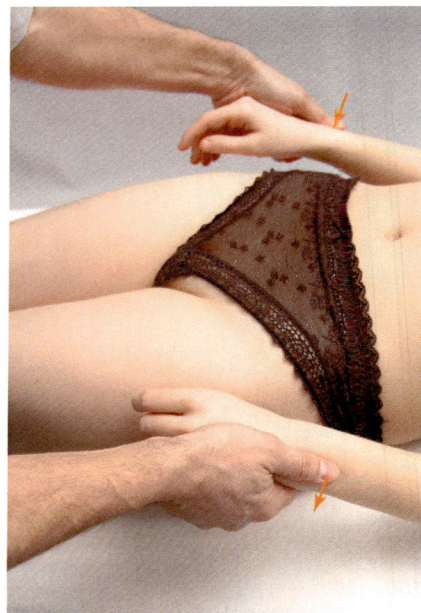

Figure 13.45. Palmar radial glide routine.   **Figure 13.46. Palmar ulnar glide routine.**

these different movements must lead you to investigate the mechanics of the elbow and the two bones of the forearm. It can signal a fixation of the interosseous membrane, a somatic dysfunction related to the ulna, the radius, or even the carpus.

NOTE

When there is a rupture of the triangular fibrocartilage complex, the movement of the ulnar styloid is distinctly larger. This exaggerated amplitude is the *piano-key sign,* revealing instability of the distal radioulnar joint.

The Wrist

Global evaluation of the possibilities of separation of the wrist provides a good demonstration of the play in the radiocarpal and the intercarpal joints. Locate the joint space all around the wrist precisely, and surround the carpals with your thumb and index finger. You are in

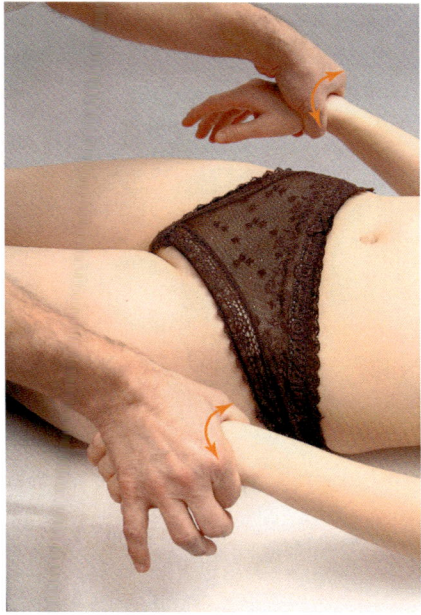

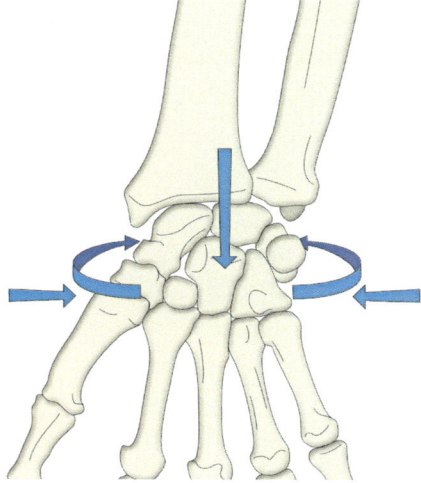

Figure 13.47. Wrist decompression routine.   Figure 13.48. Wrist decompression routine.

the right position if your thumbs and index fingers are just below the radial and ulnar styloids (fig. 13.47). Gently and gradually compress the carpal pillar along its circumference, as if delicately strangling it. In the absence of a fixation, you will feel the carpals being slightly deformed, then separating from the forearm, something like a wet bar of soap that slips away when you try to grasp it (fig. 13.48). All fixations located at the level of the hand, the wrist, or the radiocarpal joint alter or suppress this sensation. The carpal pillar seems rigid, unchanging in shape, or impacted at the wrist to the forearm.

Visceral Routines

Evaluation of Intracavity Pressures

An analysis of the prevailing pressures in the interior of the different chambers of the trunk is the preliminary general approach to visceral mechanics. The test consists of comparing the pressures that prevail in the thorax, in the supramesocolic zone, and in the inframesocolic zone (figs. 13.49, 13.50, and 13.51). To evaluate this parameter, imagine that you are verifying the degree of inflation of a balloon. It is possible to do this without necessarily crushing or even deforming the balloon. Applying slight compression to the balloon tells us instantly if it is inflated or deflated. Proceed in the same way for the different compartments of the trunk. Gently place your hand on the wall and apply a slight amount of compression with your hand to adapt to

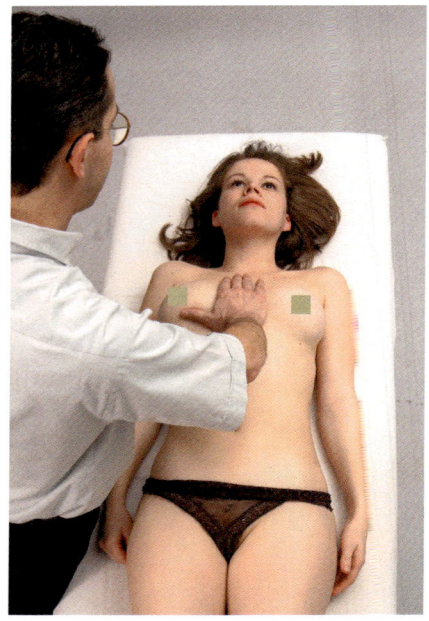

Figure 13.49. Evaluation of thoracic pressure.

that of the wall. Then, very gently compress the wall to feel for the prevailing pressure in the underlying volume. This is a very slight movement with very small amplitude. Make this evaluation at the level of the sternum, then in the supraumbilical and the infraumbilical regions. Generally, in the case of a visceral dysfunction in the zone being investigated, you will feel a clear increase in pressure.

- An increase in intrathoracic pressure can signal pleural, pulmonary, mediastinal, diaphragmatic, or pericardial dysfunction. It can also be observed when there's a dysfunction of the viscera of the neck, either the thyroid or the thymus.
- An increase in the supraumbilical pressure generally suggests dysfunctions concerning the liver, the stomach, the spleen, the gastroesophageal junction, the bile ducts, or the duodenum-pancreas.

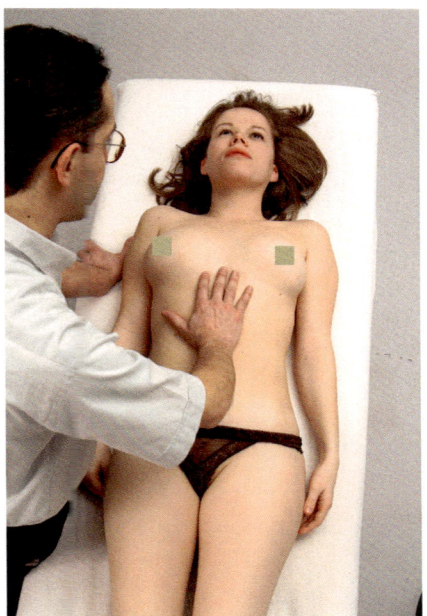 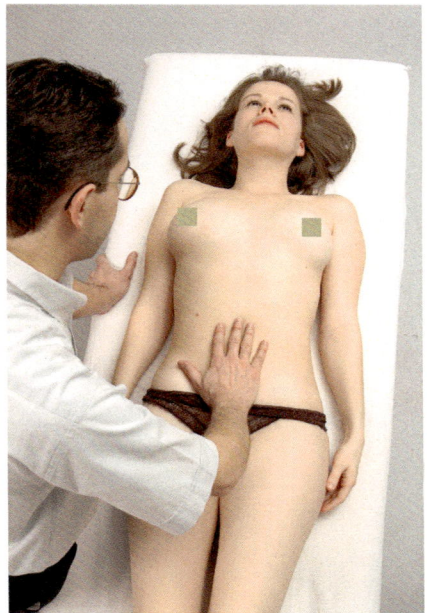

Figure 13.50. Evaluation of supra-mesocolic pressure.

Figure 13.51. Evaluation of infra-mesocolic pressure.

■ An increase in infraumbilical pressure is generally caused by dysfunction of the small intestines, the colon, the sigmoid colon, the rectum, the kidneys, the bladder, the prostate, or the uterus.

Local Listening

Originally developed by Jean-Pierre Barral, the notion of local listening has been widely practiced in recent years. Founded on the same principles as general listening, it considers a more limited area of visceral mechanics. The techniques of listening are carried out with the hand in contact with the body. According to the amount of pressure, it is possible to listen to different tissues at different levels. For visceral structures, the pressure is approximately equivalent to the weight of the hand. Each large visceral unit is heard in a key place. Visceral listenings are done from the following three observation sites:

- the sternum
- the supraumbilical region
- the infraumbilical region

You can limit yourself to listening to a zone where you have found the greatest pressure in the preceding test. Place the palm of your dominant hand on the zone that you'd like to observe. The attraction of the palm resting on the body, and not the attraction of the fingers, will tell you at which level the problem lies. If the palm moves toward the right and the fingers move toward the left, the most significant mechanical dysfunction resides to the right.

Jean-Pierre Barral (1988) has codified the different sensations obtained and their visceral correspondences. The parameters of gliding, sinking, tilting, and rotation of the listening hand have specific meanings that facilitate the diagnosis.

Viscoelastic Test of the Trunk Contents

When subjected to moderate compression, an organ changes shape at two separate times: immediate deformation is of an elastic nature, and deferred deformation has a viscoelastic nature. To call viscoelasticity into play, it is not the intensity of the compression that is important, but rather the amount of time compression has to be applied for the tissue reaction to occur. To be more precise in your diagnostic hypothesis, it is possible to make an evaluation of the visceral reaction to more localized pressure. In the case of the mechanical dysfunction of an organ, or even organ pathology, these two parameters, viscoelasticity and elasticity, change. The organ in question loses some of its ability to change shape, and its density seems to increase. It is possible to note this manually.

The abdomen is divided in nine sectors (fig. 13.52). These different topographic zones have precise limits and a specific shape. Although often represented in two dimensions on the surface of the body, these zones are, in fact, three-dimensional volumes whose contents are relatively constant. The thorax is divided into three zones: two pleuropulmonary cavities and the mediastinum, which communicates with the viscera of the neck.

It is desirable to perform tests of viscoelasticity on each of these zones. When possible, proceed by comparing symmetrical zones. For the asymmetrical zones, with experience you will quickly acquire a feel for what is normal and abnormal. It is good to be systematic, at least at the beginning. With practice, if the results of the previous test are clear-cut, you can confine yourself to exploring only the suspect zones. A problematic zone can be examined in a more specific way through

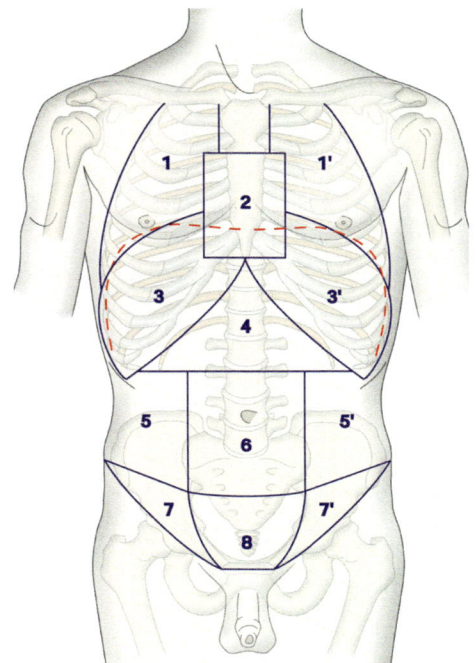

Figure 13.52. Topographic zones of the trunk.

each of the different organs it contains. We study the viscoelastic reaction of each to more limited compression inside the same zone.

The Hypochondriac Region

Begin by evaluating the viscoelasticity of the right and left hypochondrium. Apply an anteroposterior pressure on the anterior surface of each hypochondrium and compare (fig. 13.53). Next, apply pressure on the frontal plane and compare (fig. 13.54). Check the pressure by placing the heel of your hand below the inferior costal margin and pushing in the direction of the diaphragmatic pleura (fig. 13.55). Any feeling of increase in density or decrease in viscoelasticity on the right side should lead you to suspect a mechanical problem of the right lobe of the liver, the bile ducts, the right costophrenic recess, the right diaphragmatic pleura, and sometimes also the right kidney or adrenal gland. On the

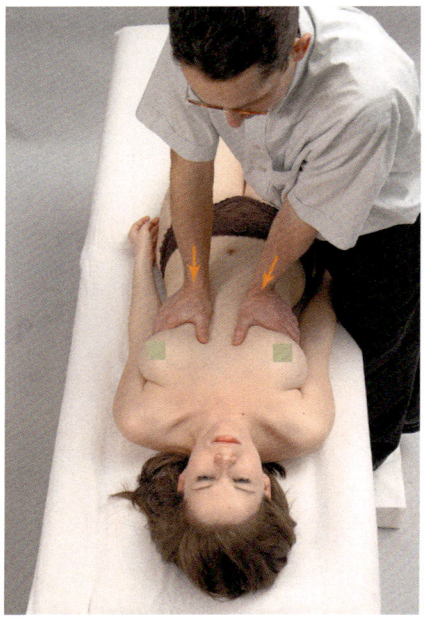

left, the cause could be at the gastroesophageal junction, the fundus or body of the stomach, the left lobe of the liver, the spleen, the left costodiaphragmatic recess, and the left diaphragmatic pleura.

The Thoracic Cavity

Place your hands on the right and left pulmonary areas, on both sides of the cardiac zone, approximately two or three finger-widths below the clavicle. Exert slight anteroposterior compression and

Figure 13.53. Anteroposterior evaluation of hypochondriac region viscoelasticity.

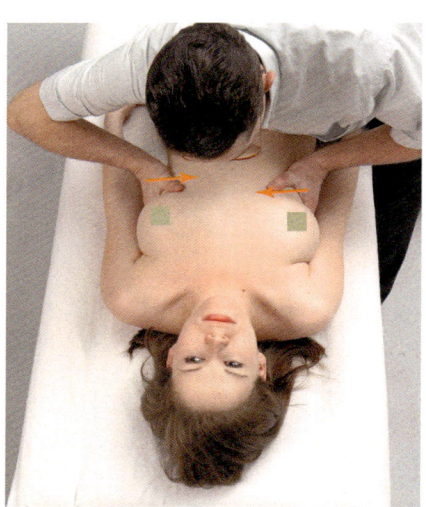

Figure 13.54. Transverse evaluation of hypochondriac region viscoelasticity.

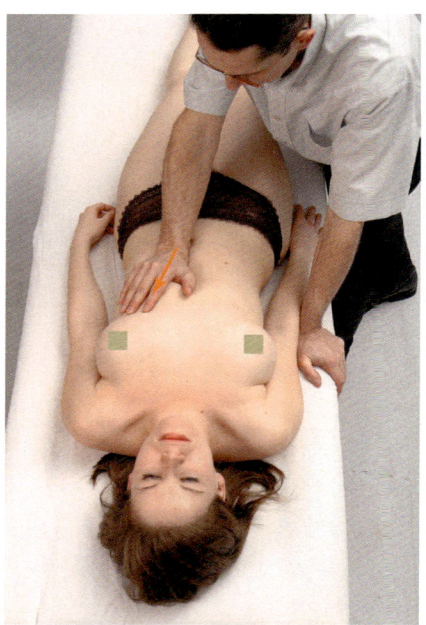

Figure 13.55. Vertical evaluation of hypochondriac region viscoelasticity.

compare. A restriction of viscoelasticity at this level could indicate a dysfunction of the middle and upper parts of the pleura, of the lung, the bronchi, or the viscera of the neck on the same side (fig. 13.56).

The Mediastinum

Place your hand on the sternum and apply slight anteroposterior compression. In the case of a restriction, we generally perceive a feeling of significant density underneath the sternum. A number of significant pulls of your hand can take place during the course of the test; the sternum is linked mechanically to multiple intrathoracic elements. A disturbance in this zone indicates dysfunction at the level of the mediastinum or the viscera of the neck. Pay attention specifically to the pericardium and its ligaments, the thymus, the thyroid, the visceral sheath of the neck, and the diaphragm (fig. 13.57).

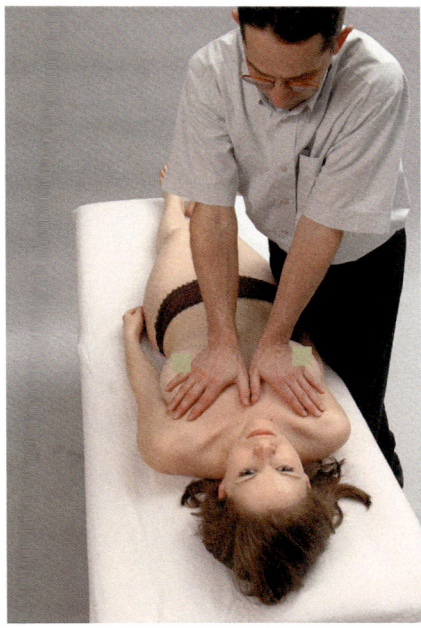 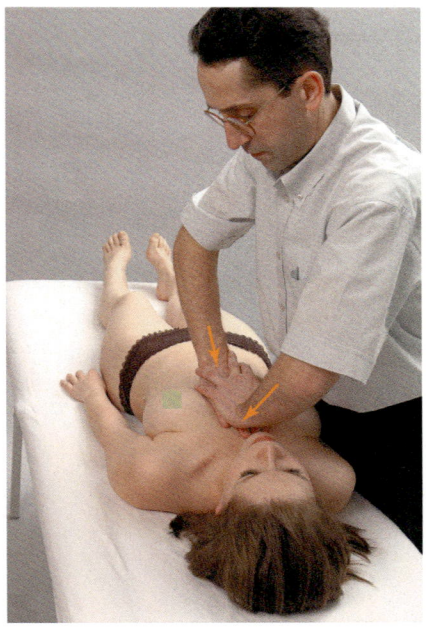

Figure 13.56. Evaluation of thoracic cavity viscoelasticity.

Figure 13.57. Global evaluation of mediastinal viscoelasticity.

NOTE

The test could also indicate problems when there is cardiac pathology or damage to the large thoracic vessels.

The Sides

Stand well above the supine patient. Place the palm of each of your hands on the anterior surface of the right side and the left side. Apply gentle compression on the side in the direction of the table. Compare by performing the maneuver either simultaneously or alternately on one side and then the other (fig. 13.58). In the case of a restriction on the right side, there could be mechanical dysfunction of the right kidney, the ascending colon, or the hepatic flexure. On the left side, the restriction concerns the left kidney, the splenic flexure, the descending colon, or the small intestine.

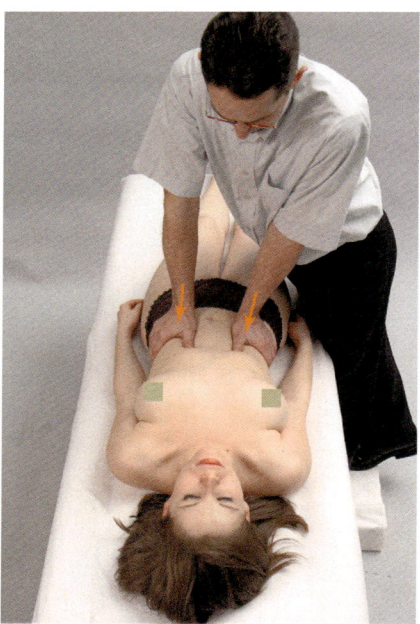

Figure 13.58. Anteroposterior evaluation of side viscoelasticity.

The Iliac Fossa

Place your right hand flat over the patient's right iliac fossa, parallel to the inguinal ligament. Gently pronate your hand to direct your compression downward, outward, and backward. Do the same on the left side and compare (fig. 13.59). For restrictions on the right side, consider the cecum, the ileocecal valve (ICV), and the appendix, as well as the right ovary. On the left side, it could be the sigmoid colon, the rectum, or the bottom part of the ileum.

The Epigastric Region

Place the heel of your hand in the epigastric fossa and provide slight compression toward the back and a little toward the cranium (fig. 13.60) Any restriction found in this test should make us suspect the central part of the diaphragm or the liver, the antropyloric region of the stomach, the duodenal-pancreatic block, the common bile duct and the sphincter of Oddi, the solar plexus, and the celiac artery.

The Umbilical Region

Place your hand flat on the umbilicus, perpendicular to the axis of the body. Slightly flex your fingers and metacarpals as you slightly compress the area in the direction of the table (fig. 13.61). A loss in viscoelasticity at this level directs us to the greater omentum, the jejunum and ileum, the root of the mesentery, or the abdominal aorta. If the

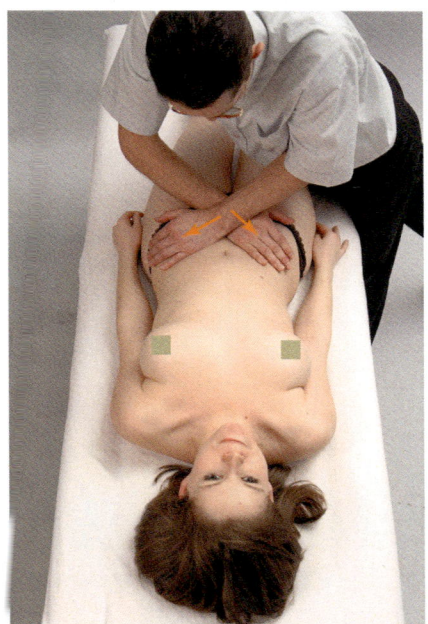

Figure 13.59. Evaluation of iliac fossa viscoelasticity.

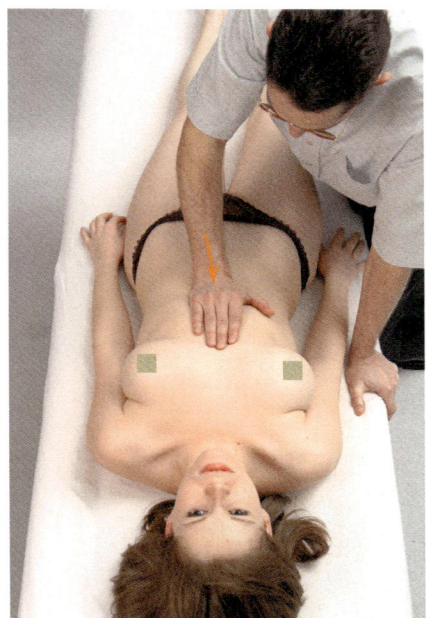

Figure 13.60. Evaluation of epigastric viscoelasticity.

337

restriction is limited to the supraumbilical region, it generally involves the hepatopancreatic ampulla, the second part of the duodenum, or the head of the pancreas.

The Hypogastric Region

Place the palm of your hand above the pubic region, between the inner edge of the two sides of the psoas muscle and a little below the projection of the sacral promontory. Exert slight pressure toward the back and in the caudal direction, at an angle of approximately forty-five degrees (fig. 13.62). A restriction in this zone should lead you to suspect the bladder, the internal genital organs (prostate and seminal vesicles or uterus, fallopian tubes, and ovaries), or the rectum.

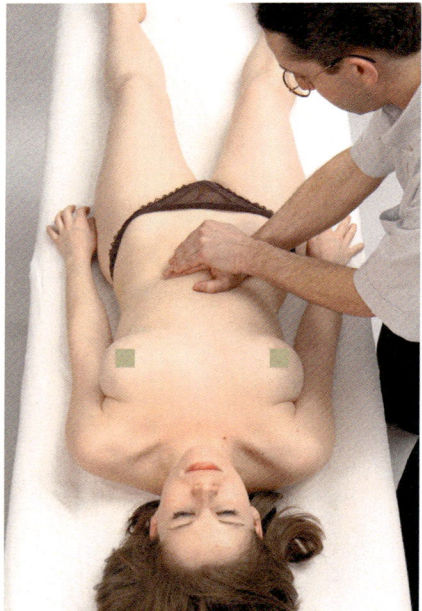 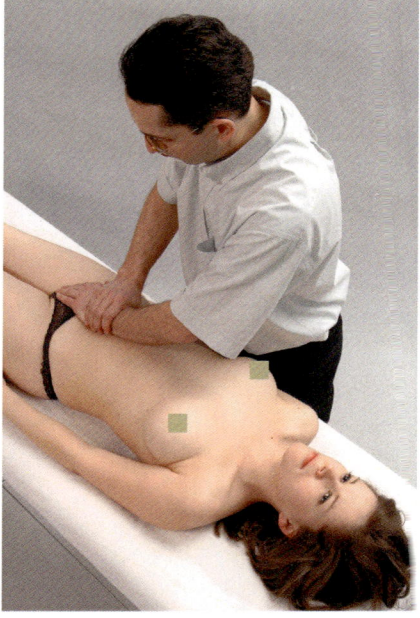

Figure 13.61. Evaluation of umbilical region viscoelasticity.

Figure 13.62. Evaluation of hypogastric viscoelasticity.

Quick Elasticity Test of the Thoracic Contents

Because of the great interdependence of the visceral container and its contents, at the thoracic level any loss of mobility necessarily affects both components. In the case of a problem, it is necessary to distinguish what arises from a somatic dysfunction from what arises from a visceral source. A good indication of the mechanical freedom of the pleuropulmonary and cardiopericardial contents is given by tests of elasticity of the thorax. Of the utmost importance is the depth at which you carry out these tests. They must not be limited to the thoracic wall but must also address the visceral elements and their envelopes, located more deeply.

Diagonal Test

Stand to the side, facing the supine patient. With your cephalic hand, contact the distal tip of the scapula with the pads of your fingers so that the heel of your hand is inside and a little above the coracoid process (fig. 13.63). With your caudal

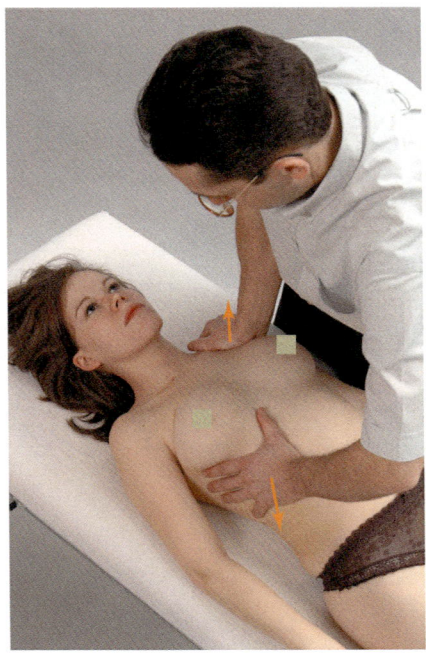

hand, contact the lower part of the contralateral hemithorax, with the shaft of your thumb and your little finger placed just above the inferior costal margin. Begin by exerting very slight pressure. Then gradually deepen the pressure so that your hands connect to the whole formed by the thoracic wall and the underlying organs. Apply traction along the axis of the diagonal formed by your hands, moving them away from each other.

Figure 13.63. Diagonal test of thoracic elasticity.

Evaluate the global elasticity of the thorax in this direction, and change to the other side to compare it with the opposite diagonal. With a little practice, you will have a very good sense, globally, of whether there is a restriction on one side or the other. It is even possible to determine where on the diagonal the majority of the fixation is located.

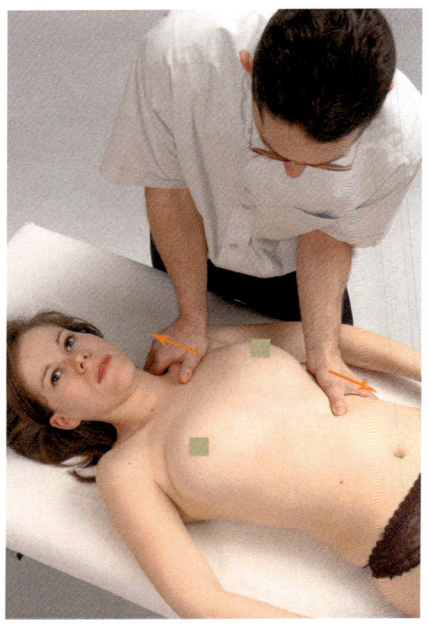

Figure 13.64. Test of unilateral thoracic elasticity.

Direct Test

This test is carried out with the same mindset as the preceding test, and it further refines those results. In the same position, place your cephalic hand on the superior part of the thorax, nestling the shaft of your thumb just below the clavicle to ensure a good hold. The rest of the hand is placed on the region of the trapezius (fig. 13.64). With your caudal hand, grasp the inferior ipsilateral costal margin between your thumb and fingers, with your thumb on the anterior surface of the thorax and your fingers and palm on the posterolateral surface of the thorax. Apply traction longitudinally, pushing in the cranial direction with the clavicle hand and in a caudal direction with the rib cage hand.

Craniosacral Routines

Local listenings of the cranium are a good way of investigating the craniosacral system and can be part of the routines. However, they are discussed with specific diagnosis since their complex decoding prematurely hinders routines. In this section I will describe simple and quick ways to evaluate the craniosacral system without necessarily listening to the primary respiratory mechanism (PRM).

The craniosacral unit is a coherent mechanical system. It is possible to evaluate its different components through tests of its structure. The cranium is a mechanical whole with the capacity to change shape; the routines that we use evaluate its response to deformation provoked by an outside force. From the purist point of view, this approach is controversial; however, it is a quick and effective way of evaluating the craniosacral system. This type of approach necessitates respect for a range of force and amplitude comparable to that of the classic cranial approach.

Evaluating the Four Parts of the Cranium

Because of its hydraulic structure, made of sutured bones, membranes, the encephalon, and liquids, the cranium has little elasticity. Like the visceral system but to a lesser extent, the craniosacral system has some viscoelasticity. With the same mindset as in the tests of visceral viscoelasticity, it is possible to begin to evaluate the cranial mechanism in four broad areas (figs. 13.65 to 13.69). Each test consists of lightly compressing the cranium along a precise line of force with the goal of evaluating the mechanics of a particular sector. The principle is to determine the elasticity perceived during compression and to assess the quality of the return movement. In the case of dysfunction in cranial mechanics, we generally feel either an increase of density with compression or a difficult return during release.

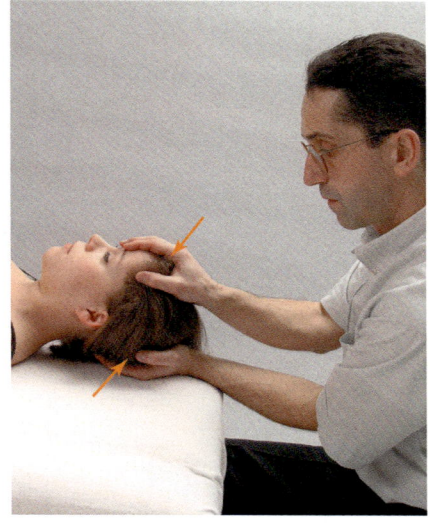

Figure 13.65. Evaluation in the glabella-inion axis.

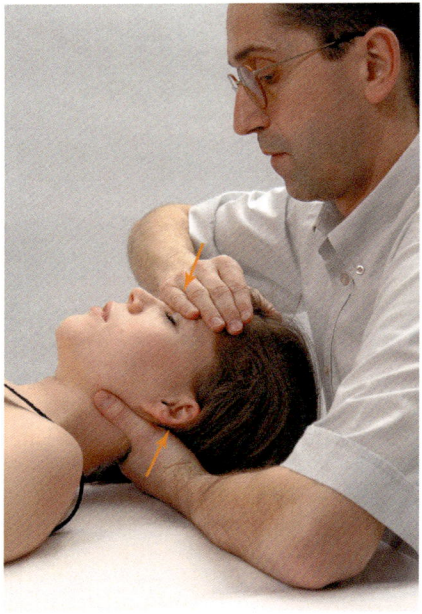

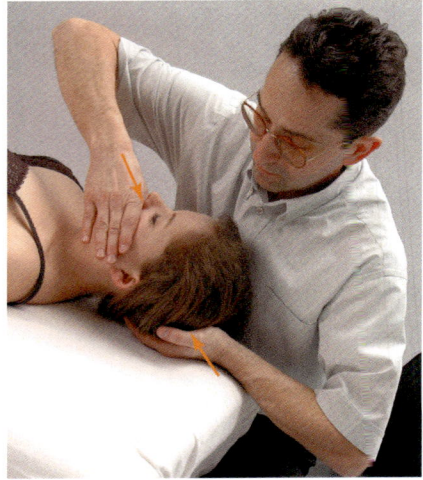

Figure 13.67. Evaluation in the incisive bone-obelion axis.

Figure 13.66. Evaluation in the nasion-opisthion axis.

Results

- The glabella-inion axis gives evidence of dysfunctions that primarily concern the cranial vault (fig. 13.70 A).
- The nasion-opisthion axis reveals dysfunctions located at the level of the base of the cranium (fig. 13.70 B).

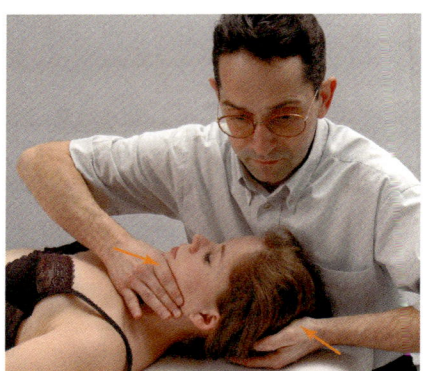

Figure 13.68. Evaluation in the gnathion-obelion axis.

- The incisive bone-obelion axis indicates dysfunctions touching the facial skeleton, the sinuses, and the maxillary teeth (fig. 13.70 C).
- The gnathion-obelion axis gives some indications of the functioning of the masticatory system: the mandible, the temporomandibular joint, the alignment of the teeth, and the temporal bones (fig. 13.70 D).

342

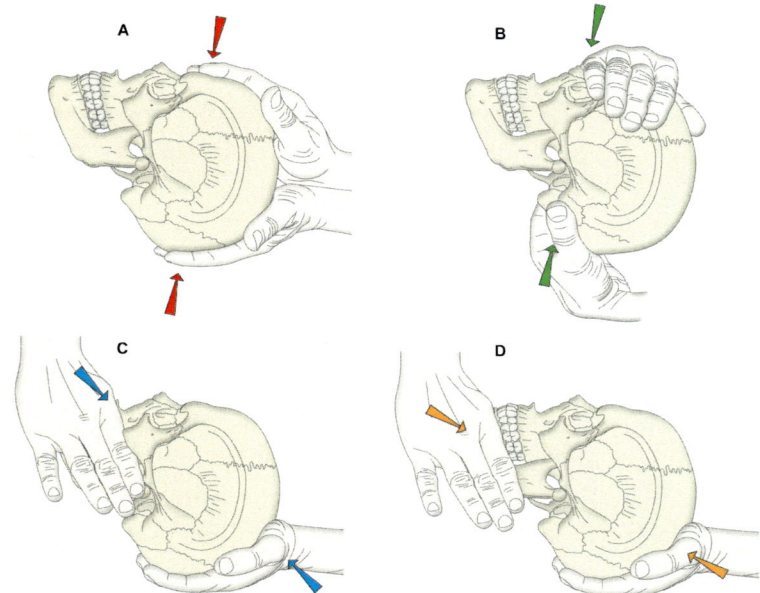

Figure 13.69. Axes of evaluating the four parts of the cranium.

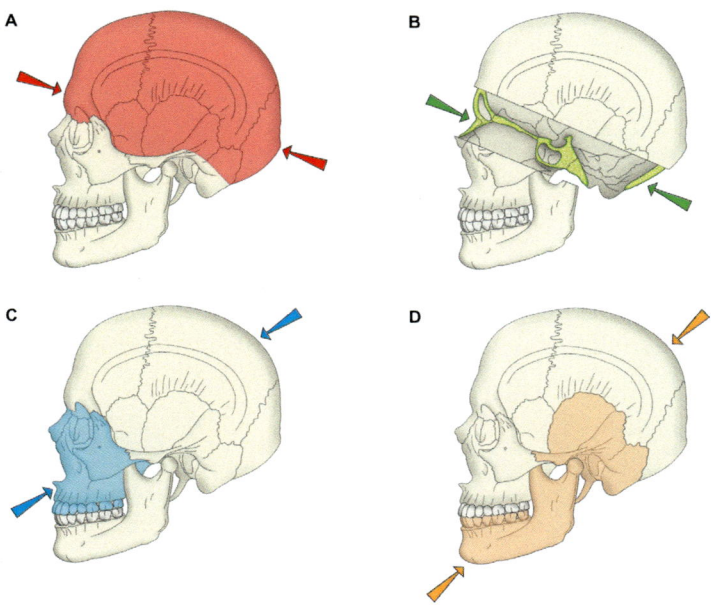

Figure 13.70. The four parts of the cranium.

Circumferential Test of Cranial Elasticity

This test is inspired by the approach to interosseous dysfunctions perfected by my excellent colleague and friend Vincent Benedetto. I have adapted and applied the principle to the entire cranium.

Principles of the Test

Osseous tissue has slight elasticity that can be perceived manually. At the level of the cranium, it is possible to assess the elasticity of a band of osseous tissue by subjecting it to longitudinal compression. If the bone has good elastic capacity, you will feel a very slight deformation as a result of the pressure. If the elastic capacity is mediocre, you will feel increased tissue density. As soon as you apply compression, the band of tissue seems to jump away from your fingers and refuses to change shape. This perception is more evident if you can compare the response of two bands of symmetrical osseous tissue (fig. 13.71). For more clarity, let's draw an analogy between the cranium and the earth. The test is performed on osseous tissue bands oriented like the earth's lines of

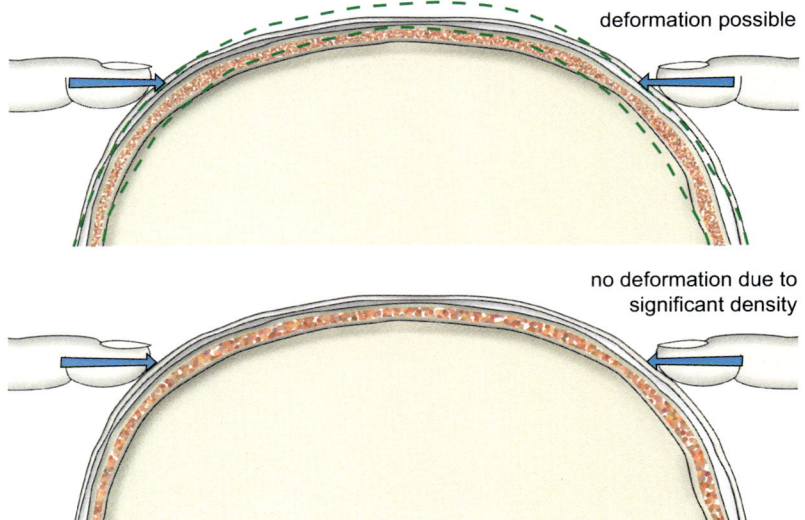

Figure 13.71. Compressing cranial osseous tissue.

344

longitude. This exploration is performed on the "northern hemisphere" of the cranium, between the vertex and the bottom part of the cranial vault. However, for reasons that are not totally clear, experience shows that this test also detects dysfunctions located in the "southern hemisphere," at the level of the base of the skull or the facial skeleton. The examination provides information about the state of an entire line of longitude, from pole to pole.

Performing the Test

Place both of your thumbs on the obelion. You will successively test several bands of osseous tissue in several directions, trying to produce a mini-bend in these bands all around the cranium. If the bend is harmonious, the cranial mechanics are free in that direction. If the osseous band resists, its direction tells you where cranial mechanics are restricted (fig. 13.72). Begin by placing your index fingers on the inner part of each orbital ridge on the frontal bone. Visualize the band of tissue between your thumbs and index fingers, and then gradually compress it longitudinally. It is a gentle and delicate test. If the contact of your fingers applies the correct pressure, adapted to the density of the osseous tissue, you will not need any force. Compare the elasticity of the right band and the left band. Notice any restrictions. Then begin again with the same procedure, moving your index fingers to the external part of each orbital ridge on the

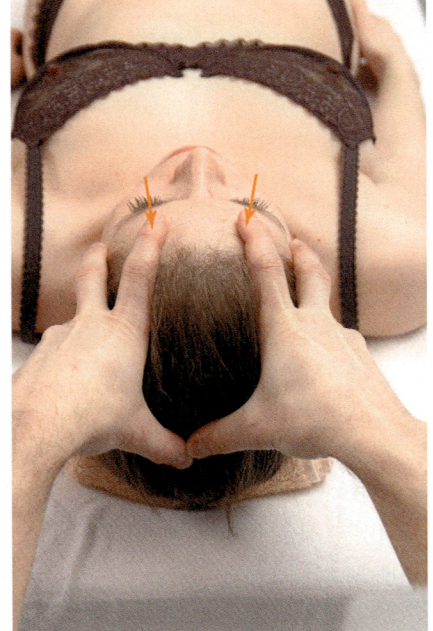

Figure 13.72. Circumferential evaluation of the cranium.

frontal bone. Do the same with your middle fingers placed on the zygomatic processes, midway between the orbital ridges and the tragi. Then proceed with your ring fingers placed on the mastoid processes. Finish with your little fingers placed on the curved plate of the occiput (fig. 13.73).

Results

Every dysfunction of cranial mechanics, wherever it is located, concerns the entire cranium and has an impact on the totality of the

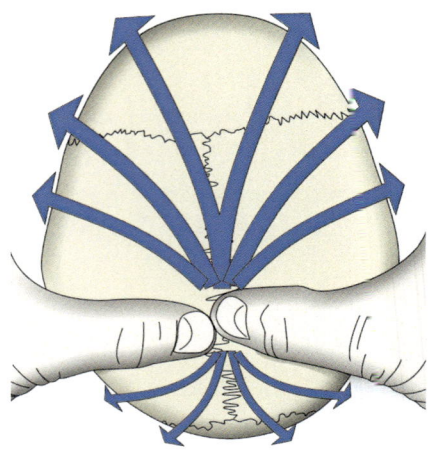

Figure 13.73. The bands in the circumferential test.

cranial bowl. If you feel that one or two bands of osseous tissue seem more rigid, and you have also found a sector of the cranium showing dysfunction in the preceding test, then you have a precise enough localization of the predominant cranial problem. Combining the results of these two tests gives you the region you need to focus on to complete your specific diagnosis. If we consider again the comparison of the cranium to the earth, we can say that the first test gives you the *latitude* of the dysfunction, while the second test tells you the *longitude*.

Micromobility and Sacral Deformability

Evaluation of the sacrum in the craniosacral relationship does not call on the same parameters as its evaluation from the osteoarticular point of view. In the physiology of the PRM, we often compare the cranium to the mechanism of a clock and the sacrum to the clock's pendulum. A more exact vision of this mechanical model is that the rod of the pendulum is equipped with little elasticity, but it is necessary to the functioning of the whole.

NOTE

- The mechanics of the sacrum and its influences are complex. A somatic dysfunction of the sacrum generally leads to a disturbance of the craniosacral system. On the other hand, absence of somatic dysfunction does not necessarily mean that the sacrum is free in its craniosacral relationship.
- Even if it is insufficient to destabilize sacroiliac joint mechanics, tissue tension can disturb the sacral play in the PRM. This is this aspect that the craniosacral routine evaluates.
- Finally, the sacrum can be ruled out as a cause only if it is free in the two facets of its mechanics: osteoarticular freedom and freedom within the craniosacral relationship.

Sacral Decompression Test

This test allows you to assess the fine balance of the sacrum. It detects the slightest tissue imbalance with great sensitivity. It clearly detects or confirms somatic dysfunctions of the sacroiliac joints and the lumbosacral and sacrococcygeal junctions.

With the patient in the supine position, stand at the right if you are right-handed. Slide your caudal hand underneath the sacrum. On the cephalic side, place your forearm on the right anterior superior iliac spine and your finger pads on the left anterior superior iliac spine. Pressing your hand against the sacrum, lift it toward the ceiling, as if to slot it in between the two iliac bones. With your forearm and cephalic hand, spread the anterior superior iliac spines apart by pushing them outward. This movement allows for the relaxation of the powerful posterior sacroiliac ligamentous system (fig. 13.74). Let the sacrum follow along with the tensions in

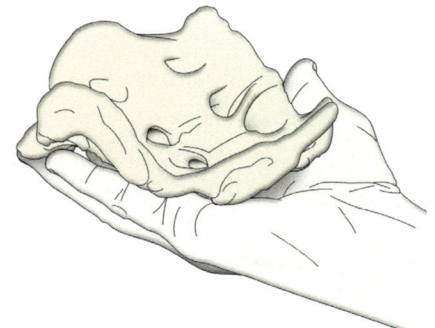

Figure 13.74. Position of the sacrum on the hand.

the tissues, if tensions exist, and make their presence known. Follow the sacral listening until it stabilizes and the sacrum reaches a point of balance.

Interpretation

In the absence of a joint fixation of the sacrum, you should feel pronounced movement without impediment; the lifting happens easily. When there is a sacroiliac joint fixation, the impression is that the sacrum rotates on the fixed side, and only the free side sinks between the two ilia. In this test you can discern a fixation at L5–S1: the apex of the sacrum sinks while the base remains solidly connected with L5. When there is a sacrococcygeal fixation, only the base sinks while the apex resists.

If the sacroiliac joints are free and there is a tissue imbalance, it will show up as a delayed, slow, and gradual movement. The more you lift the sacrum, the more the tension increases and the more the sacral listening amplifies. The position that the sacrum is pulled toward by the tensions allows you to visualize the tissue structures involved. Toward the top, it could be a tension in the spinal dura mater or a cervical or brachial plexus. This could also be a dysfunction of the base of the cranium whose influence is felt as far as the sacrum, as in spinal whiplash. Toward the bottom, it generally concerns traction imparted by the sacrosciatic ligaments, the pelvic floor, or the lower limbs. If the traction pulls laterally, we must consider a fixation of the roots or branches of the lumbosacral plexus, an asymmetrical tension of a sacrosciatic ligament, or tension in the sacrorectogenitopubic sheath.

Sacral Micromobility Tests

Once engaged in lifting the sacrum, you can fine-tune the listening of the test by inducing small movements of rotation and lateral tilt. These movements take place in tissue elasticity while calling into play real movement of the sacrum itself. Don't worry about the theoretical axes of sacrum-ilium and ilium-sacrum mobility; the range of movement is different. Test successively:

- rotation right and left
- tilt right and left
- mobility cranially and caudally
- deformability in bending and in flattening (fig. 13.75)

Pay particular attention to the study of the last two parameters of mobility. *Descent* and *ascent of the sacrum* are evaluated through caudal traction of the sacrum, followed by release. The response to the test allows you to evaluate the caudal part of the spinal dura mater as well as the lumbar and sacral plexuses. Visualize the neuromeningeal tissues as a spring inside the spinal canal. This test seeks to assess the hardness, elasticity, and symmetry of action. The traction and the release give a global idea of elasticity. Next, apply traction to the tissues to the full limit of their ability to stretch. Gently release the traction and let the hand on the sacrum follow the listening. Does the sacrum return to a balanced position? Does it make coarse movements? Does it move globally in the cephalic direction? In the caudal direction? Laterally? Analysis of each of the parameters that display themselves tell you whether the dura mater, the nerves, or again the spinal cord exert traction on the sacrum that is too strong. If some pelvic tissues limit the play of the sacrum, that could also disturb craniosacral mechanics.

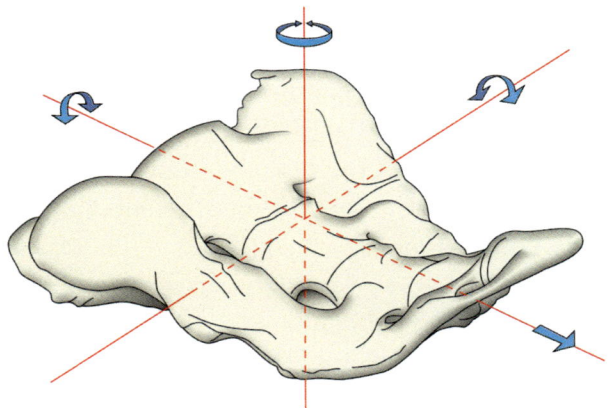

Figure 13.75. Sacrum micromobility tests.

The sacrum's *ability to deform in bending and in flattening* allows us to judge its interosseous elasticity. The late ossification of this bone gives it exceptional elasticity. In the case of a fall, shock, or considerable compression, it can change form and lose this elasticity. This is called an interosseous dysfunction, a severe lesion with mechanical repercussions because of the permanent tensions that it causes.

Suboccipital Traction Listening

This is an important maneuver to verify the freedom of the neuromeningeal contents along the entire length of the spinal canal (fig. 13.75).

The patient is in the supine position, arms next to the body, legs extended. Seated behind the head of the patient, place your palms underneath the occiput and the index finger of your nondominant hand on the inferior occipital line, immediately above the atlas. Place the index finger of your dominant hand on the other index finger in order to set up harmonious traction force on the occiput. This technique can be done with direct traction. Nevertheless, listening while creating traction during the flexion phase of the PRM increases the accuracy of the diagnosis considerably; indeed, this situation allows us to turn our focus to the neuromeningeal contents. From the beginning of the craniosacral flexion phase, apply traction to the occiput in the cephalic direction without adding another component of flexion or extension to the head of the patient. You should feel a real elongation of the dura mater. Next, gently release the occipital traction and let your index fingers follow the direction of the listening. With your eyes closed, the impression of the traction during the cranial flexion phase is almost endless. The dura mater seems to glide in a slow and harmonious way under the action of your index fingers (fig. 13.77). Begin by doing this test with your index fingers clearly at the center of the inferior occipital line in order to evaluate globally the spinal dura mater, the spinal cord, as well as the balance of the nerve roots on each side.

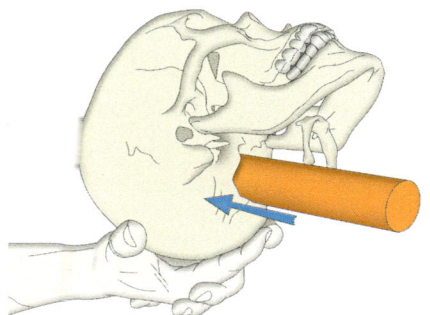

Figure 13.76. Suboccipital traction.

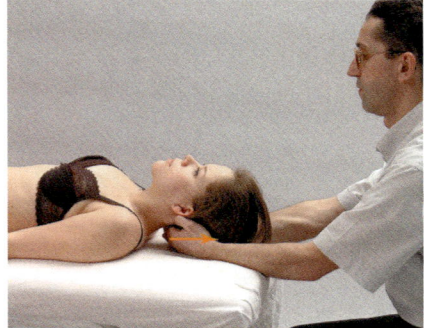

Figure 13.77. Suboccipital traction.

Interpretation

Immediate resistance to the traction indicates either:

- a very large fixation of the neuromeningeal entirety as a result of a serious trauma
- a significant fixation of the first several cervical vertebrae. In this case, immediate resistance is followed by the impression of delayed elasticity of the dura mater, underlying the vertebral blockage.

Delayed resistance to the stretching is a sign of a more limited neuromeningeal fixation. During the course of the stretching, the location of the fixation is related to how late the resistance appears; the more delayed the resistance, the lower the fixation. Lateral resistance to the traction reveals a lateral fixation of the entire neuromeninges. Generally, it is organized around tension of the roots, plexuses, and nerves on the same side. In this case, redo the test, moving your fingers underneath the occiput, slightly lateral to the right, and then to the left of the median line. You will then test the lateral portions of the dura mater and the spinal neuromeningeal contents. In comparing the healthy side to the fixed side, you should easily be able to specify the level of the problem.

Be careful of enlarged suboccipital lymph nodes that are frequently found in this region. Don't place your index finger on these little nodes;

push them aside beforehand to avoid the risk of creating an irritation that could falsify your diagnosis.

Be equally careful of the posterior branches of the large and small occipital nerves in this region, which are generally sensitive. Don't irritate them by contacting them with your fingers, as the patient will tighten and resist your listening-traction.

Positioning

For educational reasons, the general tests and procedures in this chapter have been presented system by system. In practice, it is desirable for the patient not to change position for each test. For the examination, practitioners arrange these routines as best they can in successive positions:

- standing
- seated
- supine
- prone

Routines and general tests can be combined in each position. Nevertheless, your attention should be to "variable geometry": at each moment you must precisely measure the significance of each test within the clinical context of the patient to know what kind of information you can gather.

In conclusion, let me repeat that it is desirable in any given position to begin with the listening tests before carrying out the other mechanical tests. Listening is more reliable if the structures have not yet been disturbed by extrinsic mechanical pulls.

Chapter 14

Tools of Differential Diagnosis

Not doubt, certainty is what drives one insane.

— FRIEDRICH NIETZSCHE

Differential diagnosis has two goals:

- *determining contraindications,* absolute and relative, for certain techniques that the patient cannot support or that must be abandoned
- *determining pathology,* the most probable scenario that organizes identified dysfunctions during general diagnosis. This part of the consultation prepares the subsequent element, *specific diagnosis.*

It is impossible to envisage exhaustively all the probabilities that these two aspects of diagnosis present. However, it is possible to describe some general concepts necessary for their accomplishment.

Determining Contraindications

Semiological Knowledge

Knowledge of classical medical semiology allows osteopaths to avoid some common clinical pitfalls. As I said in the first part of this book, osteopaths do not seek to identify an illness at the base of the nosological frame. In the course of diagnosis, we seek to determine whether our actions can be beneficial for the patient. Once again, we are not concerned with determining the nature of the pathological entity but with knowing if support is justified, if it involves any risks, and if specialized advice is necessary. In current practice, with only the perspectives of a clinical examination and an interview, the information gathered allows us to make ninety percent of decisions. The possible remaining contraindications are detected in the course of specific diagnosis thanks to more precise tests.

Imaging

The renowned Jean-Pierre Barral points out that a photo of a motor in working order and a photo of one that is broken down are hardly different; the difference is in function. Using radiology to objectify osteopathic dysfunctions has been an area of much investigation and study. Such an approach seems somewhat irrelevant to me. How can we use a static image to detect an anomaly that affects the movement of a structure? So imaging is only of minimal interest in obtaining a positive diagnosis. However, it is of primary importance to establish a differential diagnosis and to determine contraindications. Radiological imaging allows us more easily to discern the risks of manipulation, especially at the spinal level. In the case of trauma, imaging is often the best means to remove any suspicion of a fracture. Generally, medical imaging allows us to detect certain tumors, osteoporosis, and osseous angiomas.

Supplementary Examinations

For osteopathic diagnosis, biological tests naturally have the same value as imaging. Even better, they allow us to confirm clinical suspicion of a contraindication. The existence of an inflammatory syndrome or an endocrine pathology can only be verified with certainty by biological assays.

Determining Pathogenesis

The Notion of Dysfunctional Chains

A mechanical dysfunction never remains isolated. The body always adapts itself to imbalance. Step by step, through successive compensations, the dysfunction spreads far from its place of origin. With the emergence of secondary dysfunctions, different from the primary dysfunction, a mechanical dysfunction creates what we call a *dysfunctional chain.*

Note: the term *osteopathic lesion* has been replaced by *dysfunction;* it appears logical to change the terms *lesional pattern* and *lesional chain* to *dysfunctional pattern* and *dysfunctional chain.*

Patterns of Dysfunction

The same initial dysfunction does not necessarily create the same cascade of dysfunctions in everyone. The pattern of dysfunction is defined as a particular sequence of imbalances. Generally, we look to muscular and fascial chains to explain the results of mechanical imbalances. I think the creation of a dysfunctional chain can develop in a variety of ways according to four main aspects:

- fascial
- neuromuscular
- barometric
- physiological

Fascial Tension

Propagation of a dysfunctional chain can be through tension in a membrane or a tendinomuscular or fascial element. Theoretically, an infinite number exist, but in practice we have established the existence of favored axes. Certain anatomical elements are preferential mechanical vectors. Characterized by distortion of the myofascial chain, disequilibrium slowly progresses to various lengths, and its propagation can follow an ascending or descending path.

Examples

- Twisting an ankle can produce an ascending fascial tension along the fibular or posterior tibial muscles. This tension destabilizes the fibula, then the knee, and finally unbalances the pelvis and lumbar spine.
- A ptosis of the small intestine pulls on the mesentery. The insertions of the mesenteric root are against the lumbar wall between L2 and the base of the sacrum. Mesenteric tensions can spread and pull the lumbar spine into lordosis. This state can create pain in the lumbar region or at the lumbosacral junction. Parietal dysfunction is then a consequence of a visceral dysfunction.

Neuromuscular Skeletal Reactions

Here a postural response to a nociceptive or proprioceptive stimulus is created by the dysfunction, or by the intermediary of neuromuscular hyperactivity. Certain dysfunctions operate with positive pressure, and others operate with negative pressure. With the interplay of pressures and the synergy of the unity of some diaphragms, an imbalance can spread to any other section of the body.

Examples

Tension, irritation, or inflammation of the meninges can elicit a strong paravertebral muscle response. The result can be a global mobility restriction of the back or reduced mobility at a localized spinal cord level. Meningeal tension can result from meningitis, and spinal dural tension can stem from trauma or epidural anesthetic.

Any visceral dysfunction or pathology sends nociceptive impulses along the splanchnic nerves. These nerves in turn deliver their charge to the spinal segment corresponding to the affected organ. Such nociceptive information is the underlying cause of hypertonic muscular response or spasm. Eventually, postural adaptation sets in as the body attempts to protect the organ involved.

This type of phenomenon creates numerous secondary somatic dysfunctions at the spinal cord level. Here again is a case of somatic disturbance resulting from visceral dysfunction. Adaptive shortening of the psoas muscle accompanying appendicitis or abdominal tension commonly found with peritonitis are examples of this type of defense mechanism.

Pressure Imbalance

Although invisible, pressure constitutes a considerable and omnipresent mechanical force. A primary dysfunction can have widespread repercussions because it can alter the pressure systems of different cavities and components. The human body is compartmentalized into manometric chambers that are closely linked to the various anatomical and functional diaphragms. Some areas have positive pressure systems, and others operate under negative pressure. Owing to the synergy among diaphragms, an imbalance can be transmitted from one area of the body to another.

Examples

After a stress, total hypertonia of the diaphragm can involve abdominal hypertension. This preferentially disturbs the organs already affected by a loss of mobility or motility. Thus visceral symptoms appear that are as varied as gastroesophageal reflux or urinary stress incontinence.

The pleural cavity and epidural space are some of the virtual spaces where negative pressure rules. The pleural cavity is situated between an osteoarticular wall and a visceral element, and the epidural space is between an osteoarticular wall and a neural element. All modifications of pressure gradients within these spaces have some consequences for the static and dynamic state of the parietal container and the visceral or neural contents.

Physiological Repercussions

A mechanical dysfunction obviously disturbs the proper functioning of the affected element. In turn, weakening or disappearance of this function causes an overload or impediment to another complementary or connected function.

Examples

A hepatic dysfunction often causes an increased work load for the kidneys to eliminate metabolic wastes. The fragility of the kidneys is thus augmented by deficient hepatic dysfunction.

A somatic dysfunction of the back of the foot inevitably creates a loss of elasticity in the arch of the foot. This induces diminished cushioning capacity, not only at the level of the foot but also in the whole lower limb. The superior articulations are strained, necessitating a degree of fascial tension. This hyperattraction can be the origin of pain or discomfort, and it may precipitate the deterioration of an articulation. Thus, certain decompensations of arthrosis in the hip or knee suddenly occur after a small injury.

Repercussions can also occur in the opposite way. There is often somatic dysfunction of the hip in the case of heel pain, a bone spur on the calcaneus, or Sever's disease (calcaneal apophysitis). Most often this dysfunction is homolateral, with a general tendency to sacral verticalization. From the biomechanical point of view, in this position the sacrum is hyperstable and then loses much of its cushioning capacity. All the cushioning structures of the lower limb are also pulled, and the heel suffers with each impact on the ground. The calcaneus is then the seat of the pain and undergoes different processes, more or less inflammatory, of histological modification.

A complex vertebral dysfunction can affect the balance of the spinal nerves and sympathetic ganglia, and in fact the spinal cord. It creates what Irvin M. Korr (1982) calls a *facilitated segment.* This facilitation corresponds to a disturbance of the neurovegetative equilibrium in the territory of the segment. Viscera that depend on that segment can see their functions upset, with weakened immune defenses and their regulatory systems disturbed. A visceral dysfunction is then the consequence of a somatic dysfunction.

A somatic dysfunction may restrain a vascular axis. The vascularized territory is affected, and the tissues have diminished perfusion. Functions in the concerned region are perturbed.

Determining the Hierarchy

Patients generally come for consultations with symptomatology situated at the end of a dysfunctional chain that they are unaware of. Usually they have no problem describing their symptoms, but in the course of differential diagnosis, it is momentarily necessary to refuse to listen to their complaints so as to not be influenced by the symptoms.

The general diagnosis inventories all of the mechanical dysfunction of the patient. The osteopath calls attention to the components of one or several dysfunctional chains but establishes no responsibility, causality, or hierarchy in the observed dysfunctions. At the end of this diagnostic stage, various paths can be envisioned. It is then necessary to arrange the different possibilities in series before rushing into all the possible specific investigations.

The art of differential diagnosis—really more an art than a science—consists of following the diverse elements of the unbalanced chain to establish the proper pathogenesis of the patient. In practice, determining the pathology of the patient means finding where to begin his or her treatment. This is not the desire for intellectual satisfaction but the search for efficacy and innocuousness, because in large part the results directly depend on it. The order we follow when we manipulate a dysfunctional chain is very important. In following it, we reduce the manipulative risk at the vertebral level and diminish the patient's apprehension, avoiding a good number of painful reactions after treatment. This is a great reason to focus carefully on this diagnostic process.

There is no unique procedure to select and create a hierarchy of the dysfunctions found. Each case requires considerable adaptability to organize our investigations. However, determining the origin of a mechanical imbalance depends on *diagnostic convergence.*

Elucidating the hierarchy first requires determining what the most important mechanical system is in the organization of the dysfunctions. What appears first—the musculoskeletal system, the craniosacral system, or the mechanical visceral system? Responsibility can be shared; implicating a system does not automatically preclude the involvement of others. Next, it is necessary to elaborate a probable outline of dysfunctions, regrouping the principal symptoms and the different functional signs associated with a *coherent mechanical clinical picture*. Of course, there are limitations and difficulties in attaining this ideal goal. Determining the hierarchy hardly explains everything. It is very rare that all the symptoms are easily integrated in an explanatory outl ne.

Framework for Determining the Hierarchy

There are two main scenarios:

- The patient has symptomatology that is expressed at the time of consultation.
- The patient consults for a problem that is not manifested at the time of consultation.

Expressed Symptomatology

Whatever the causative symptom (pain, articular limitation, ringing in the ears, or another manifestation), their presence and what patients say during the appointment provide important information in determining the dysfunctional scheme. This includes cases where the pathology is set off by active movement or a specific maneuver, for example during a straight leg raise test. From there, we take the symptom as a point of reference and observe its evolution in tests, which can make it increase, decrease, or disappear. The use of aggravating tests, relief tests, and inhibiting tests allows us to weigh the different dysfunctions and determine which is most probably responsible.

Unexpressed Symptomatology

When the symptoms do not manifest during an appointment, generally this indicates a chronic or subacute case. The investigative field is vast, and generally we must keep in mind other tools of selection and the process of creating a hierarchy to determine the impact of different dysfunctions.

Tools for Determining the Hierarchy

The tools for determining the hierarchy are numerous. Certain tools depend on analysis by the practitioner, and others depend on the patient. None are in systematic usage.

The Outcome of Listenings

General and local listening provide primary information to put the patient's different problems into perspective. Listening detects major instances of imbalance as they are expressed in the deepest tissues. All zones of attraction revealed by manual listening give particular importance to the dysfunctions found. It is where the principal imbalance of the patient is situated at the time of the clinical examination. Conversely, a dysfunction situated outside of that zone is less important to the imbalance we are dealing with.

The Qualities of Dysfunctions

Routines use some essentially binary tests; with a bit of practice, however, these tests also provide information on the dysfunction of a qualitative nature.

Tactile information differs depending on the severity and intensity of a dysfunction. Slightly limited mobility, or by contrast a massive fixation without any mobility, provide clues as to the degree of damage of the anatomical element evaluated. We may also perceive differing sensations when movement stops. It can be sharp and harsh, or gentle and progressive. This qualitative assessment is significant in determining the hierarchy.

Marked qualitative differences are called *disparities*. They give us an idea of differing gravity, significance, and severity. Generally, the more significant and massive the loss of mobility is, the greater the probability that it is the primary dysfunction. Conversely, perception of restriction of full mobility is often synonymous with a secondary dysfunction. For example, a somatic vertebral dysfunction can be encountered in several situations. It can be a primary injury, secondary to a visceral dysfunction, adaptive to another vertebral dysfunction, or even due to tension within the dura mater. Each of these possibilities is accompanied by a specific sensation in the mobility test.

The Pathogenicity of Dysfunctions

Dysfunctions do not all have the same pathogenic value. Some are much more unbalancing for the organism than others. The pathogenicity of a dysfunction depends on several factors: type, nature, localization, or complexity.

Type

An anatomical element can have its mobility disturbed in a variety of ways. In Chapter 4 I defined the notions of physiological and nonphysiological dysfunctions; their pathogenicity is not the same. Some examples:

- At the *vertebral level,* not all somatic dysfunctions have the same value. Physiological somatic dysfunctions respect the laws of vertebral movement. They are less pathogenic than nonphysiological somatic dysfunctions, which create much more significant mechanical attractions. These nonphysiological dysfunctions, considered the third degree of transfer, are by far the most severe, and have the most significant pathogenic effect. They are detected in routine vertebral tests by the sensation of bilateral fixation. These are generally very "loud," creating significant neurovegetative disturbances.
- At the *level of the pelvis,* all traumatic dysfunctions of the sacrum, especially those in lateral flexion, should be considered much more carefully than physiological dysfunctions. These dysfunctions induce imbalances locally and at a distance, and they can have grave static and dynamic consequences.
- At the *level of the cranium,* a dysfunction in compression of the sphenobasilar synchondrosis creates such a disturbance that it constitutes an obstacle to all treatment. Compression or traumatic impaction of this joint without a doubt represents one of the highest degrees of pathogenicity.

Nature

According to the tissue affected by a mechanical dysfunction, the severity of consequences for the whole body varies. Certain organs or tissues insure predominant functions. Also, mechanical disturbances generate numerous proprioceptive and nociceptive influxes, which themselves may generate secondary dysfunctions.

In general, fixations of the dura mater and meninges as well as protective elements of the central nervous system produce multiple postural adaptations, thus contributing to creating many somatic dysfunctions along the vertebral axis. Consequently these tensions or meningeal dysfunctions should be considered primary dysfunctions when compared to spinal somatic dysfunctions, especially at the upper cervical level.

Certain organs, such as the liver, kidneys, pleuropulmonary system, and cardiopericardial system, are also generators of especially severe or expressive secondary spinal dysfunctions. Through their ligamentous connections, the richness of their vascular systems, or the complexity of their neurovegetative innervation, these elements easily produce somatic dysfunctions that can be expressed acutely. To some degree, the uterus and the prostate also belong in this category.

In practice, all visceral and neuromechanical dysfunctions should be considered as potentially primary. Because of the nociceptive influx and proprioceptive misinformation that generate them, we should always place significance on manipulating them before manipulating vertebral dysfunctions. Vertebral dysfunctions that are not resolved by treating visceral and neuromechanical dysfunctions then become the object of specific manipulations. When vertebral somatic dysfunctions are non-physiological, there is a greater chance that they are primary; we can then deviate from this rule.

Localization

Vertebral somatic dysfunctions have different pathogenicity according to their placement. Anatomical connections and biomechanical conditions are the determining parameters.

At the spinal level, the richness of the interactions with the autonomic nervous system is fundamental. In these terms the vertebral zone between C7 and L2 is without doubt most significant. Remember that the principle neurovegetative centers are found along the intermediolateral tracts of this segment of the spinal cord. It is also from this region that the white communicating nerve branches emerge at each vertebral level.

The type of sagittal curve in which the dysfunction is situated also has an impact on its pathogenic value. Experience shows that dysfunctions situated in the primary kyphotic curves require more attention than those situated in the secondary or lordotic curves. Thus somatic dysfunctions situated at the cervical or lumbar level are usually adaptive to dysfunctions in adjacent kyphotic zones. At first glance, manipulating these areas is rarely indicated.

Complexity

According to the degree of complexity of the dysfunction, determining primarity can be difficult. For example, the complex picture of the sequelae of whiplash associates somatic, visceral, and craniosacral dysfunctions. In such a context, it is necessary to consider that the soft elements are more primary than the hard elements. Thus the meninges, spinal nerves, and other nerves act as true brakes on vertebral mechanics. Ligamentous visceral systems likewise generate significant tensions. All these elements must be considered responsible for the chronic aspects of spinal imbalances and recurring pain. When it is necessary, manipulation of somatic dysfunctions is only done after the treatment of neuromeningeal and visceral structures.

Odor

An attribute of clinical diagnosis is that it rests on sensory perceptions. The hand is the primary tool, but other senses are also important, notably olfaction. Odor is a good reflection of metabolism and lifestyle, revealing visceral functioning, general physiology, and toxicity. Modifications in body odor accompany certain dysfunctions or illnesses. The consumption of alcohol or tobacco, absence of hydration, or even an unbalanced diet equally influence odors.

In my practice, the body odors of certain patients frequently orient me toward a diagnosis. A patient presenting renal dysfunction does not have the same odor as a patient with irritable bowel syndrome or a patient with hepatic problems. Anyone who has worked in neurological medicine knows that the pronounced odor of a hemiplegic is not soon forgotten. In women, simple changes in the estrogen-progesterone balance over the course of the menstrual cycle can create specific odors, noticeable in the hair.

How do you describe an odor? How do you transmit your own observations? I do not have a specific answer, but I can encourage you to try to smell and identify the unpleasant odors of your patients. Remember specific odors that you find in different individuals with similar afflictions. Rapidly and with a degree of reliability you will be able to associate certain odors with specific dysfunctions.

Supplementary Tests

Certain tests allow us to evaluate the mechanical impact of a dysfunction at the base of a myofascial-articular chain:

- aggravating tests
- relief tests
- inhibiting tests

Aggravating Tests

These are tests of "mechanical accumulation": they augment the mechanical influence of a dysfunction to measure the impact on a given symptom. To conduct these tests, we can:

- weigh down an anatomical element in order to implicate it more strongly in a chain of dysfunctions
- stretch the dysfunctional mechanical chain to increase its influence at a distance

Example: your visceral routines reveal a loss of viscoelasticity of the umbilical region. Palpation determines that the loops of the small intestine are ptosed and fixed. To conduct an aggravating test, the patient is seated, and you stand behind. Make contact with the superior part of the small intestinal mass and push it down toward the hypogastric region. As a point of reference, ask the patient about the development of a symptom: lumbago, pelvic pressure, or another. An increase in the test's reference symptom indicates the mechanical responsibility of the element tested in generating the symptom (fig. 14.1).

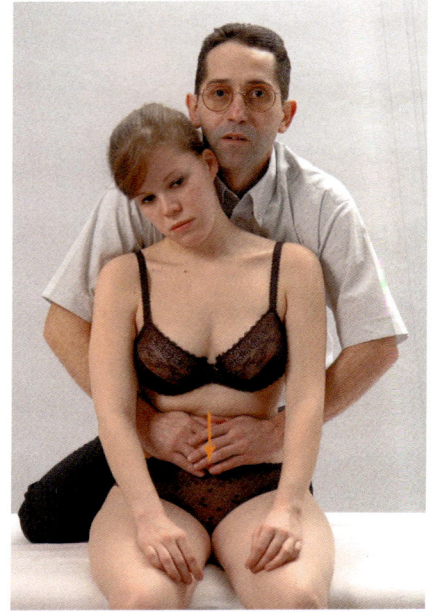

Figure 14.1. Aggravating test at the umbilical level.

Relief Tests

These are tests of "mechanical removal": They diminish the mechanical influence of a dysfunction to see if the symptomatology disappears. To conduct these tests, we can:

- take away an element of the pressure in order to relieve the chain mechanically
- progressively relax the chain in order to observe whether the symptom lessens with the maneuver

Example: your visceral routines show a fixation of the right hypochrondrium, which you attribute to ptosis of the liver. To conduct a relief test, make contact with the inferior surface of the liver and delicately lift it to push against the diaphragm. There are two main means to verify the efficacy of relief:

- ask the patient about the evolution of a reference symptom, such as a sensation of abdominal weight, respiratory discomfort, or even pain in the cervical spine or right shoulder. Improvement of the symptom due to the maneuver implicates the liver mechanically in the imbalance.
- as a point of reference, make a limited articular movement, and observe whether there is an amplitude gain with increased comfort. If relief of the liver allows improved active mobility of either abduction of the scapulohumeral joint or cervical rotation, the mechanical responsibility of the liver is established (fig. 14.2).

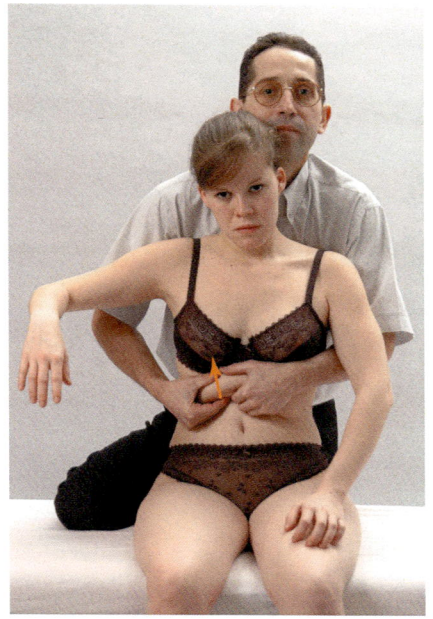

Figure 14.2. Relief test on the right hypochrondrium.

Inhibiting Tests

Inhibiting tests are often confused with relief tests. They are very different, however, being more in the mind than in the execution. Their mechanics are not yet known; we think that they put the nervous system into play, certainly by proprioceptive or nociceptive information bias. These tests play on the tissular listening of the element in dysfunction. Manually following the listening of a structure in primary dysfunction through a maneuver called *induction* allows us to observe a reaction of instantaneous liberation of the secondary dysfunctions.

Example: you have found a loss of viscoelasticity in the hypogastric region and a somatic dysfunction of the sacrum. The most precise tests show you that the uterus is fixed. To determine whether it is the

367

uterus or the sacrum that is in primary dysfunction, you can utilize an inhibiting test (fig. 14.3). With the patient in the supine position, place one of your hands on the sacrum and the other on the hypogastric area facing the uterine fundus. Test minute movements of the sacrum or listen to its respiratory mobility, and note the disturbed parameters. Then do a tissular listening of the uterus. Do an induction, raising and following its listening. Again, verify the movement possibilities of the sacrum. Have they improved? If this is the case, uterine inhibition improving sacral mobility is a sign of primary dysfunction of the

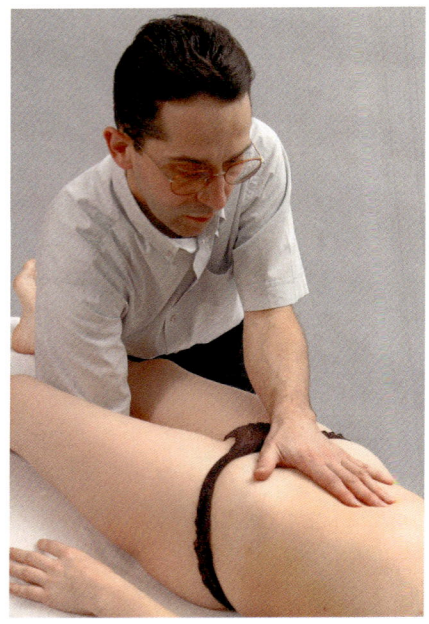

Figure 14.3. Sacrum-hypogastric inhibition.

uterus; the sacrum is really only a secondary dysfunction. If this is not the case, do an induction on the sacrum, meaning listening, and observe whether the listening of the uterus changes. If so, it is the sacrum that is in primary dysfunction and not the uterus. This principle of inhibition can be generalized in order to compare dysfunctions two by two.

General Impact Tests

These tests measure the reverberation of a dysfunction globally in an individual.

Arterial Pressure

We have seen that measuring blood pressure must be systematic in patients who present cardiovascular risk factors. Outside these cases, taking systolic pressure on both arms can aid in seeing the pathology of a patient more clearly. Any difference of more than one point of systolic pressure between the right and left sides is significant. Such an inequality is called *anisotension*. There is generally a *predominance of dysfunctions on the side with the lowest pressure*. As examples, we find:

- retraction or tissular fibrosis at the level of the upper limb, at the level of the superior thoracic aperture, or at the cervical vertebrae
- somatic dysfunction of the clavicle, the lower cervical vertebrae, or the first ribs
- visceral fixation, most often homolateral

Modified Adson's Test

Adson's test (fig. 14.4) studies possible variations in the radial pulse. It is done by placing the upper limb in extreme abduction: the shoulder is rotated externally with the elbow bent ninety degrees, and then the impact of this position on the homolateral radial pulse is verified. In this position, closure of the costoclavicular stricture and of the subpectoral tunnel is produced, which allows us to check for thoracic outlet syndrome.

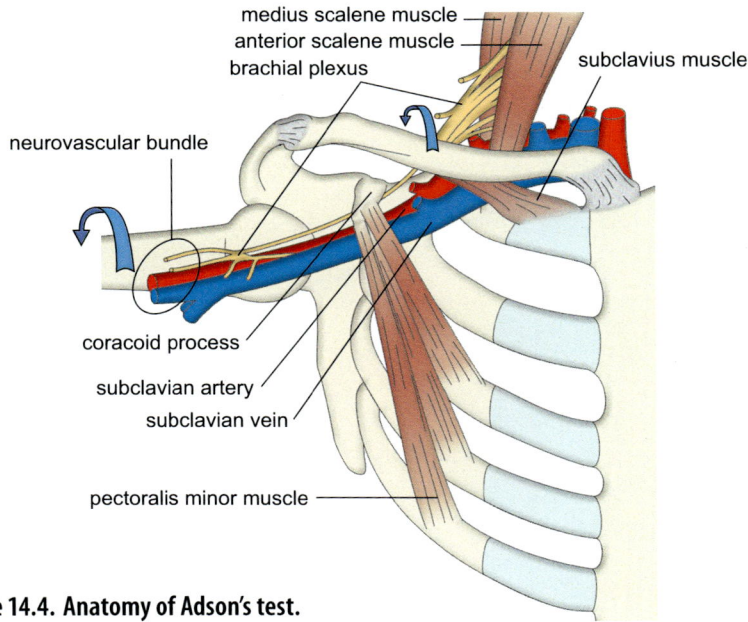

medius scalene muscle
anterior scalene muscle
brachial plexus
subclavius muscle
neurovascular bundle
coracoid process
subclavian artery
subclavian vein
pectoralis minor muscle

Figure 14.4. Anatomy of Adson's test.

A variant of this test proposed by Jean-Pierre Barral and Pierre Mercier (2004) adds a lateral side-bend and opposite rotation to the cervical vertebrae. This test, sometimes called the Soto-Hall test, checks for a diminished or missing radial pulse (fig. 14.5). The primary dysfunction is situated on the side where the radial pulse disappears. It is possible to use this test to triage several dysfunctions (fig. 14.6). Suppose that the test was positive on the right side and that you have found several mechanical problems:

- a fixation of the liver
- a fixation of the right diaphragmatic pleura
- a fixation of the right clavicle

To find out which is the most troubling for the patient, use this technique: place the arm in the exact position where the radial pulse disappears. Then do a hepatic inhibition, gently pushing the organ superior and anterior, and verify whether the radial pulse reappears. Next, make an inhibiting or relief maneuver of other dysfunctions, verifying each time whether the radial pulse reappears. The inhibiting maneuver that is most effective in restoring the radial pulse indicates the location of the most primary dysfunction.

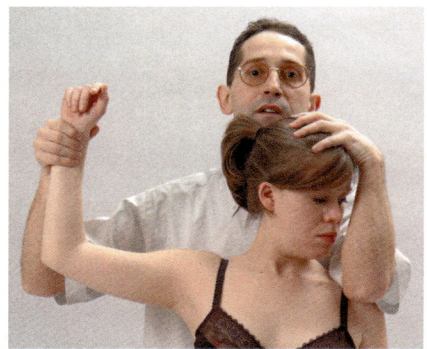

Figure 14.5. Modified Adson's test.

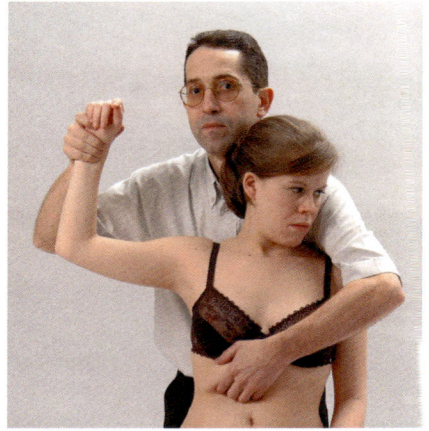

Figure 14.6. Completed Adson's test.

Logical Links

Reasoning allows us to establish logical links as well as cause-and-effect relationships. As part of diagnosis, it is then necessary to bring out the obvious facts. To do so, some knowledge of anatomy, biomechanics, articular physiology, physiology, and physiopathology are indispensable. The elements called *osteopathic links* are common shortcuts that designate these different logical links.

NOTE

Logical links must rely on dysfunctions detected manually. They should not in any way be used to shore up a deficit of manual perception to construct a purely intellectual diagnosis.

Analogical Links

Analogies establish a connection or similarity among several different elements. They are a way of reasoning founded on highlighting resemblances. They are a way of thinking that can consider form, function, situation, or appearance. Analogies deal with the mind, which is always partial and sometimes fortuitous. With their size and limitations, analogies can sometimes help to arrange dysfunctions with apparently little connection among them. Examples of analogical relationships:

- The kidney, the ear, and the foot have a shape almost identical to a bean. They have *analogous morphology*. In functional pathology, we often find that the kidney can produce pain on the sole of the foot, and that it may even be implicated in tinnitus (fig. 14.7).
- The temporomandibular and scapulohumeral articulations likewise present a *structural analogy* with the coxofemoral articulation. These three articular complexes have comparable mechanical functions, and the temporal bone, scapula, and coccyx are often tied to craniosacral dysfunctions.
- The surface of the brain is visually very similar to the surface of the small intestine. The two structures present an *analogy of appearance*.

371

In physiology, it is surprising to see that numerous neurotransmitters are created or used jointly by both.

The doctrine of the five elements in traditional Chinese medicine is mostly founded on analogical relations. Practitioners sometimes use surprising correlations. For example, the wood element is connected to the liver, the spring season, the color green, anger, and the eyes and tendons. Similarly the symbolic dimension of illnesses and symptoms is at the level of analogies. Practitioners who use somatoemotional techniques are served by this kind of decoding every day.

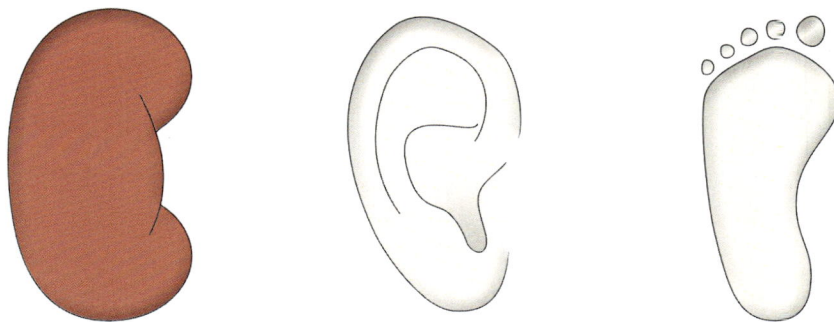

Figure 14.7. Morphological analogy of the kidney, ear, and foot.

The Chronology of Antecedents

The age and order of appearance of lesions, dysfunctions, or symptoms are of great significance for diagnosis as much as for prognosis. These elements, gathered from the interview, allow us to organize dysfunctional sequences into a specific time frame. Traumatic surgical or obstetric antecedents are dated. They group different factors together, some of them disturbing the mechanics of the patient. They constitute precious etiological indicators that must be confirmed by the clinical examination.

We do not treat a patient with a dysfunction of several days in the same way as a patient who has had a dysfunction for many years. When a patient has manifested the pathology for a long time, recuperation will take longer.

Biotype and Environment

According to their biotype, patients have their own weaknesses and strengths.

- Weaknesses have considerable diagnostic significance. They allow us to understand how the decompensation is established in the body.
- Knowledge of strengths allows us to guide the treatment to better favor healing.

Knowledge of biotypes allows us to foresee the most likely pathological patterns.

Underlying Pathologies

Similar to the environment, the existence of a known pathology is a determiner. It indicates how the organism has been able to evolve in its most recent imbalances. Pathology likewise weakens certain elements and creates an environment conducive to decompensations.

Semiological Knowledge

There is a classical semiology of diverse organic pathologies. In the same way, we find true clinical pictures, more or less complete and typical, in certain functional injuries. Knowledge of this semiology is fundamental to understanding the connections in certain dysfunctions. For example, the sequelae of whiplash provide to the osteopath a functional symptomatology that constitutes a good example of a proper clinical picture.

Experience

When reconsidering an ongoing issue, the experience of the practitioner is significant in determining the hierarchy of dysfunctions. Having confronted many cases strongly influences the analytical capacities of the therapist. It is necessary, however, to remain sufficiently flexible and not to be anchored by any ideas that might be erroneous.

Intuition

Intuition is one of the most ancient faculties that human beings have. It belongs to a higher instinct that predates language. Today it is often hidden behind rationality. According to Cappon (1994), "intuition grasps in a flash the total picture and the relations between the elements rather than the elements themselves." This intuitive intelligence, attached to our primitive brain, has a certain degree of experience and unsuspected resources. It is global and instantaneous, using an immediate-response system that is independent of thought and clear of hesitation and doubt.

Logical thought has developed some defense mechanisms to avoid intrusions by intuition. These mechanisms become permeable in dreaming, defective in the case of mental illness, and can completely collapse with senility. Intuition has nothing to do with spirituality or religion. It is an intelligence that is not fastened to a field of theoretical knowledge but that depends directly on experience. In order to approach it, it cannot be considered as an external reality; rather we must turn toward ourselves. This personal and subjective process does not preclude rigor and judgment. As indicated by its Latin root, *intueri,* meaning "to look inside," intuition is a profound experience of inner certainty.

In many scientific disciplines, such as physics, intuition plays a fundamental role. Sometimes it is a unique way of knowing. Many discoveries, paradigm shifts, and major scientific contributions have been intuitive. The history of the discovery of relativity by Albert Einstein illustrates this phenomenon. He literally saw himself riding a ray of light in his process of examining the universe and imagining its workings from this point of view. His discoveries stemmed from that image. The physicist John Archibald Wheeler, who worked with Einstein for twenty-five years, continually told his students never to make the smallest calculations before knowing the answer. "If you don't know the answer in advance," he said, "it is completely useless to do the calculation" (Wheeler 1988). Even in the simplest discoveries, the mark of intuition often resides in the elegance and beauty of the solutions.

Techniques and years of practice have nothing to do with intuition. Techniques serve to express and formulate intuition. If Einstein had never studied physics and mathematics, he never would have discovered relativity. Although he had the same tools as physicists of his day, he probably possessed something more. The thing that allowed him to have an unencumbered perspective also allowed him to have his clear insights.

Intuition's place in diagnosis is undeniable. All intuition should be respected and verified by thorough examination. While it is necessary to learn to develop confidence, it would be dangerous to blindly base diagnosis on this parameter alone. *Intuition is both a form of intelligence and a sense to be developed.*

Conditions at Consultation

Even the reason why patients seek consultation helps determine the hierarchy of their dysfunctions (fig. 14.8). The goals of treatment should be presented clearly so as not to stray from the correct path.

- If the reason for the consultation is simple, with a cause or precise point of departure, generally it involves a rather recent acute event of traumatic origin. Diagnosis must include your assessment of lesions and dysfunctions while also determining the state of the patient just before the traumatic event. The objectives of treatment are to correct the consequences of the traumatic event that led the patient from this previous state as well as to prevent recurrences.
- If the reason for the consultation is complex, with an imprecise origin yet to be determined, it most often concerns a chronic affliction or a problem of older origin. Diagnosis should determine where the patient's loss of adaptation is situated. We need to group the symptoms and signs in a coherent outline of dysfunction to approach it from the most probable etiology.

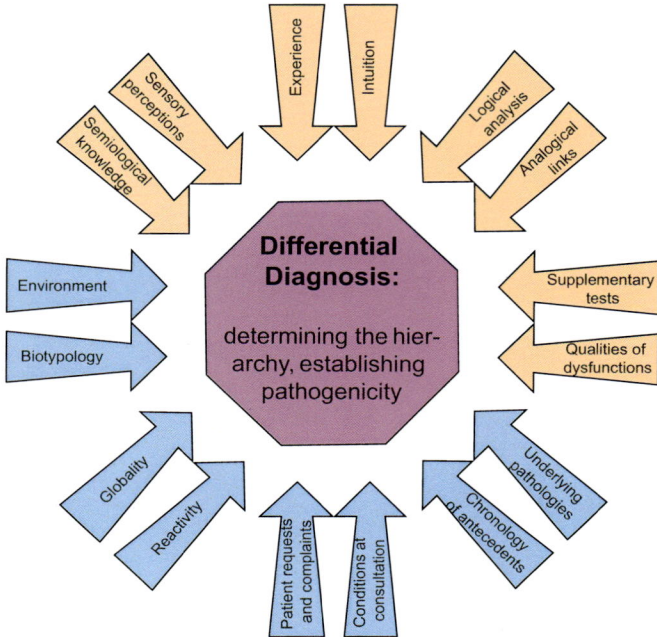

Figure 14.8. Elements used to determine the hierarchy of dysfunctions.

NOTE

Patient complaints and requests sometimes necessitate reconsidering treatment priorities. This must not cause you to reconsider your manual diagnosis. What your hands detect and what your mind analyzes are objective elements of your diagnosis. Patient requests may influence your therapeutic decisions, but they do not change the mechanical reality.

Osteopathic Indications

What is a good osteopathic indication? Is it based on separating a contraindication from an indication? Surgeons do not offer surgical indications unless they consider that there is a good chance of improving the sick person. Osteopaths should only treat patients if they consider that there is a good chance of improvement. The stakes and the risks are not the same for surgery and osteopathy: the limitations of indications are necessarily less clear for osteopaths. The evolution of certain patients can be surprising, and we should not be too modest nor too presumptuous.

When an indication does not appear evident to us, we need to be pragmatic (fig. 14.9). If you do not have the experience to manage a rare or unknown (to you) pathology, it is completely appropriate to suggest to the patient that management of its evolution can be revisited. Depending on the situation, you can make two or three appointments before judging the results. If your treatment is efficacious, the indication was good. Conversely, inefficacy of treatment is a sign of a bad indication. This attitude, in which clarity and transparency are predominant, allows you to establish a relationship of trust based on achieving results.

> Birth and the perinatal period
> Pain and imbalance from growth
> Injuries
> Functional pathologies
> Sequelae of illnesses or surgery
> Stress and emotions

Figure 14.9. Common indications in osteopathy.

Remember that osteopaths do not specifically treat the illness or the pathology; we treat the patient. Take care not to think that the only reason for a consultation is to find an indication. Be vigilant: treatment that is customarily effective for a given reason for consultation signifies neither systematic success nor a general osteopathic indication. Finally, every time we determine an indication, we should not be swayed by our failures or our successes. Consider every possibility when making a decision. In current practice, there are several reasons for consultation that can be misleading. Even in the absence of formal contraindications, a good indication cannot be assumed.

Using homeopathic terminology, there are a certain number of *barriers* that can hinder osteopathic treatment. Vaccination sequelae, dental amalgams, and malocclusion are common examples. The excellence of an indication rests on identifying a *mechanical etiology* that explains the appearance of the symptomatology. A good osteopathic indication can be proposed when the patient presents a significant *sum of mechanical dysfunctions*. The more mechanical dysfunctions we find, and the more these dysfunctions appear fixed, the better the indication. Conversely, the rarer and less intense these dysfunctions are, the less favorable the osteopathic indication. In this last case, we need to know when to refer the patient to another therapist. To know how to recognize our own limits is not an easy thing; it is not an admission of inability, however, but rather an expression of our competence.

Conclusion

The different themes developed in this book should never make you forget that an osteopathic diagnosis is not intellectually contrived. On the contrary, it is determined by what the hand detects in every patient. So it is established from *perception* and becomes *known,* not the reverse. In no situation can speculation and intellectual construction augment deficiencies in perception. *Perceived feeling* is the basis of diagnosis. If the hand remains the essential tool of the osteopath, very good clinical knowledge will be developed. It is in this sense that diagnosis constitutes true *knowledge.* Finally, diagnosis requires exact organization of the different investigations. Even if practitioners arrange them at their own convenience, osteopathic diagnosis still requires the *method.*

Every day, osteopathic manipulative techniques become more precise and more codified. Originally, the osteoarticular sector represented the essential tissular techniques, but progressively visceral, craniosacral, and neuromeningeal manipulations have gained much importance. Osteopathy remains one and indivisible, however, with the diversification of our therapeutic actions imposing respect for the original concepts more than ever.

Faced with the plethora of techniques, we risk gradually being inundated by too many therapeutic tools. The danger then lies in specializing in a style of techniques or searching for ready-made therapeutic recipes. This is far removed from osteopathic principles. Only a well-developed diagnosis allows us to respect osteopathy's concepts and resist being scattered.

Glossary

acrocyanosis: A syndrome characterized by permanent cyanosis of the hands, sometimes the legs, and more rarely the ears, nose, cheeks, and posterior surfaces of the arms, observed especially in young girls. Exaggerated by cold and humid weather, it seems to be due to sympathetic endocrine problems.

amphotony: Hypertonia of the sympathetic and parasympathetic autonomic nervous system.

anabolism: See *metabolism.*

anamnesis: Information gathered by the physician by asking specific questions of the patient or other people who know the person and can give relevant information, with the aim of obtaining information useful in formulating a diagnosis and providing medical care to the patient.

anisotension: Inequality of the blood pressure of the two arms. Generally the weaker side is the side of predominant dysfunction.

belief: To place trust in a statement that has not been or cannot be verified or demonstrated. Belief is founded on evidence or personal intuition.

cacochyme: In a bad mood, often pleasurably. Used to describe individuals, usually older men, who are weak and in poor health.

catabolism: See *metabolism.*

cenesthesia: Vague internal sense of bodily existence based on weak organ sensitivity, independent of the sense organs.

cenesthopathy: Trouble with the internal sense of bodily existence, consisting of an abnormal bodily sensation, more annoying than painful. It is not accompanied by depression or delirium, and resists therapeutic and psychiatric medications. It is considered to be a sensitivity hallucination.

clinical: From the Greek *klinē*, "bed." Concerns what may be established or accomplished by the doctor, at the bedside, without the help of any apparatus or laboratory methods.

coarctation of the aorta: Congenital narrowing of the aortic isthmus, provoking arterial hypertension of the upper limbs and arterial hypotension of the lower limbs.

concept: An explicit, abstract, and general representation that results in the elaboration of a coherent theory.

constitution: The physical and psychic structure of an individual.

constraint: Also called effort; the internal resistance of a material when submitted to external stimulus. There are three fundamental types of constraint:

- traction, which produces elongation of the object
- compression, which tends to reduce the dimensions of the object
- shearing, which corresponds to forces applied like scissor blades

craniosacral mechanism: Structural elements supporting the primary respiratory mechanism.

dysfunction: Any trouble with the functioning of a system.

elasticity: The ability of certain bodies to return to their original shape when the deforming force ceases.

ERS: Extension rotation side-bend, used to designate a vertebral somatic dysfunction presenting a chronic fixation in these three parameters.

facilitation: Clinical concept used by osteopaths to describe neuro-physiological mechanisms that accompany a vertebral somatic dysfunction. Lowering the threshold of neuronal excitability in the medullary segment concerned causes reinforcement of neural activity.

fixation: In a general sense, the loss of mobility of a mechanical system. A fixation can affect an articular unity or can concern a tissular system that loses its mobility, gliding, extensibility, or elasticity.

FRS: Flexion rotation side-bend, used to designate a vertebral somatic dysfunction presenting a chronic fixation in these three parameters.

fulcrum: A point of support or pivot, situated where tissular tensions balance themselves.

holism A doctrine that leads to knowledge of the whole from individual specifics, where knowledge of the whole is recorded.

holistic Of or relating to holism.

homeostasis: Tendency of an organism to maintain itself in relative stability.

humor An affective, emotional, and instinctive state of mind, giving spiritual states an agreeable or disagreeable tone.

iatrogenic: Provoked or induced by the doctor.

lesion: From the Latin *laesio,* "wrong" or "damage." Alteration of anatomical and histological characters of tissue due to accidental or morbid cause (injury, parasitic action, defective functioning of an organ, etc.). The study of lesions is pathological anatomy.

metabolism: The whole of the transformation undergone by substances absorbed by an organism: synthesis reactions leading to storage (anabolism) and to freeing energy (catabolism).

morbic: Pertaining to an illness.

morbidity: The state of an illness; sum of the illnesses that have struck an individual or a group of individuals in a given time.

nocebo effect: The appearance of undesirable effects, generally benign, after the administration of a medication that is inactive or incapable of producing these effects.

nosogenesis: The study of causes and development of diseases.

nosography: Methodical classification of diseases.

nosology: The study of distinctive characters that allow definition and classification of diseases.

paradigm: A theoretical model of thought oriented toward research and reflection.

pathogenesis, pathogenic, pathogenicity: Mechanism by which the causes of disease act to unleash its development.

penetrance: The frequency with which a discomfort manifests its effects.

placebo effect: A positive effect caused by treatment devoid of scientifically recognized therapeutic activity. In a wider sense, all therapeutic action of psychological origin.

primary respiratory mechanism (PRM): A physiological system

comprising the inherent movement of the central nervous system, the fluctuation of the cerebrospinal fluid, the action of the intracranial and intraspinal membranes, the micromobility of the cranial bones, and the involuntary movement of the sacrum. It is manifested by two phases: inspiration and expiration.

sign: All manifestation of an injury that the practitioner can objectively ascertain or intentionally provoke for a diagnostic goal.

somatization: Process in which physical symptoms appear resulting from psychological conflicts.

SPECT: Single-photon emission computed tomography. A method of calculated tomography that employs radionuclides emitting single photons at a given energy level. It can be used to observe biochemical and physiological processes as well as the size and volume of an organ or the brain.

steppage: A gait abnormality of people affected by paralysis of the extensors of the toes and the flexors of the foot. With the foot strike of each step, they strongly flex the thigh at the pelvis so as not to scrape their toes against the ground.

sthenia: The energetic capacity of reaction and metabolic adaptation of an individual.

symptom: All manifestations of a pathological state perceived by the patient (subjective symptom) or discovered by the practitioner (objective symptom).

syntonic: A psychiatric term for the harmonious fusion of a subject's behavior in the ambient environment. It is one of the characteristics of cyclothymic temperament (as opposed to schizothymic).

thymic: A psychiatric term from the Greek *thymos,* "mind." The external behavior of individuals, seen specifically in relation to their positive or negative moods.

trauma: All the corporal lesions sustained by a subject in the course of an external aggression.

volition: An active phenomenon of the encephalon that determines will. In a wider sense, will itself.

References

Abehsera, Alain. 1986. *Traité de medecine ostéopathique.* Charleroi, Belgium: OMC.

Albe-Fessard, Denise. 1996. *La douleur. Ses mécanismes et les bases de ses traitements.* Paris: Masson.

Amen, Daniel G. 2000. *Images into Human Behavior: A Brain SPECT Atlas.* New York: Mindworks Press.

———— 2002. *Healing the Hardware of the Soul.* New York: Simon & Schuster.

Barral, Jean-Pierre. 1984. *Manipulations uro-génitales.* Paris: Maloine.

———— 1988. *Visceral Manipulation.* Vista, CA: Eastland.

———— 1994. *Diagnostic thermique manuel.* Paris: Maloine.

———— 2004. *Manipulations viscérales 2.* 2nd edition. Paris: Elsevier.

———— 2005. *Le thorax: Manipulations viscérales.* 2nd edition. Paris: Elsevier.

Barral, Jean-Pierre, and Alain Croibier. 1997. *Approche ostéopathique du traumatsme.* Saint-Étienne, France: Editions ATSA, CIDO & Actes Graphiques.

———— 2004. *Manipulations des nerfs périphériques.* Paris: Elsevier.

Barral, Jean-Pierre, B. Ligner, D. Paoletti, D. Prat, L. Rommeveaux, and D. Triana. 1993. *Nouvelles techniques uro-génitales.* Aix-en-Provence, France: Editions CIDO & De Verlaque.

Barral, Jean-Pierre, Jean-Paul Mathieu, and Pierre Mercier. 1992. *Diagnostic articulaire vertébral.* 2nd edition. Aix-en-Provence, France: Editions CIDO & De Verlaque.

Barral, Jean-Pierre, and Pierre Mercier. 2004. *Manipulations viscérales 1.* 2nd edition. Paris: Elsevier.

Bates, Barbara. 1993. *Guide de l'examen clinique.* 3rd edition. Paris: Arnette.

Benoit, Odile, and Jean Forêt. 1995. *Le sommeil humain: Bases expérimentales, physiologiques et physiopathologiques.* Paris: Masson.

Blétry, Olivier, Julie Cosserat, and Rachid Laraki. 1995. *Redécouvrir l'examen clinique, clé du diagnostic, fascicule 2.* Paris: Doin.

Bonnel, François, and Michel Georgesco. 1985. "Voies anatomiques et physiologie de la douleur." In *La douleur chronique,* edited by L. Simon, 1–22. Paris: Masson.

Bossy, Jean, et al. 1990. *Neuro-anatomie.* Collection Anatomie Clinique. Paris: Springer-Verlag France.

Boureau, François, J. F. Doubrère, and M. Luu. 1985. "Les méthodes d'évaluation de la douleur clinique." In *La douleur chronique,* edited by L. Simon, 37–42. Paris: Masson.

Boureau, François. 1988. *Pratique du traitement de la douleur.* Paris: Doin.

Bourhis, A., and J. M. Spitalier. 1970. "La Douleur maladie en carcinologie." *Biol. Med.* 59:427–58.

Brasseur, Louis, Marcel Chauvin, and Gisèle Guilbaud. 1997. *Douleurs: Bases fondamentales, pharmacologie, douleurs aiguës, douleurs chroniques, thérapeutiques.* Paris: Maloine.

Bruxelle, Jean. 1994. "La douleur: aspects neurophysiologiques et neuropsychologiques." In *Souffrances corps et âme, épreuves partagées,* edited by Jean-Marie von Kaenel, 18–33. Paris: Autrement.

Cappon, Daniel. 1990. *Intuition.* Toronto: Bedford House.

———. 1994. *Intuition & Management.* Westport, CT: Greewood.

Cassano, C., and F. Tronchetti. 1955. "Le cadre metabolique des différents types constitutionnels." In *Traité de médecine biotypologique,* edited by Nicola Pende, 347–85. Paris: Doin.

Corman, Louis. 1988. *Nouveau manuel de morphopsychologie.* Paris: Stock.

Cyr, Michele G., and Steven A. Wartman. 1988. "The Effectiveness of Routine Screening Questions in the Detection of Alcoholism." *JAMA* 259:51–4.

De Doncker, Émile, and Marius Lacheretz. 1977. "Traitement du pied plat." *Rev. Chir. Orthop.* 63:731–88.

Debray, Quentin, Bernard Granger, and Franck Azaïs. 1998. *Psychopathologie de l'adulte.* Paris: Masson.

Delaunoy, P. 1983. *Introduction à la médecine ostéopathique.* Maidstone, UK: ESO.

Delchambre, Nadine, Marie-Rose Lefevre, Anne Ligot, and Nicole Mainjot. 2000. *Guide d'observation des 14 besoins de l'être humain: Orientation diagnostique.* Brussels: De Boeck.

Di Giovanna, Eileen L., Stanley Schiowitz, and Dennis J. Dowling, editors. 1997. *An Osteopathic Approach to Diagnosis and Treatment.* Philadelphia: Lippincott Williams & Wilkins.

Dubos, René, and Maya Pines. 1966. *Sante et maladie.* New York: Time-Life.

———. 1971. *Health and Disease.* New York: Time-Life.

Duval, Jacques Andreva. 2004. *Techniques osteopathiques d'équilibre et d'échanges réciproques*. Rennes, France: Sully.

Epstein, Owen, David de Bono, and John Cookson. 2000. *Examen clinique: Eléments de sémiologie médicale*. Translated by Bernard Devuld from *Clinical Examination*. 2nd edition. Brussels: De Boeck.

Frymann, Viola L. 1998. *The Collected Papers of Viola M. Frymann: Legacy of Osteopathy to Children, Presented by the American Academy of Osteopathy*. Indianapolis: Hollis Heaton King.

Garnier, Marcel, and Jacques Delamare. 1995. *Dictionnaire des termes médicaux*. 24th edition. Paris: Maloine.

Goldcher, Alain. 2001. *La podologie*. 4th edition. Paris: Masson.

Greenman, Philip E. 1996. *Principles of Manual Medicine*. 2nd edition. Baltimore: Lippincott Williams & Wilkins 1996.

Grossinger, Richard. 1995a. *Planet Medicine: Modalities*. Berkeley, CA: North Atlantic Books.

———. 1995b. *Planet Medicine: Origins*. Berkeley, CA: North Atlantic Books.

Harrison, T. R. 1995. *Médecine interne*. 13th edition. Paris: McGraw-Hill–Arnette.

Hoerni, Bernard. 1996. *Histoire de l'examen clinique, d'Hippocrate à nos jours*. Paris: Imothep-Maloine.

Hogstel, Mildred O., and Rhonda Keen-Payne. 1995. *Evaluation clinique du patient*. Collection Memento de l'infirmière. Paris: Maloine.

Israel, Lucien. 1995. *Cerveau droit, cerveau gauche: Cultures et civilisations*. Paris: Plon.

Issartel, Lionelle, and Marielle Issartel. 1983. *L'ostéopathie exactement*. Paris: Laffont.

Jackson, Adam J. 1996. *The Ten Secrets of Abundant Health*. New York: Harper.

——— 1999. *Les dix secrets de la sante*. Translation of *The Ten Secrets of Abundant Health*. Thonex, Switzerland: Vivez Soleil.

Jouvet, Michel. 1991. "Le sommeil paradoxal: Est-il le gardien de l'individuation psychologique?" *Rev. Canad. Psychol.* 45(2): 148–68.

Julian, Othon André, and Marc Haffen. 1981. *Homéopathie*. Paris: Masson.

Klotz, H. P. 1955. "Les biotypes en médecine psychosomatique." In *Traité de médecine biotypologique*, edited by Nicola Pende, 775–80. Paris: Doin.

Korr, Irvin M. 1982. *Bases physiologiques de l'ostéopathie*. Paris: SBO-RTM-Maloine.

Kretschmer, Ernst. 1925. *Körperbau und Charakter: Untersuchungen zum Konstitutionsproblem und zur Lehre von den Temperamenten.* Berlin: Julius Springer.

Kretschmer, W. 1955a. "Les biotypes et les états mentaux." In *Traité de médecine biotypologique,* edited by Nicola Pende, 789–800. Paris: Doin.

———. 1955b. "Le somatopsychisme." In *Traité de médecine biotypologique,* edited by Nicola Pende, 105–17. Paris: Doin.

Laborit, Henri. 1979. *L'inhibition de l'action: Biologie, physiologie, psychologie, sociologie.* Paris: Masson.

Lapidus, P. W. 1963. "Kinesiology and Mechanical Anatomy of the Tarsal Joints." *Clin. Orthop.* 30:20–4.

Laurent, B. 1994. "Données physiopathologiques concernant douleur et antalgiques." In *Le médecin, le patient et sa douleur,* edited by Patrice Queneau and Gérard Ostermann, 11–28. Paris: Masson.

Lazorthes, Guy. 1981. *Le système nerveux périphérique: Description, systématisation, exploration.* 3rd edition. Paris: Masson.

Le Corre, François, and Emmanuel Rageot. 2001. *Atlas pratique de médecine manuelle ostéopathique.* Paris: Masson.

Lelord, François, and Christophe André. 1996. *Comment gérer les personnalités difficiles.* Paris: Odile Jacob.

Lemperière, Thérèse, André Féline, Jean Adès, Patrick Hardy, and Frédéric Rouillon. 1977. *Psychiatrie de l'adulte.* Paris: Masson.

Lévy-Soussan, Pierre. 2002. *Psychiatrie.* Collection Med-Line. Paris: Estem.

Littlejohn, John Martin. 1974. *Notes sur les principes de l'ostéopathie* Maidstone, UK: Editions du Centenaire.

Magoun, Harold I. 1951. *Osteopathy in the Cranial Field.* Indianapolis: The Cranial Academy.

Marié, Eric. 1997. *Précis de médecine chinoise: Fondements historiques, théorie et pratique.* Saint-Jean-de-Braye, France: Dangles.

Martiny, Marcel. 1955. "Biotypologie et prosopologie statique"; "Le comportement general des biotypes de base devant les agressivités morbides"; "Quelques réflexions sur le choix des techniques psychométriques en biotypologie." In *Traité de médecine biotypologique,* edited by Nicola Pende. Paris: Doin.

Mayfield, Demmie, Gail McLeod, and Patricia Hall. 1974. "The CAGE Questionnaire: Validation of a New Alcoholism Screening Instrument." *Am. J. Psychiatry* 131:1121–3.

Mitchell, Fred, Sr. 1979. "Towards a Definition of 'Somatic Dysfunction.'" *Osteopathic Annals* 7:12–25.

Myers, David G. 1997. *Psychologie.* Paris: Flammarion Médecine Sciences.

Njølstad, Inger, Ivar Aaraas, and S. Lundevall. 1992. "Look at the Patient, Not the Notes." *Lancet* 340:413–4.

Novey, Donald W. 1999. *Guide de l'examen physique.* Paris: Maloine.

Pende, Nicola. 1955. "Introduction à la science de la constitution"; "Le concept du biotype"; "Les biotypes de base." In *Traité de médecine biotypologique,* edited by Nicola Pende. Paris: Doin.

Pouget, Régis. 1995. *Précis de psychologie médicale et de psychiatrie.* Montpellier, France: Sauramps Médical.

Queneau, Patrice, and Gérard Ostermann. 1994. *Le médecin, le patient et sa douleur.* Paris: Masson.

Quevauvilliers, Jacques, and Abe Fingerhut. 1997. *Dictionnaire medical.* Paris: Masson.

Richard, Jean-Pierre. 1987. *La colonne vertébrale en ostéopathie.* Aix-en-Provence, France: De Verlaque.

Ricoeur, Paul. 1994. "La souffrance n'est pas douleur." In *Souffrances corps et âme, épreuves partagées,* edited by Jean-Marie von Kaenel, 58–69. Paris: Autrement.

Salomon, Paule. 1997. *La brûlante lumière de l'amour.* Paris: Albin Michel.

Sarembaud, Alain. 1991. *Homéopathie.* Paris: Masson.

Schiowitz, Stanley. 1997. "Static Symetry." In *An Osteopathic Approach to Diagnosis and Treatment,* edited by Eileen L. Di Giovanna, Stanley Schiowitz, and Dennis J. Dowling, 37–47. Philadelphia: Lippincott Williams & Wilkins.

Schneider, Kurt. 1959. *Clinical Psychopathology.* New York: Grune and Stratton.

Seidel, Henry M., Jane W. Ball, Joyce E. Dains, and G. William Benedict. 2001. *Guide de l'examen physique.* 2nd edition. Paris: Berti.

Servan-Schreiber, David. 2003. *Guérir le stress, l'anxiété et la dépression sans médicaments ni psychanalyse.* Paris: Laffont.

Sheldon, William H. 1954. *Atlas of Men: A Guide for Somatotyping the Adult Male at All Ages.* New York: Harper.

Sigaud, Claude. 1890. *Étude de Psycho-Physiologie.* Repr. Kila, MT: Kessinger Legacy Reprints, 2009.

Simon, Lucien, B. Roquefeuil, and Jacques Pélissier. 1985. *La douleur chronique.* Paris: Masson.

Solano, Raymond. 1988. *Guide pratique en ostéopathie.* Toulouse, France: Erès.

Sournia, Jean-Charles. 1995. *Histoire du diagnostic en médecine.* Paris: Editions de Sante.

Steiner, Rudolf. 1938. *Imagination, inspiration, intuition; etudes psychologiques.* Repr. Geneva: Editions Anthroposophiques Romandes, 1986.

Stengers, Isabelle. 1995. "Le médecin et le charlatan." In *Médecins et sorciers,* Collection Les Empêcheurs de Penser, edited by Tobie Nathan and Isabelle Stengers, 115–61. Paris: Synthélabo.

Still, Andrew Taylor. 1892. *The Philosophy and Mechanical Principles of Osteopathy.* Repr. Kirksville, MO: Osteopathic Enterprise, 1986.

———. 1897. *Autobiography of Andrew T. Still.* Kirksville, MO: A. T. Still.

———. 1899. *Philosophy of Osteopathy.* Kirksville, MO: A. T. Still.

———. 1910. *Osteopathy, Research and Practice.* Repr. Seattle: Eastland Press, 1992.

Sutherland, William G. 1939. *The Cranial Bowl.* Repr. Kirksville, MO: Free Press, 1994.

Swartz, Mark H. 1991. *Manuel de diagnostic clinique anamnèse et examen.* Paris: Maloine.

Thomas, M. 1999. "Réflexions sur la définition du diagnostic." *Info-Afdo* 25(3): 6–7.

Thooris, A. 1955. "Les types humains selon l'école de morphologie française." In *Traité de médecine biotypologique,* edited by Nicola Pence, 575–99. Paris: Doin.

Tribolet, Serge, and Mazda Shahidi. 2000. *Précis de sémiologie des troubles psychiques.* Thoiry, France: Heures de France.

Tricot, Pierre. 1992. *Ostéopathie, une technique pour libérer la vie.* Paris: Chiron.

Trifaud, André. 2001. "Les énigmes scientifiques des guérisons miraculeuses." *Acta Med. Cathol.* 70:213–21.

Truhlar, Robert E. 1950. *Doctor A. T. Still in the Living: His Concepts and Principles of Health and Disease.* Cleveland, OH: privately published.

Tubiana, Raoul. 1980. *Traité de chirurgie de la main. 1: Anatomie, physiologie, biologie, méthodes d'examen.* Paris: Masson.

Upledger, John E. 1987. *Craniosacral Therapy II: Beyond the Dura.* Seattle: Eastland Press.

Upledger, John E., and Jon Vredevoogd. 1983. *Craniosacral Therapy.* Seattle: Eastland Press.

Vague, Jean. 1955. "Biochimie de la constitution." In *Traité de médecine bio-typologique,* edited by Nicola Pende, 87–103. Paris: Doin.

Vannier, Léon. 1965. *La typologie et ses applications thérapeutiques. Premiere partie: Généralités et constitutions.* Revised and corrected 4th edition. Paris: Doin.

———. 1979. *La pratique de l'homéopathie.* Paris: Doin.

Verdun, M. 1955. "Méthode et techniques anthropométriques." In *Traité de médecine biotypologique,* edited by Nicola Pende, 231–84. Paris: Doin.

Von Hayek, H. 1953. *Die menschliche Lunge* 1st edition. 2nd Edition 1970. Berlin: Springer.

Wernham, John. 1985. "Mechanics of the Spine." In *The Maidstone College Year Book,* edited by John Wernham, 20–33. Maidstone, UK: Maidstone College of Osteopathy.

———. 1995. "Technique and Performance." In *Lectures on Osteopathy,* edited by John Wernham, 97–8. Maidstone, UK: Maidstone College of Osteopathy.

Wheeler, John Archibald. 1988. *Between Quantum and Cosmos: Studies and Essays in Honor of John Archibald Wheeler.* Princeton, NJ: Princeton University Press.

Willem, Georges. 2001. *Manuel de posturologie: Approche clinique et traitements des pathologies rachidiennes et céphaliques.* Paris: Frison Roche.

Winckler, W, and E. Vagel. 1949. "Insulinschockbehanlung u. Konstitution." *Arch. f. Psychiatr. u. Neur.* 182.

World Health Organization. 1946. Preamble to the Constitution of the World Health Organization, adopted by the International Health Conference, New York, 1946. *Official Records of the World Health Organization* 2:100.

Zetlaoui, Paul. 1995. "La douleur." In *Redécouvrir l'examen clinique, clé du diagnostic, fascicule 2,* edited by Olivier Blétry, Julie Cosserat, and Rachid Laraki, 69–88. Paris: Doin.

Index

About the Author

ALAIN CROIBIER, DO, MRO(F), is a highly regarded osteopath in France and has been in private practice since 1990. Together with the esteemed osteopath Jean-Pierre Barral, Croibier developed the modalities of Neural Manipulation, New Manual Articular Approach, and Visceral Vascular Manipulation, based on their ongoing clinical research. A professor of Visceral Manipulation and osteopathic diagnosis at the Osteopathic College of the A. T. Still Academy in Lyon, he is also an international teacher of Visceral Manipulation, Neural Manipulation, Visceral Vascular Manipulation, and New Manual Articular Approach for the Barral institute, where he holds the title of curriculum codeveloper.

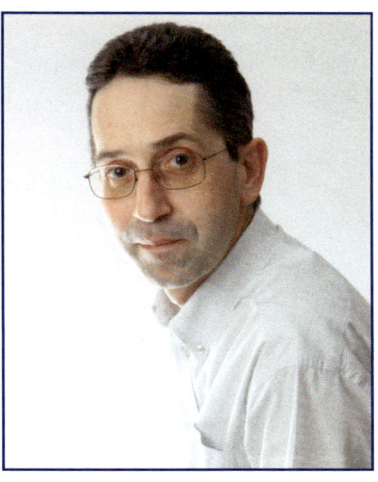

About North Atlantic Books

NORTH ATLANTIC BOOKS (NAB) is an independent, non-profit publisher committed to a bold exploration of the relationships between mind, body, spirit, and nature. Founded in 1974, NAB aims to nurture a holistic view of the arts, sciences, humanities, and healing. To make a donation or to learn more about our books, authors, events, and newsletter, please visit www.northatlanticbooks.com.